MW00635321

VALIDATED!

THE MAKEUP OF

VAL GARLAND

WORDS BY KARL PLEWKA

LAURENCE KING

Published in 2018
by Laurence King Publishing Ltd
361–373 City Road
London EC1V 1LR
Tel +44 20 7841 6900
Fax +44 20 7841 6910
enquiries@laurenceking.com
www.laurenceking.com

© Val Garland 2018
Executive producer: Joey Choy

ISBN 978 1 78627 308 6

Art direction: Angus Hyland
Interviews and text by Karl Plewka
Commissioning editor: Camilla Morton
Senior editor: Gaynor Sermon
Design: Amira Prescott
Picture researcher: Tory Turk
Production manager: Sian Smith

Front cover: © Sølve Sundsbø; model Karen Elson
Back cover: © Sølve Sundsbø; model Erin O'Connor

Printed in China

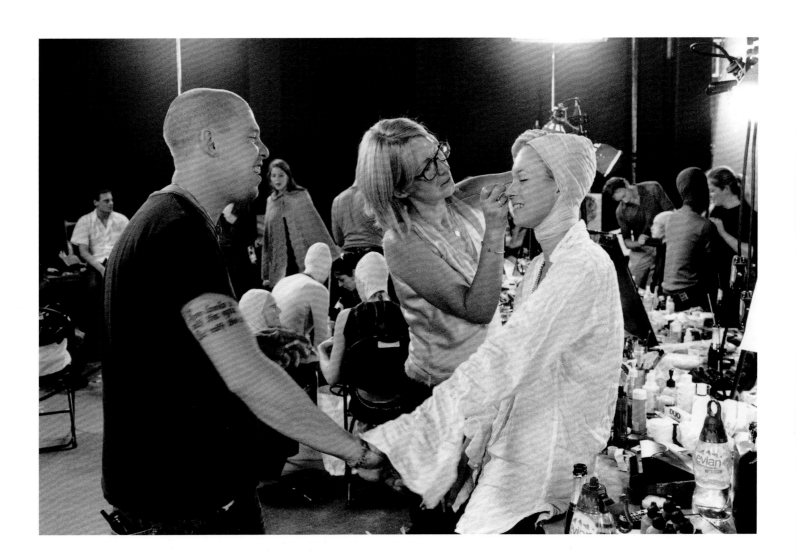

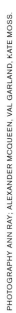

Val can make me look like the sexy kind of girl I want to look like when I go out. She does that really well, as well as doing the weirdness – like when they wrapped my head at McQueen and I said, 'Please give me some mascara, Val, I want some mascara!' She said, 'it's not in the look, dear.' I was like, 'Lee! Lee!' And he just said, 'Oh, FFS Val, give her some mascara.'

KATE MOSS

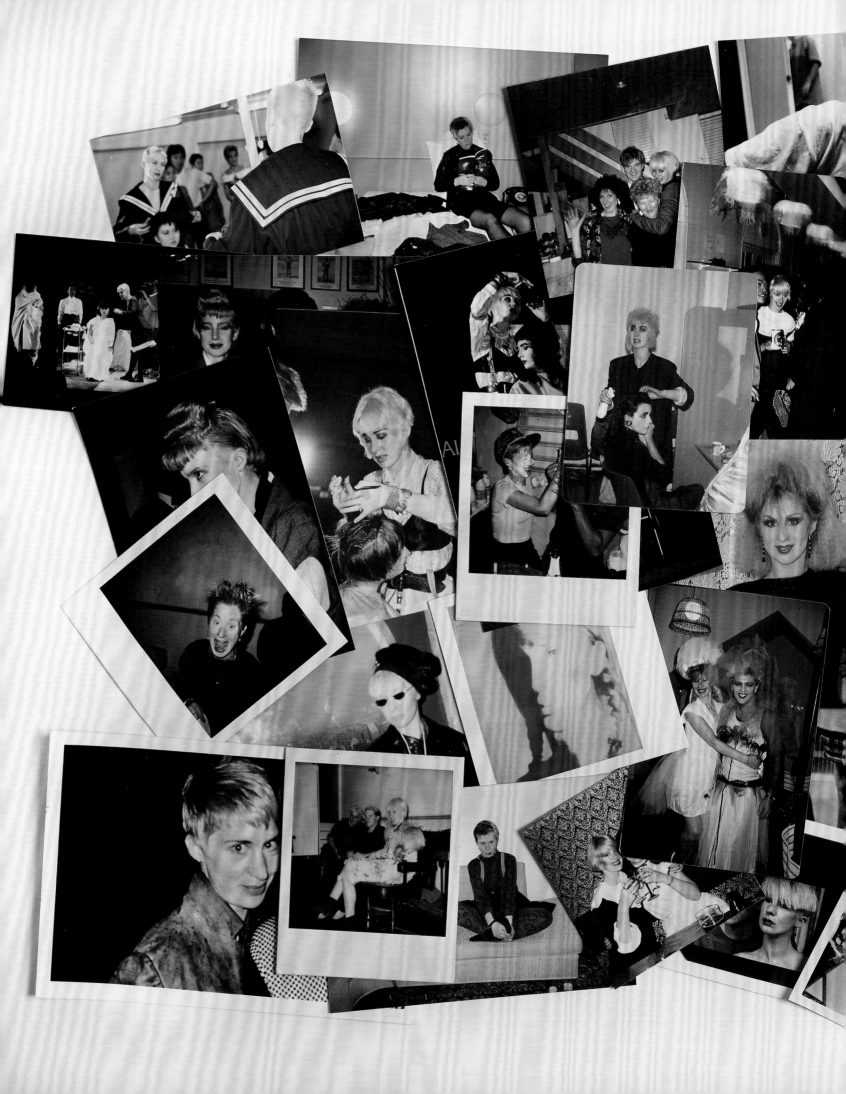

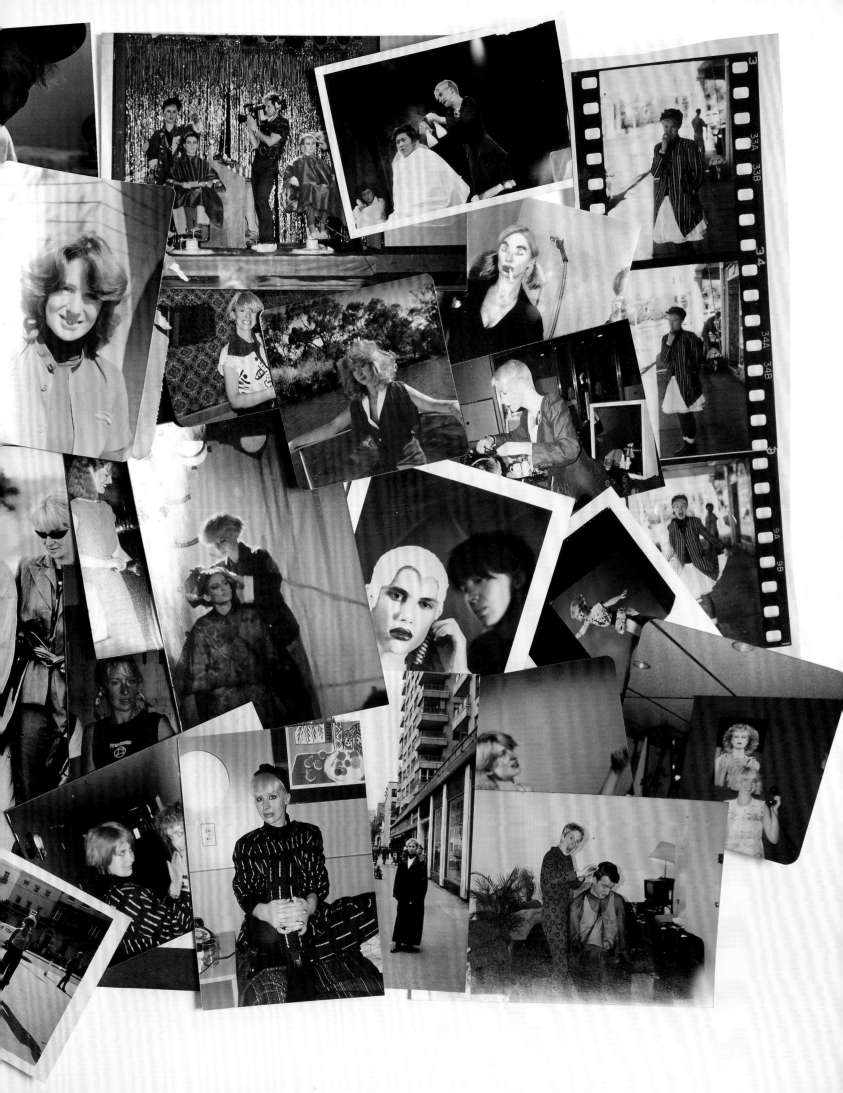

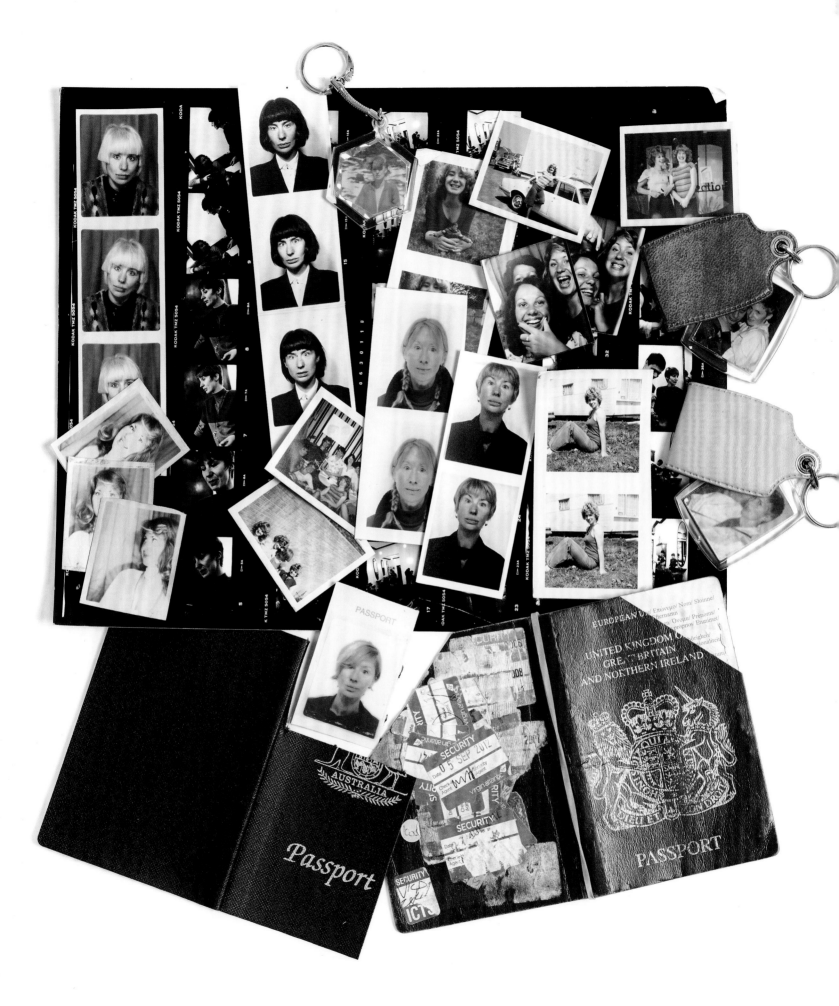

'I NEVER PLANNED TO BE A MAKEUP ARTIST.
IT WAS SOMETHING THAT JUST HAPPENED.
I ALWAYS THOUGHT I WAS NOT GOOD ENOUGH,
NOT WORTHY OF SUCH ACCOLADES.

THIS IS MY JOURNEY.
IF I CAN DO IT, SO CAN YOU.'

VAL GARLAND

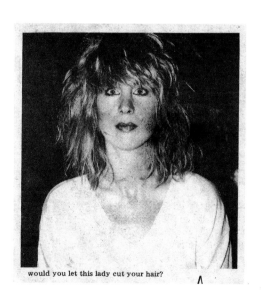

would you let this lady cut your hair?

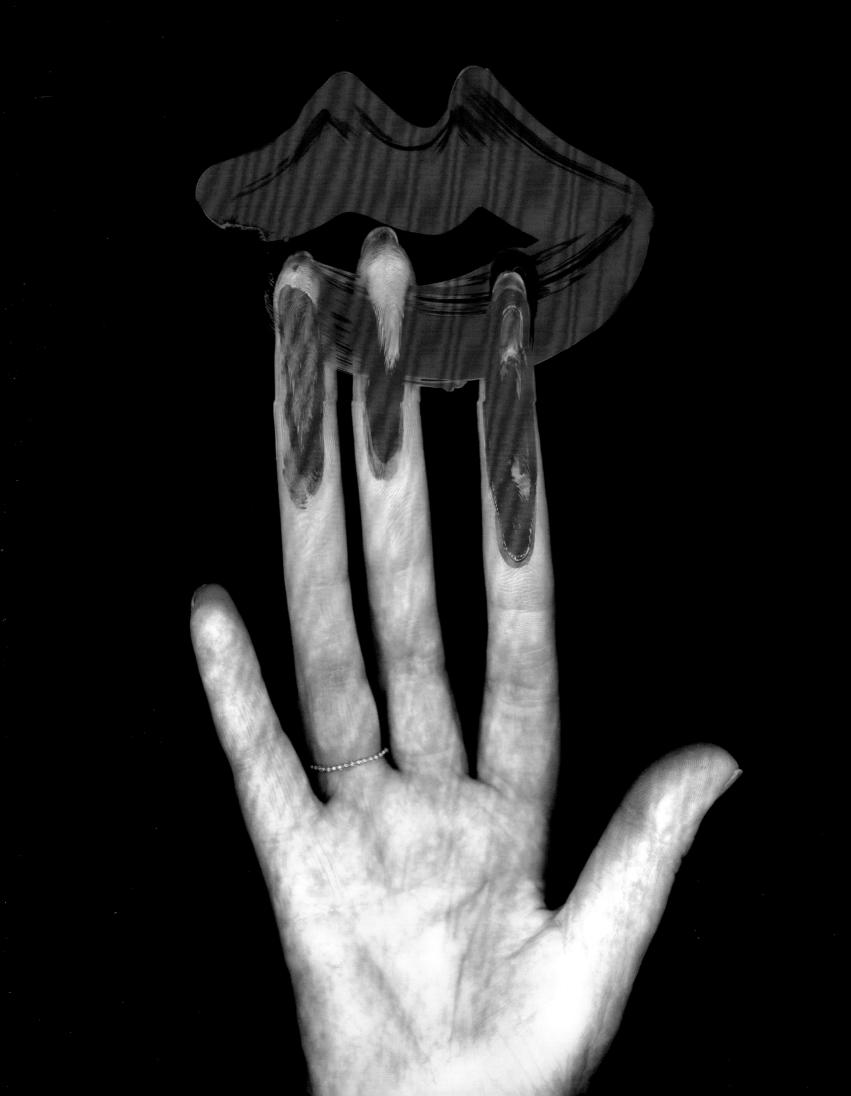

A TRULY RADICAL IMAGE-MAKER

Val Garland could not be invented. She is not the classic version of the creative eccentric, for she is multi-layered and complex, spontaneous and unpredictable, a stranger to both the banality of formula and the tiresome self doubt that might plague some creatives. Her life's work – ranging from beautiful masks, indolent and kittenish, to subversive, visceral daubings – proves this time and again.

Val Garland is a dichotomy between authority and rebellion. She has the appearance and calmly confident demeanour of an elegant gallery owner, but one who eyes the world with the scrutiny of a truly radical image-maker. Makeup can be a dramatic device, and much of Val's work has the power to make the audience mentally sit up straight and pay attention. The images collected in this book demonstrate how a true artist's vision can endlessly propagate ideas through many mediums and across multiple genres.

Val's work transports us over fantastical terrains, from the intricacy of William Morris-like patterns to psychedelic paisley print swirls, from raw hypermodernity to dewy, erotic veils and savage, graphic contours. This is a book that showcases the incredible art of the makeup artist, whose eye can travel the face and body and ultimately effect a transformation, and, at times, a transfiguration. What is always most surprising is how these many makeup visions, in all their diversity, somehow all come from the same source: Val Garland's apparently limitless imagination and extraordinary psyche.

This isn't just a book about makeup or the artist who created these outstanding images, it is a monument to the myriad forms and interpretations of true beauty.

Karl Plewka

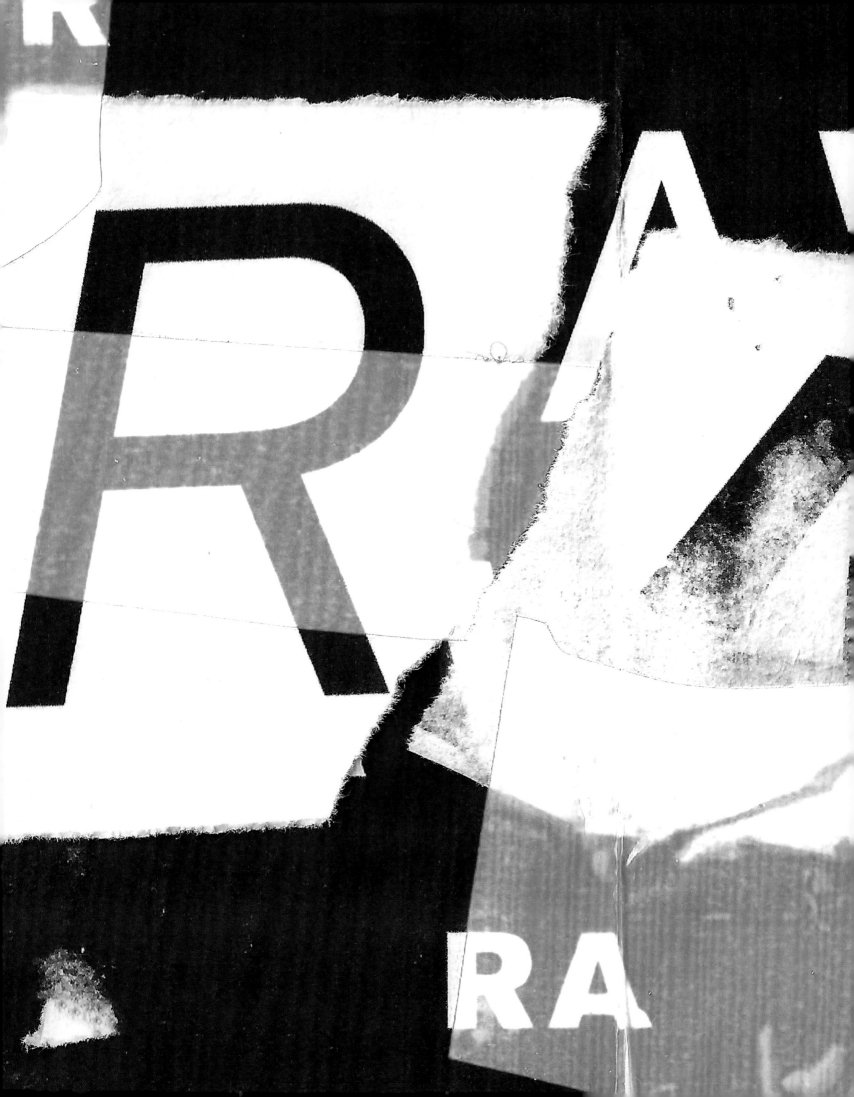

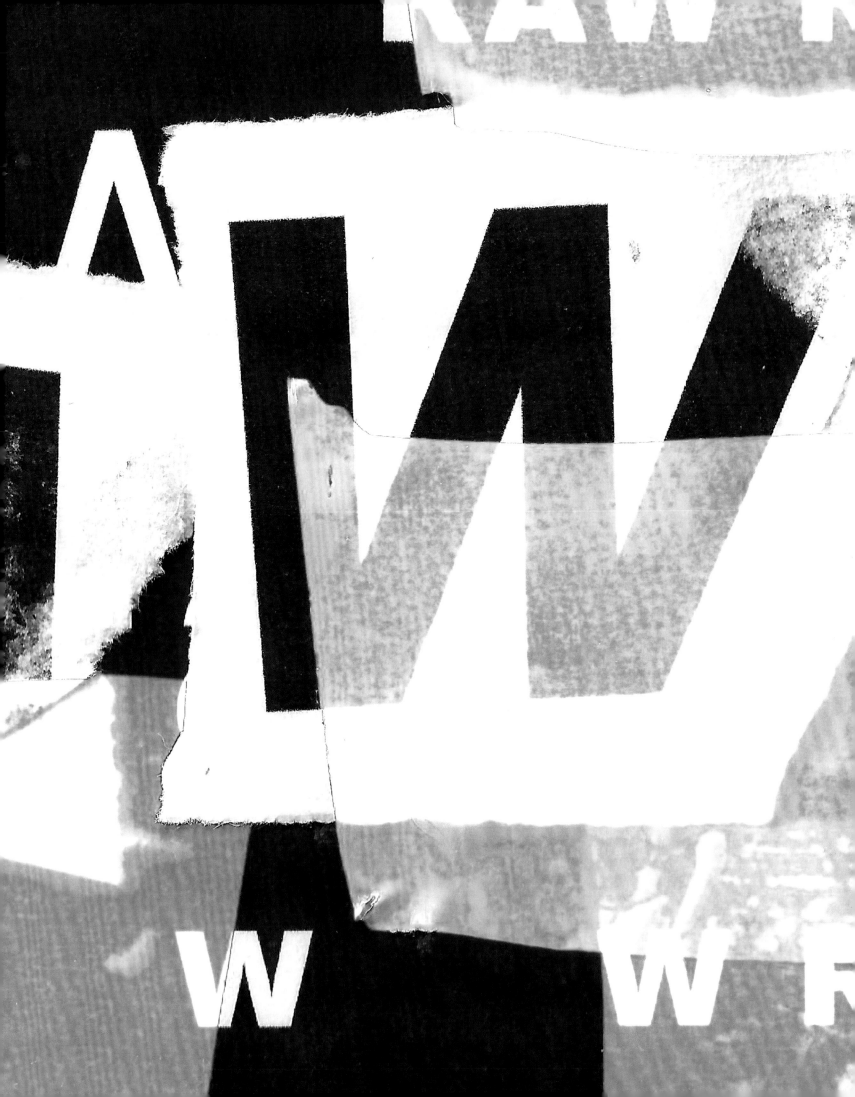

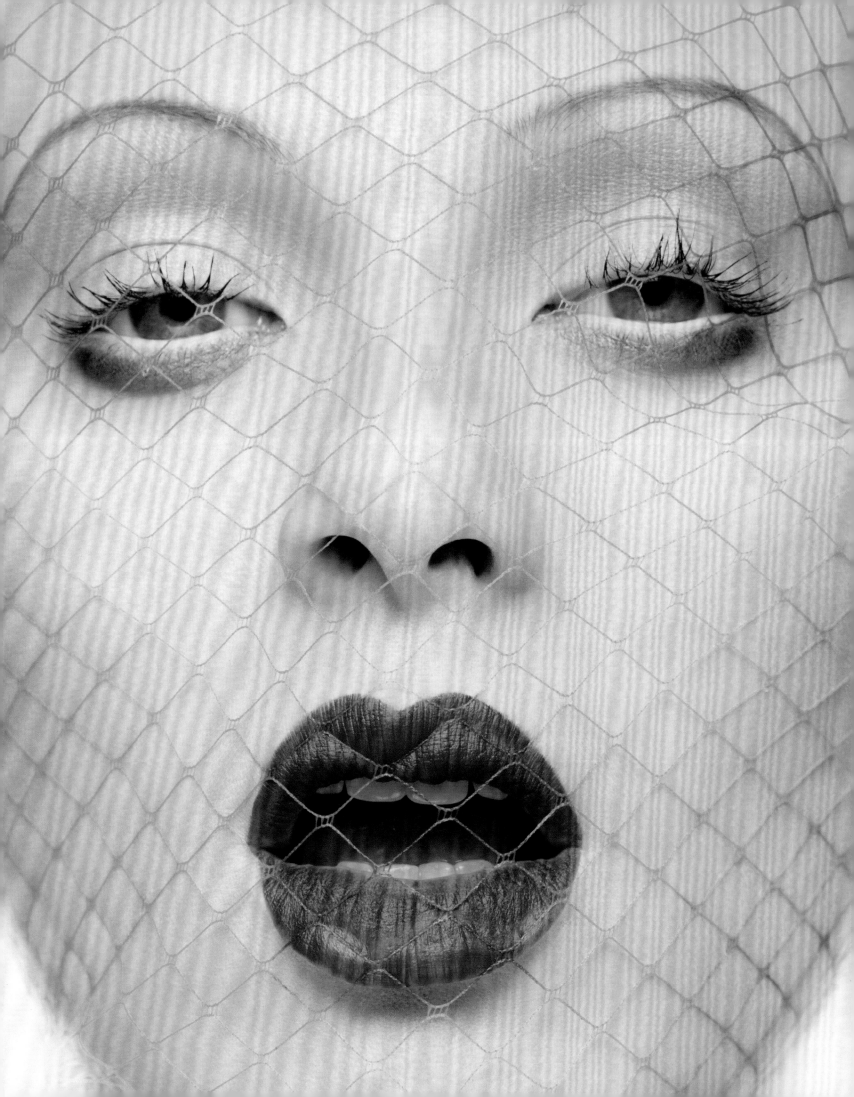

In the early nineties, Val's makeup career was just beginning in a London where fashion had jettisoned the glamorous Amazonian beauty of the eighties and was now associated with the violent chic of the post-Reagan era and the makeup-free waif, who never appeared to wash, let alone wear lipstick, as she lay indolent among the demi-squalor of her inner-city flat. True to form, Val didn't play by the grunge rules, and took her own stance when it came to creating inventive but modern makeup. At a time when makeup was often sneered at by her fashion contemporaries, Val's approach was to learn the alchemy of the perfect skin so treasured by her new collaborators, such as Nick Knight, who were shooting on expensive 10x8 film that gave only one chance to capture the perfect image. Val took up the challenge and ran with it. So the star of this chapter is ultimately the beautiful skin that, since her early makeup days, Val has so often been called upon to create. Although well known for her avant-garde work, she claims this is only 10 per cent of what she does. 'It all goes back to the fact you've got to "feel" the skin' she says, and these words sum up the 'raw' makeup looks here perfectly. By creating the perfect parchment, her typically spontaneous final flourishes, like an eye, a lip, a brow, even freckles, become almost iconic in their solitude. But certain canvases are better than others when it comes to raw makeup. Kate Moss, who is Val's raw makeup muse, particularly inspires her – something she puts down to the supermodel's extraordinary bone structure – and to this end Moss is notably prolific in these images. As the famous adage goes, 'Nature in the raw is seldom mild', and this is true of the makeup in this chapter. These are also makeup looks that require a sense of confidence in the wearer, as 'raw' is often about the beauty of baring more as opposed to hiding away any imperfections. Exposure is not always easy in a world so obsessed with artifice, but in this chapter Val utilizes purity to create maximum impact.

SKIN
UP

NUMÉRO 58, NOVEMBER 2004; PHOTOGRAPHY SØLVE SUNDSBØ; FASHION EDITOR JONATHAN KAYE; HAIR PETER GRAY; MODEL KAREN ELSON.

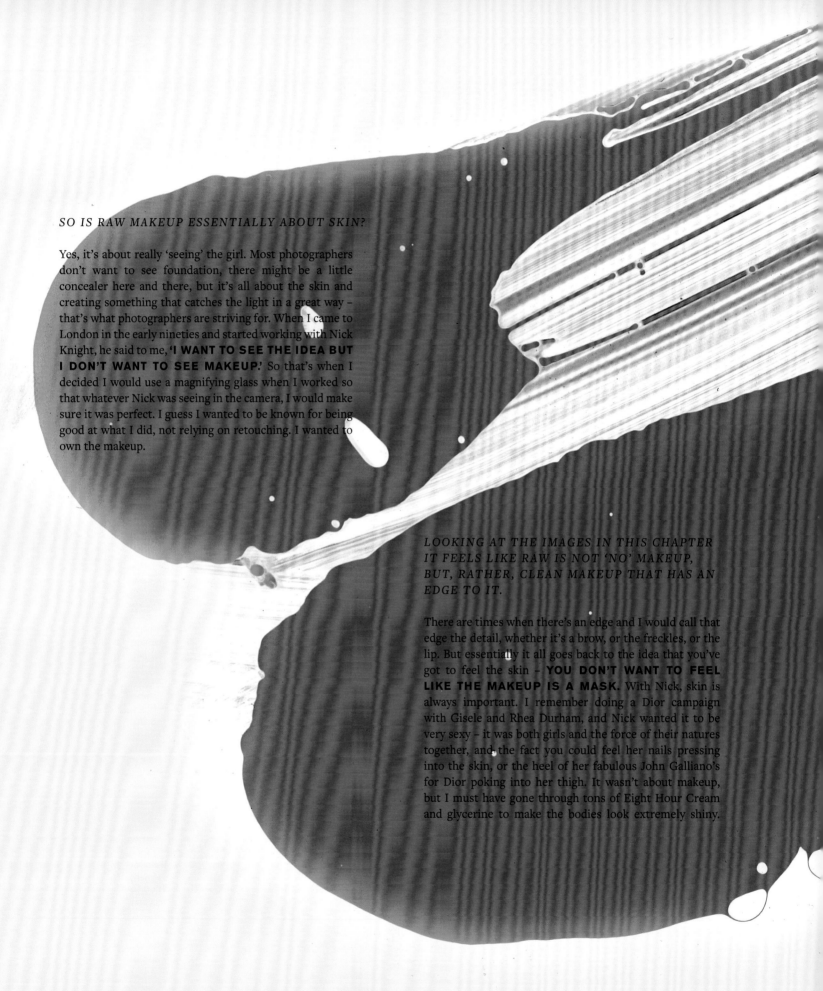

SO IS RAW MAKEUP ESSENTIALLY ABOUT SKIN?

Yes, it's about really 'seeing' the girl. Most photographers don't want to see foundation, there might be a little concealer here and there, but it's all about the skin and creating something that catches the light in a great way – that's what photographers are striving for. When I came to London in the early nineties and started working with Nick Knight, he said to me, **'I WANT TO SEE THE IDEA BUT I DON'T WANT TO SEE MAKEUP.'** So that's when I decided I would use a magnifying glass when I worked so that whatever Nick was seeing in the camera, I would make sure it was perfect. I guess I wanted to be known for being good at what I did, not relying on retouching. I wanted to own the makeup.

LOOKING AT THE IMAGES IN THIS CHAPTER IT FEELS LIKE RAW IS NOT 'NO' MAKEUP, BUT, RATHER, CLEAN MAKEUP THAT HAS AN EDGE TO IT.

There are times when there's an edge and I would call that edge the detail, whether it's a brow, or the freckles, or the lip. But essentially it all goes back to the idea that you've got to feel the skin – **YOU DON'T WANT TO FEEL LIKE THE MAKEUP IS A MASK.** With Nick, skin is always important. I remember doing a Dior campaign with Gisele and Rhea Durham, and Nick wanted it to be very sexy – it was both girls and the force of their natures together, and the fact you could feel her nails pressing into the skin, or the heel of her fabulous John Galliano's for Dior poking into her thigh. It wasn't about makeup, but I must have gone through tons of Eight Hour Cream and glycerine to make the bodies look extremely shiny.

RAW DOESN'T HAVE TO BE ABOUT JUST THE MAKEUP – IT CAN ALSO BE AN ATTITUDE.

KATE MOSS IS QUITE PREVALENT IN THIS CHAPTER.

The thing about Kate is she has an incredible bone structure. Kate is one of those people you can put absolutely no makeup on and she looks incredible. She's a chameleon. You can also pile it on and she looks like Catherine Deneuve crossed with Charlotte Rampling, Brigitte Bardot and Suzie Wong – she can be all of those characters. It just comes down to the canvas, and she's a great canvas to paint on. There's a shoot I did with Mario for British *Vogue*, and when Sam and I walked into the studio, Lucinda and Mario both said to me, 'Don't unpack your kit'. I said, 'Pardon?' And they said, 'No don't, just take out your cleanser and your moisturizer and that's it, because today we don't want you or Sam to do anything. Just brush up her eyebrows, moisturize her, that's it.' And that's exactly what we did, and because Kate is so powerful it worked. There's not a scrap of makeup on her and she just looked incredible. It's one of my all-time favourite moments.

KATE LOOKS INCREDIBLY SEXY IN THESE IMAGES. WOULD YOU SAY THERE'S A SEXUAL TRIGGER IN RAW MAKEUP?

IT'S ALL ABOUT THE PURITY. It's the flower coming into bloom, like she's almost ready to explode. I love all of that. Sometimes I just don't want to do any makeup at all because 'raw' looks so much more now. Raw doesn't have to be about just the makeup – it can also be an attitude.

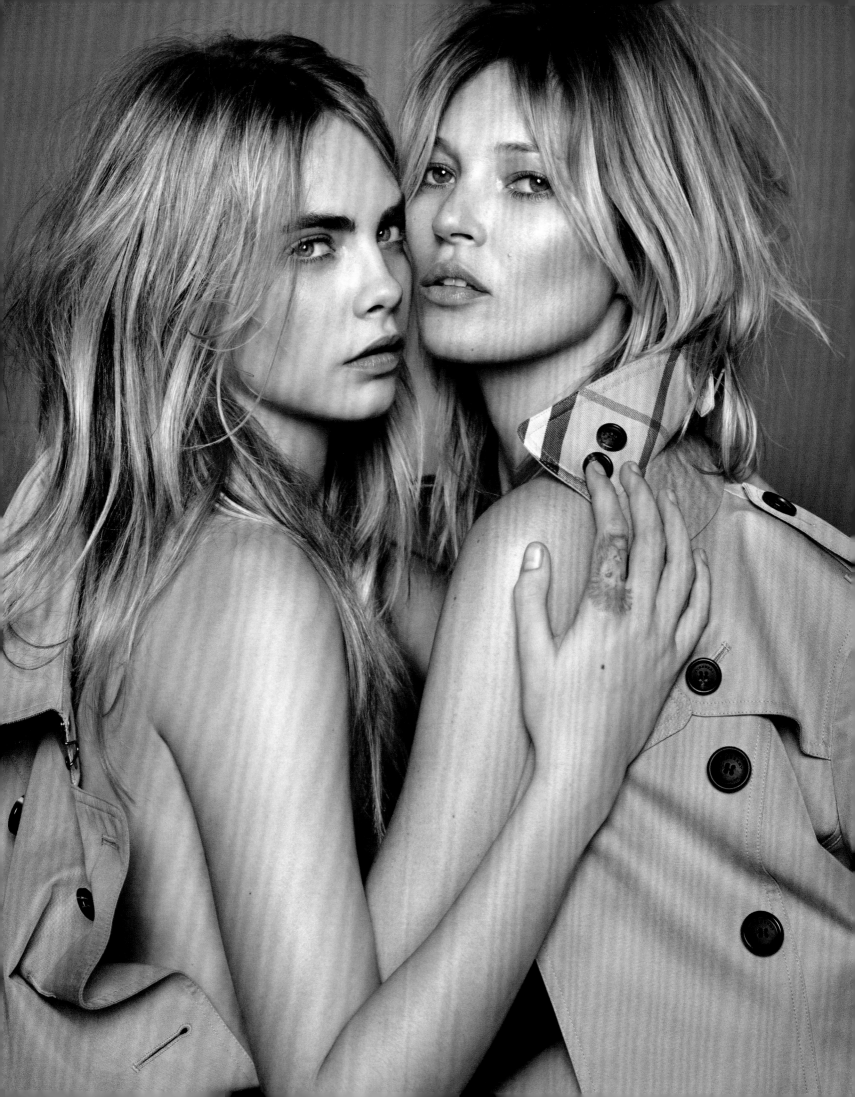

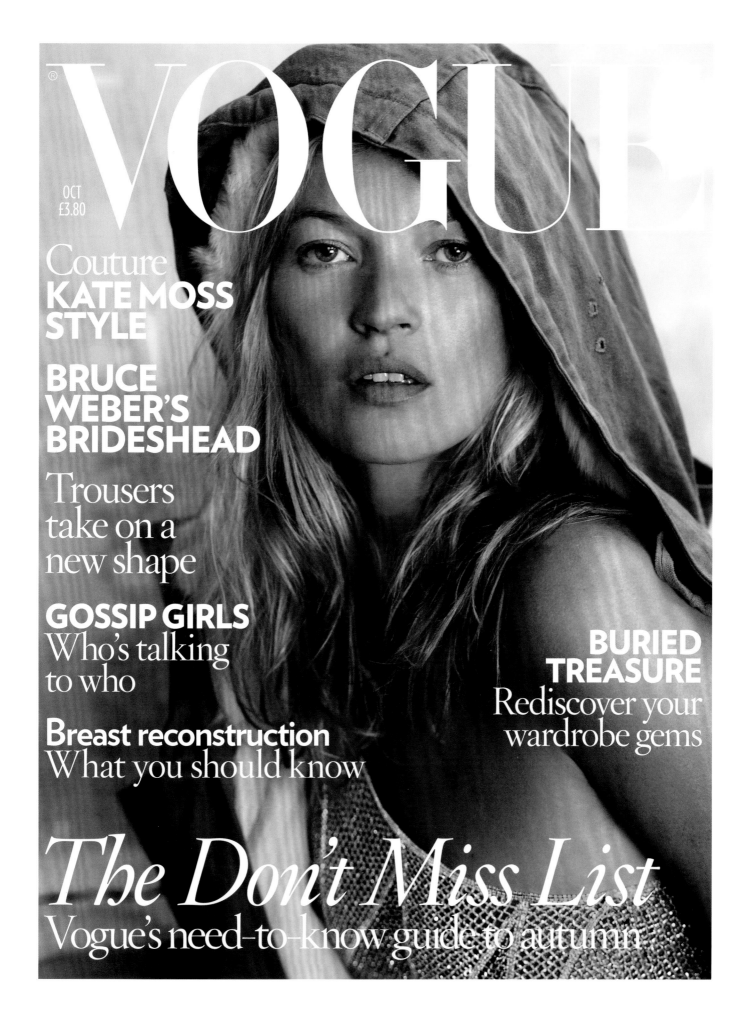

VOGUE

OCT
£3.80

Couture
**KATE MOSS
STYLE**

**BRUCE
WEBER'S
BRIDESHEAD**

Trousers
take on a
new shape

GOSSIP GIRLS
Who's talking
to who

Breast reconstruction
What you should know

**BURIED
TREASURE**
Rediscover your
wardrobe gems

The Don't Miss List
Vogue's need-to-know guide to autumn

BURBERRY CAMPAIGN 2014; PHOTOGRAPHY MARIO TESTINO; CREATIVE DIRECTION CHRISTOPHER BAILEY; FASHION EDITOR ELLIOTT SMEDLEY; HAIR SAM MCKNIGHT; MODELS KATE MOSS, CARA DELEVINGNE. BRITISH VOGUE OCTOBER 2008; PHOTOGRAPHY MARIO TESTINO; FASHION EDITOR LUCINDA CHAMBERS; HAIR SAM MCKNIGHT; MODEL KATE MOSS.

'That's how I want to be in real life. It was a really natural one for Val and Nick. That's how I'd like to look every day.'

KATE MOSS

BRITISH VOGUE SEPTEMBER 2005; PHOTOGRAPHY NICK KNIGHT; FASHION EDITOR KATE PHELAN; HAIR SAM MCKNIGHT; MANICURIST MARIAN NEWMAN; MODEL KATE MOSS.
BRITISH VOGUE MAY 2003; PHOTOGRAPHY NICK KNIGHT; FASHION EDITOR KATE PHELAN; HAIR SAM MCKNIGHT; MANICURIST MARIAN NEWMAN; MODEL KATE MOSS.

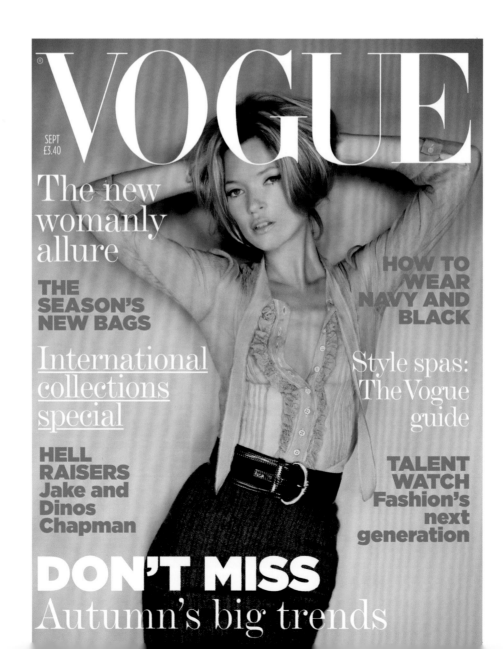

VOGUE

SEPT
£3.40

The new womanly allure

THE SEASON'S NEW BAGS

International collections special

HELL RAISERS Jake and Dinos Chapman

HOW TO WEAR NAVY AND BLACK

Style spas: The Vogue guide

TALENT WATCH Fashion's next generation

DON'T MISS Autumn's big trends

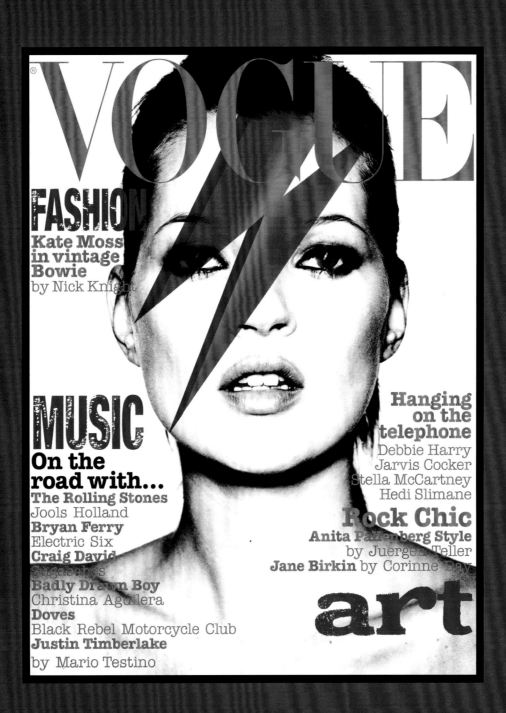

IT'S ABOUT THE PURITY.
PURE BLACK

This was a Nick Knight shoot for *The Independent* magazine and the funny thing was we shot Kate in the studio and it was a simple, natural makeup. Nick said 'I wonder if we should make the shot very monochrome, take Kate's skin to a platinum black.'

When the shot was published there was an enormous outcry in the media about painting Kate Moss black. But it's about purity. Pure black. Black as a colour.

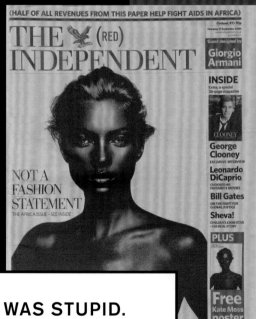

'[THE CONTROVERSY IT CREATED] WAS STUPID.
I DON'T REALLY SEE IT LIKE THAT. I LOVE IT. I THINK
IT'S AMAZING. AND IT'S ALMOST LIKE PLATINUM.
YOU KNOW, IT'S JUST AN IMAGE.'

KATE MOSS

THE INDEPENDENT SEPTEMBER 2006; PHOTOGRAPHY NICK KNIGHT; HAIR SAM MCKNIGHT; MANICURIST MARIAN NEWMAN; MODEL KATE MOSS.

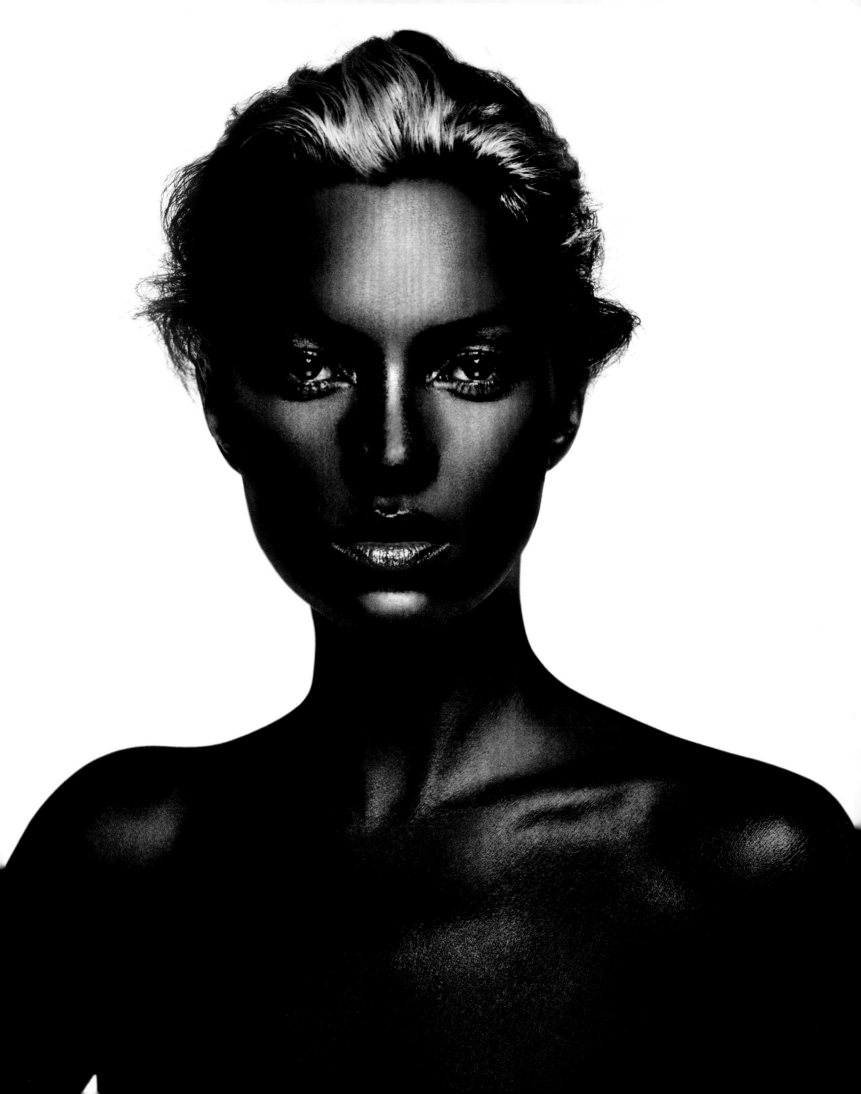

I BELIEVE YOU USED PART OF THE WARDROBE FOR THIS IMAGE OF EMMA WATSON FOR INTERVIEW?

Francesca, the stylist on this shoot, had a piece of flesh-coloured tulle with an embroidered lip on it. We had talked about doing a red lip – and that would have been great – but the spontaneity of putting the tulle in front of Emma's lips just felt much more *Interview* magazine.

INTERVIEW MAGAZINE MAY 2009; PHOTOGRAPHY NICK KNIGHT; FASHION EDITOR FRANCESCA BURNS; HAIR SAM MCKNIGHT; MANICURIST MARIAN NEWMAN; MODEL EMMA WATSON.

'A lot of people try to do what she does

BUT THEY CAN'T.

Val's quite raw and there are people who try to do that, but only Val keeps the beauty in it.'

SAM MCKNIGHT

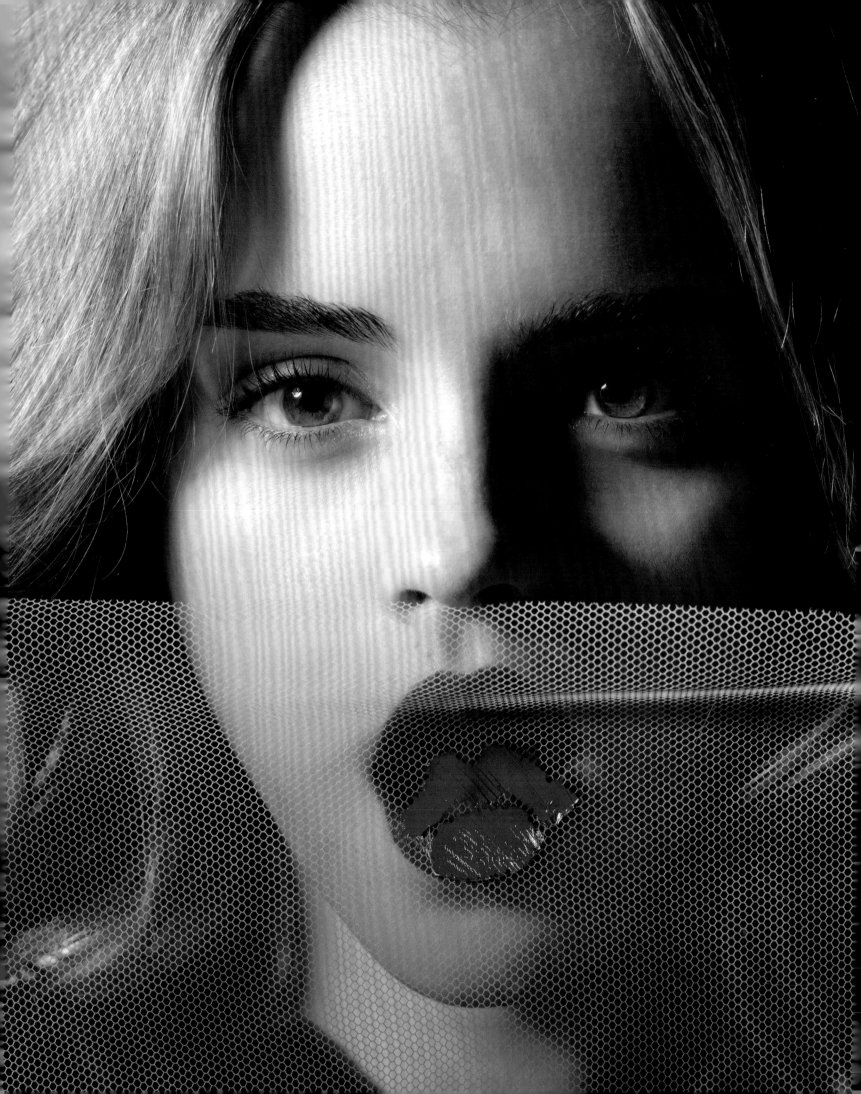

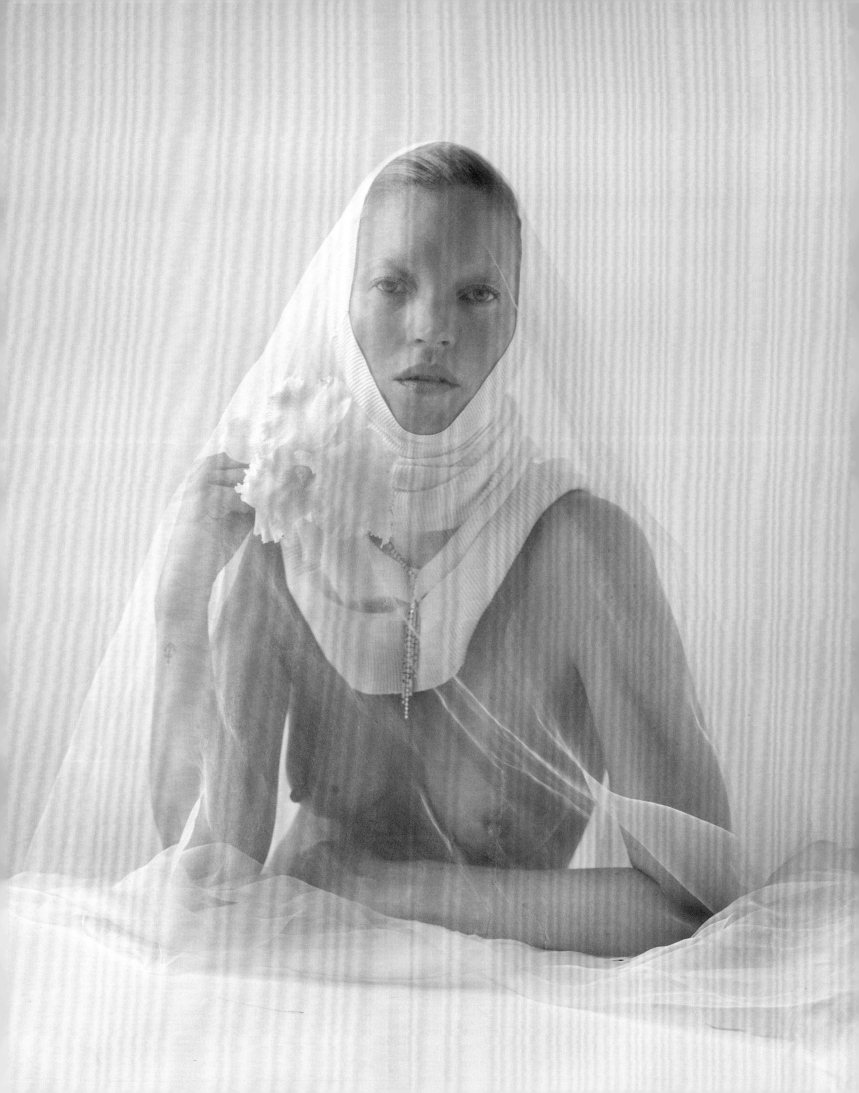

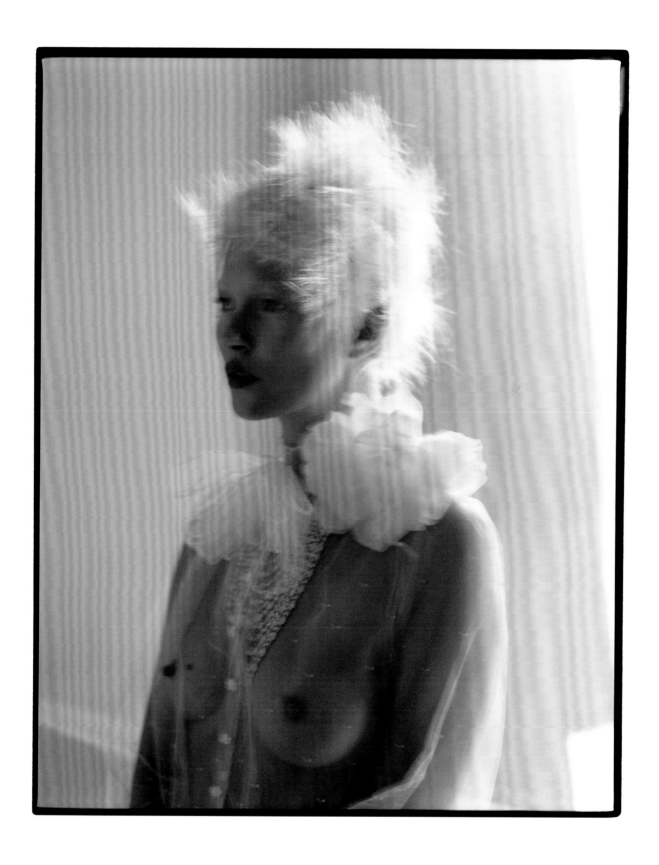

LOVE MAGAZINE NO. 8 FALL 2012, 'WALTZ DARLING'; PHOTOGRAPHY TIM WALKER; FASHION EDITOR KATIE GRAND; HAIR MALCOLM EDWARDS; MODEL KATE MOSS.

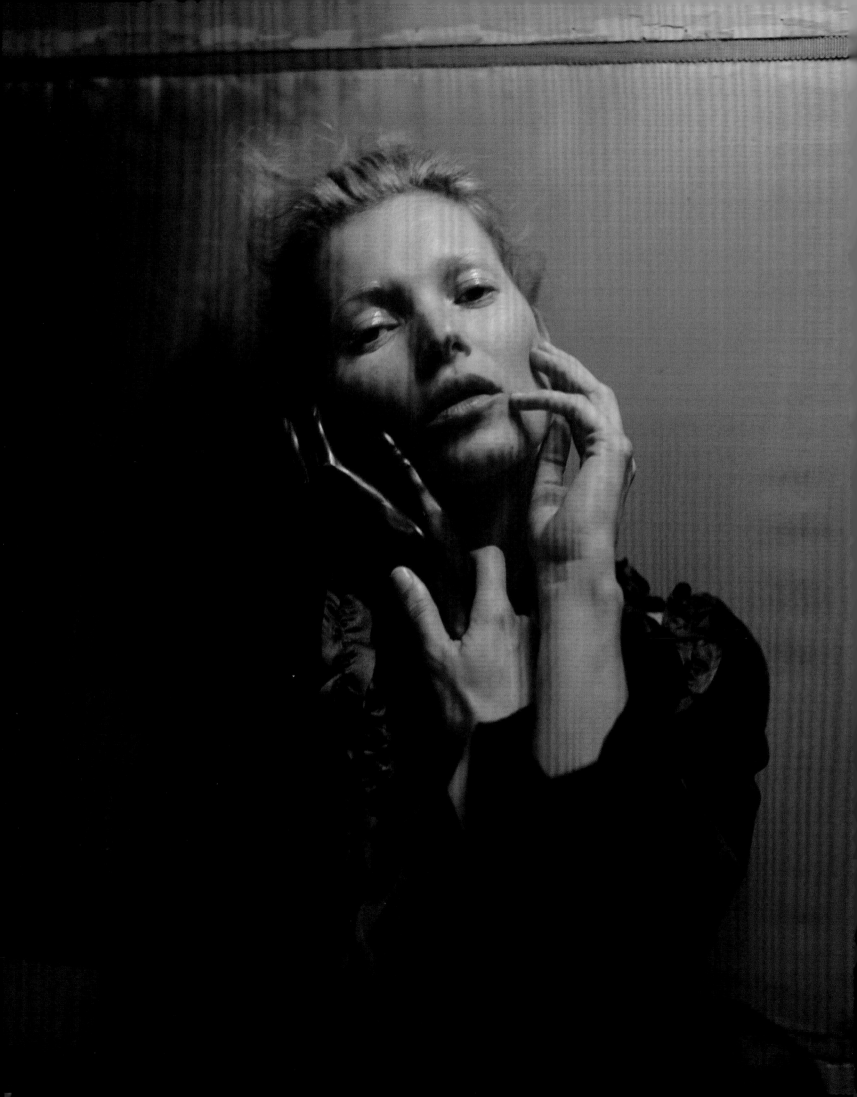

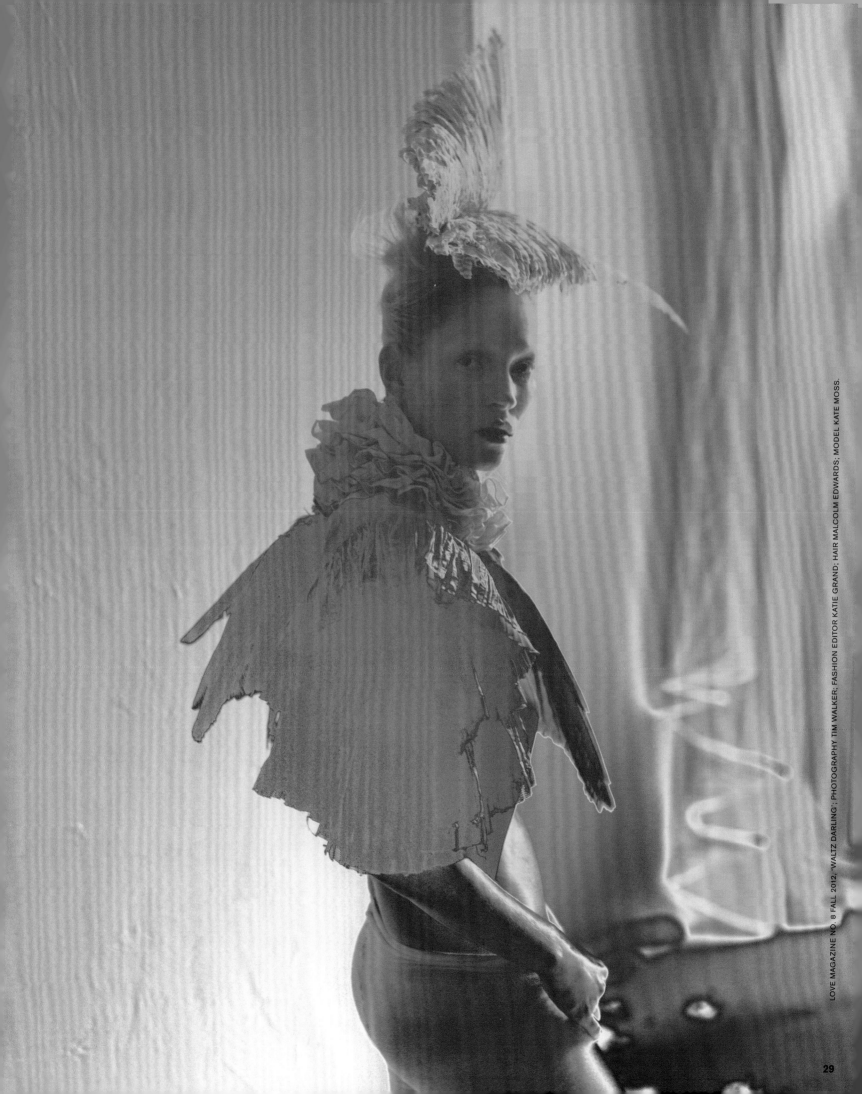

LOVE MAGAZINE NO. 8 FALL 2012, 'WALTZ DARLING'; PHOTOGRAPHY TIM WALKER; FASHION EDITOR KATIE GRAND; HAIR MALCOLM EDWARDS; MODEL KATE MOSS.

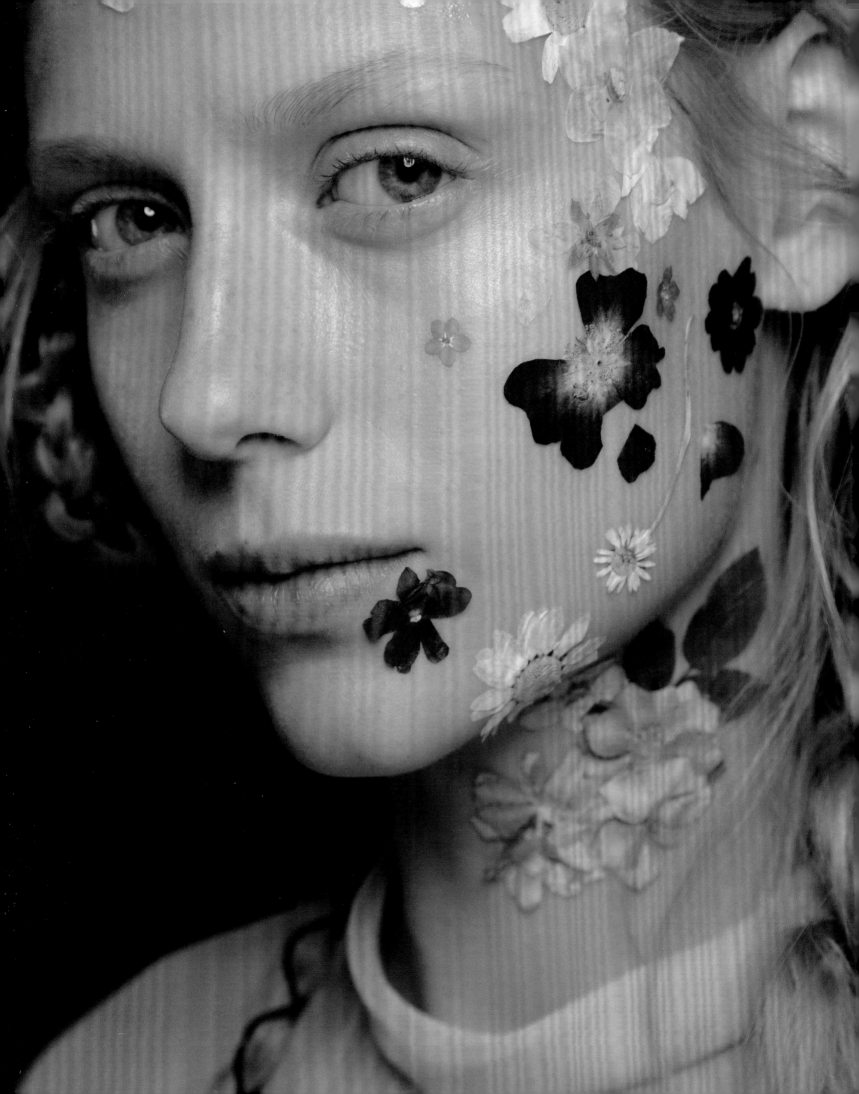

*WHICH DESIGNERS DO YOU GO DOWN THE RAW
ROUTE WITH?*

There was one Preen show I did and Justin and Thea wanted it to feel
like the girls had gone into the woods and laid down and fallen asleep
on a flower bed. I thought it was good to 'flower power' the girls' lips,
because from a distance it could look like an Irving Penn photograph;
you wouldn't realize until they got close that it was not in fact lipstick,
it was flowers. It was quite poetic.

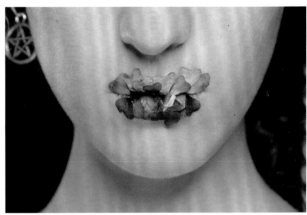

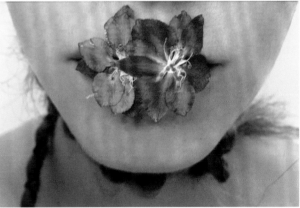

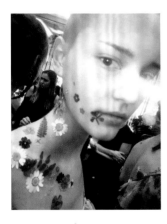

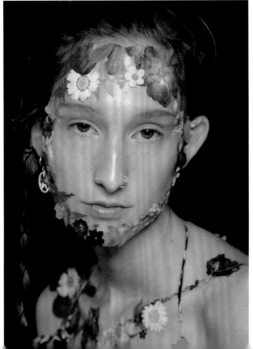

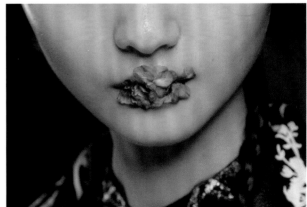

PREEN SS17; PHOTOGRAPHY LUCA CANNONIERI; MODELS SOFIE HEMNET, LINA HOSS, JAY WRIGHT, LORNA FORAN, HE CONG.

THE MAKEUP CAN CHANGE DIRECTION AT ANY MOMENT

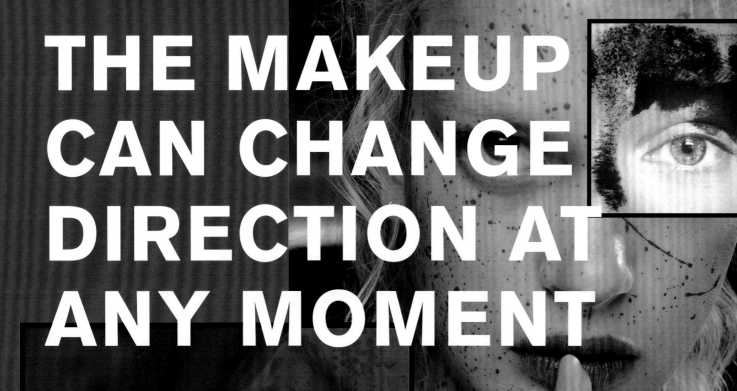

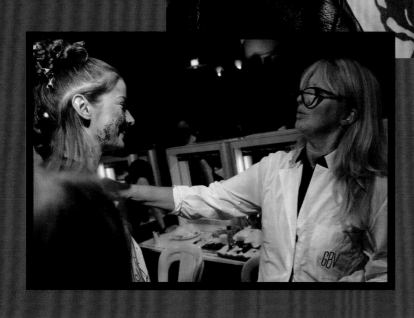

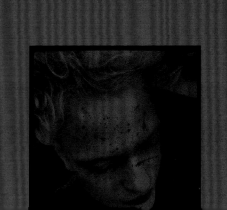

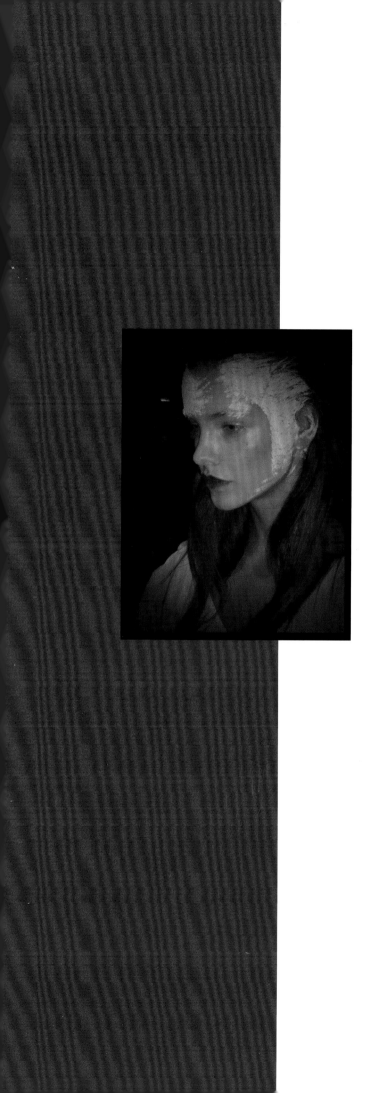

YOU'VE DEFINITELY DONE MANY RAW IDEAS AT VIVIENNE WESTWOOD'S SHOWS.

There was a Gold Label show in Paris where Vivienne and Andreas [Kronthaler] said, 'We really don't want any make-up; we want to feel the skin. We're feeling Frida Kahlo, but the charity-shop version. She's futuristic but she needs to look weathered, dusty.' And I thought, 'She's running for the number 52 bus in South London, and she's running, running, running, so she's a bit out of breath, she stops, puts her hand out for the bus, and then a big old truck goes by and she gets splattered with mud.'

DO YOU EVER EXPLAIN IT LIKE THAT TO THE DESIGNER?

It's best not to, because invariably what happens is **THE MAKEUP CAN CHANGE DIRECTION AT ANY MOMENT**, and something like a Westwood show is a journey – you won't know what it looks like until it comes out on the catwalk, as it may even change after the rehearsal, or in the line-up. This sounds like beauty coming out of chaos. Vivienne loves chaos. Another example of raw at Westwood is where Sam did very simple hair and I did a very beauteous face, then I took clay masks and painted around the edges of the face. Just before the show I put my hands onto it so it cracked a bit and I really liked that – peeling off, cracking, decaying – and then inside there's the beauty, like a butterfly, the beautiful nucleus of her.

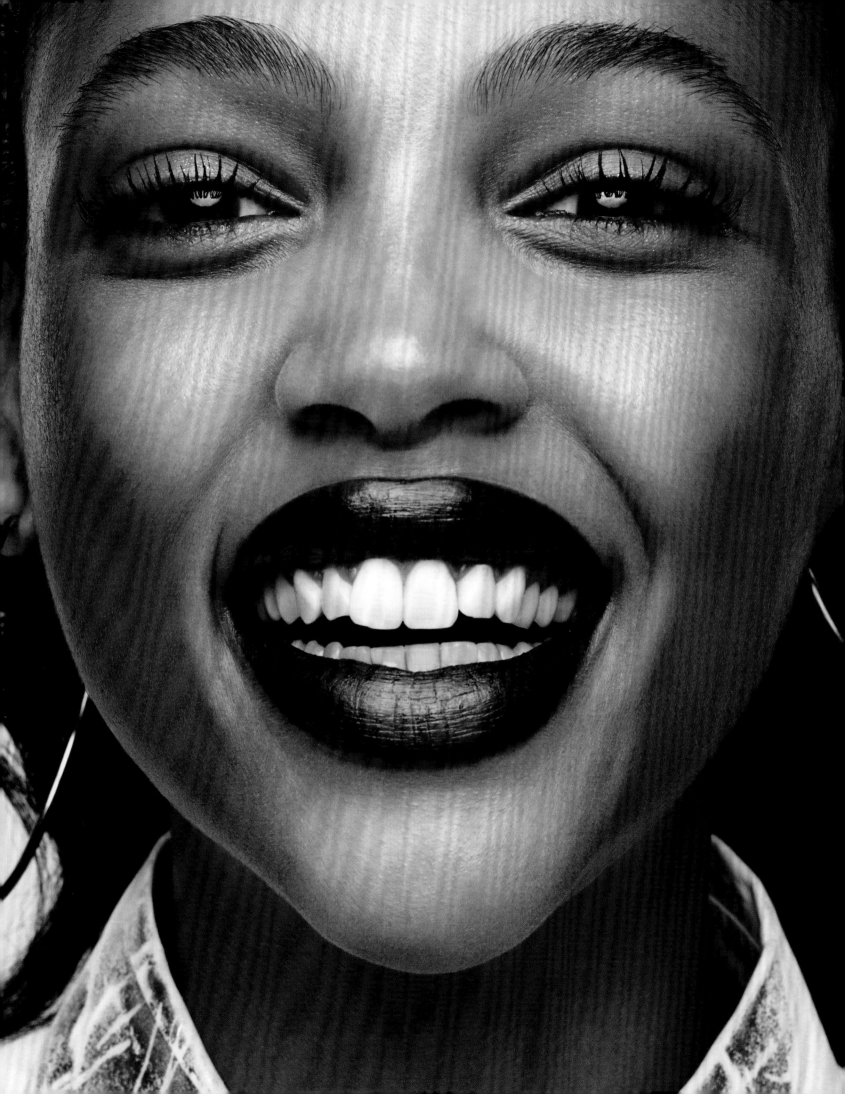

'THE FOCUS WITH VAL IS ALWAYS, "I DON'T GIVE A DAMN, AS LONG AS IT LOOKS AMAZING." THERE ARE NO RULES WITH HER. THERE'S NO, "OH, THAT'S NOT COOL ENOUGH." OR, "THAT'S NOT WHAT'S HAPPENING NOW."'

SØLVE SUNDSBØ

I'd say I am avant-garde
10% of the time.

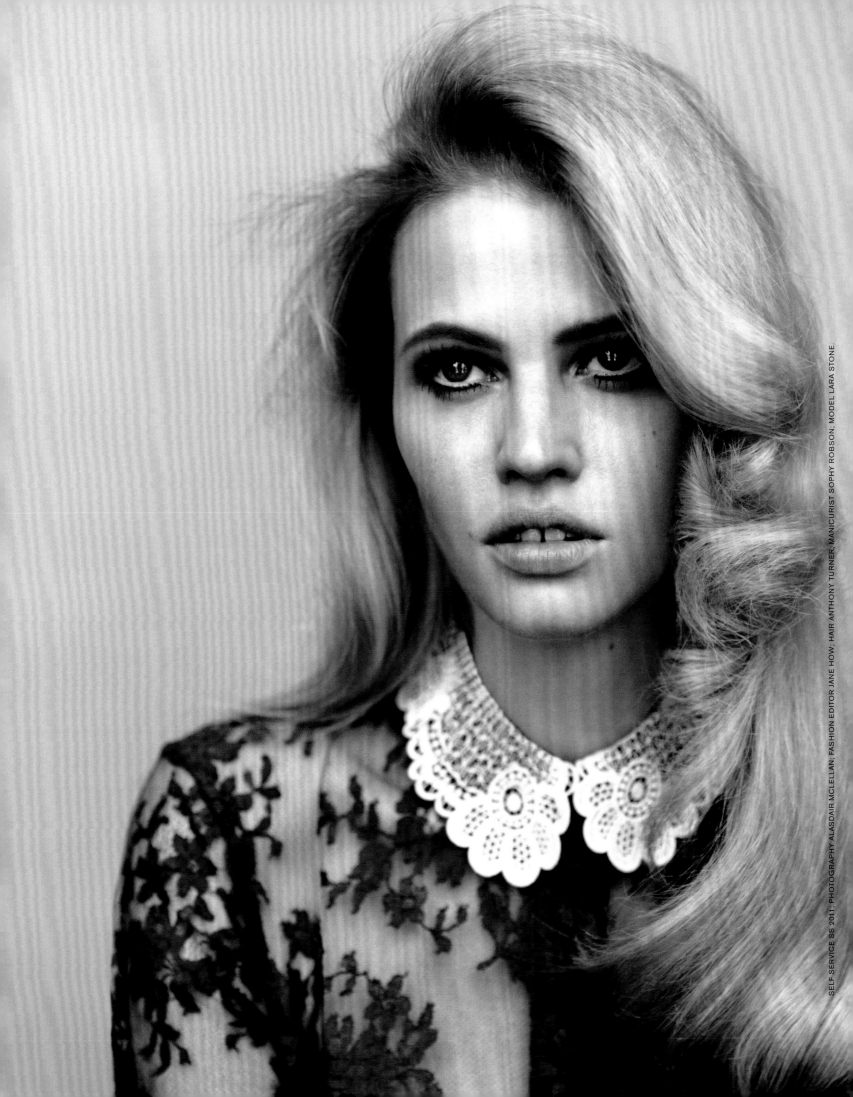

'I REMEMBER HE WAS HOLDING A ROSE.

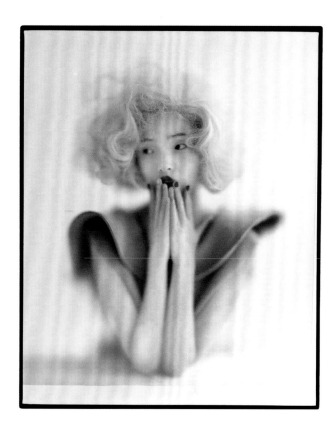

VAL SAID,

"I JUST WANT TO GET IN AND DO HIS FACE YELLOW.

LEAVE IT TO ME.

I JUST NEED FIVE MINUTES."

AND SHE WENT IN AND DID IT, AND THAT SORT OF MADE THE PICTURE. IT ACCENTUATED THE THREE THINGS YOU NEED IN A PICTURE. IT WAS

THE YELLOW FACE, THE YELLOW ROSE, THE YELLOW DRESS.'

TIM WALKER

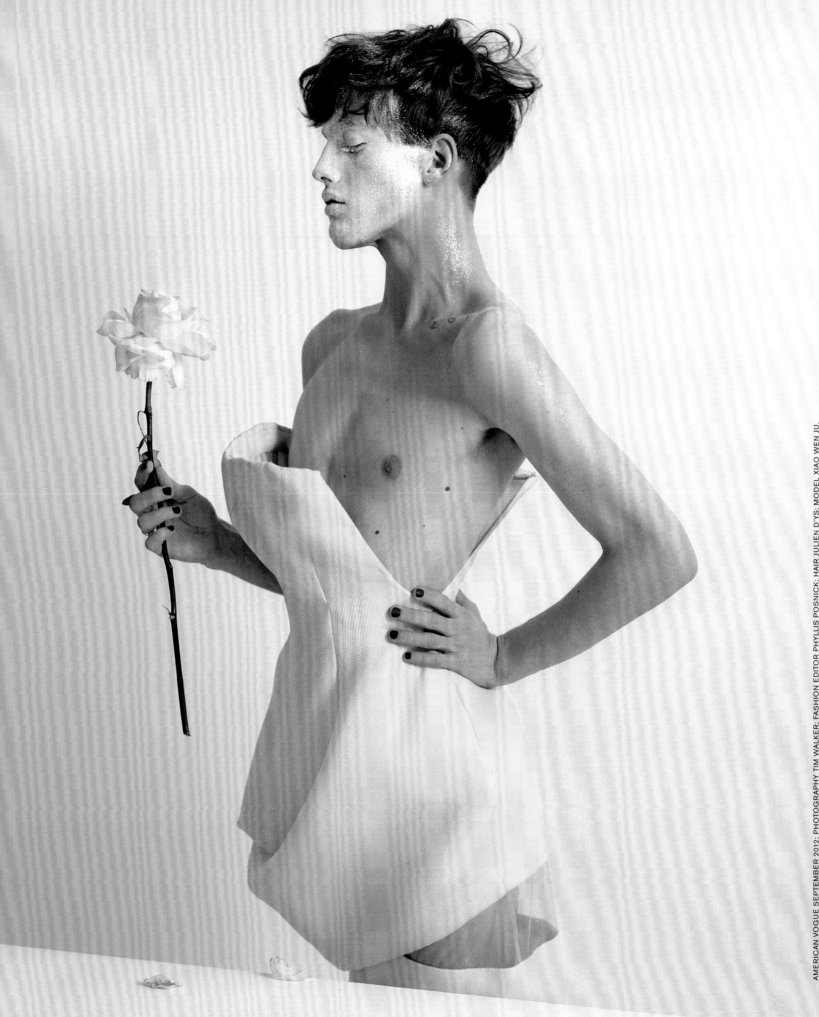

AMERICAN VOGUE SEPTEMBER 2012; PHOTOGRAPHY TIM WALKER; FASHION EDITOR PHYLLIS POSNICK; HAIR JULIEN D'YS; MODEL XIAO WEN JU.
W MAGAZINE APRIL 2013; PHOTOGRAPHY TIM WALKER; FASHION EDITOR EDWARD ENNINFUL; HAIR MALCOLM EDWARDS; MANICURIST TRISH LOMAX; MODEL SYLVESTER ULV HENRIKSEN.

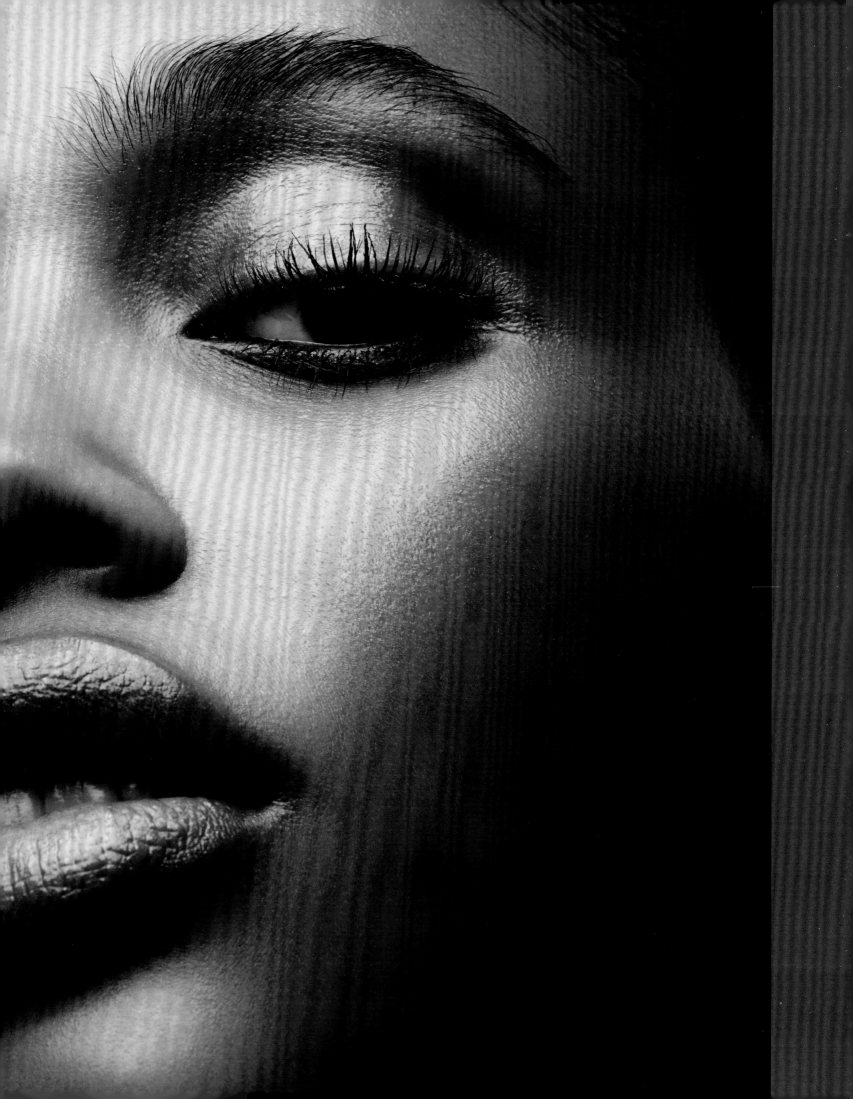

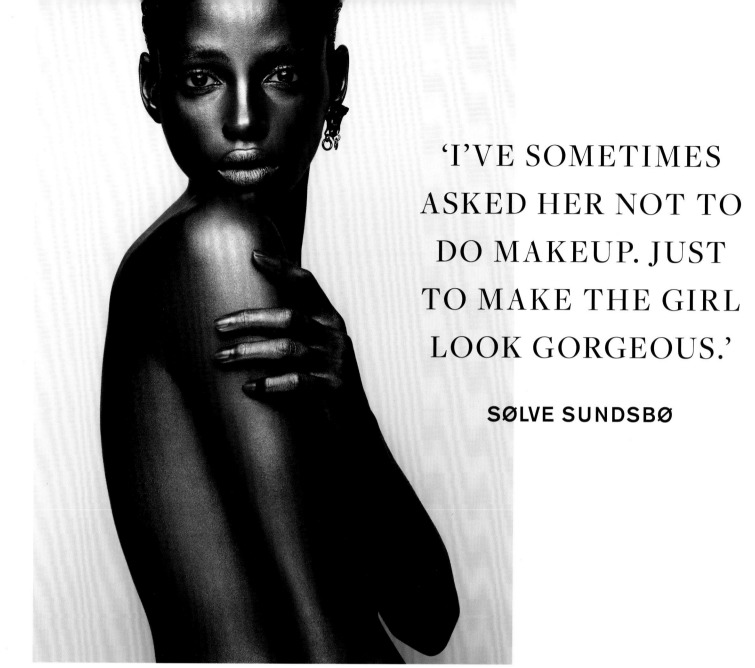

'I'VE SOMETIMES ASKED HER NOT TO DO MAKEUP. JUST TO MAKE THE GIRL LOOK GORGEOUS.'

SØLVE SUNDSBØ

ALLURE OCTOBER 2016; PHOTOGRAPHY SØLVE SUNDSBØ; FASHION EDITOR BEAT BOLLIGER; HAIR RUDI LEWIS; MANICURIST MARIAN NEWMAN; MODEL AYA JONES.

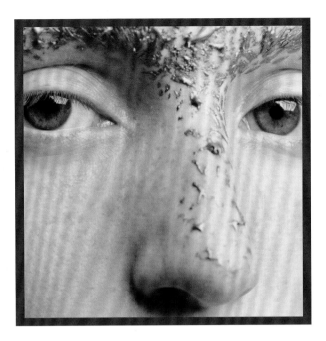

CRÈME MAGAZINE; PHOTOGRAPHY RICHARD BUSH.
I-D OCTOBER 2001 (UNPUBLISHED) 'MCDONALDIZATION'; PHOTOGRAPHY RICHARD BUSH; FASHION EDITOR JANE HOW; HAIR EUGENE SOULEIMAN.

This was a shoot with Richard Bush (above) for a magazine that no longer exists called *Crème*, and it would have been Richard and I going to a studio somewhere in East London, not even having a hairdresser, and Richard just letting me play and recording it. I loved the idea of the 10x8 close-up so you can see the texture of the skin. The product I put on here was gold-coloured icing. I guess this image relates to how I love medieval paintings when they're so old that the paint's literally cracking.

This is an unpublished picture (opposite) that was shot for *i-D* magazine by Richard, with Jane How and Eugene Souleiman. I think we all felt like this was an iconic moment, and we were so excited for it to be published. Then 9/11 happened and the story just could not be published, it was politically incorrect. It was a very sensitive time.

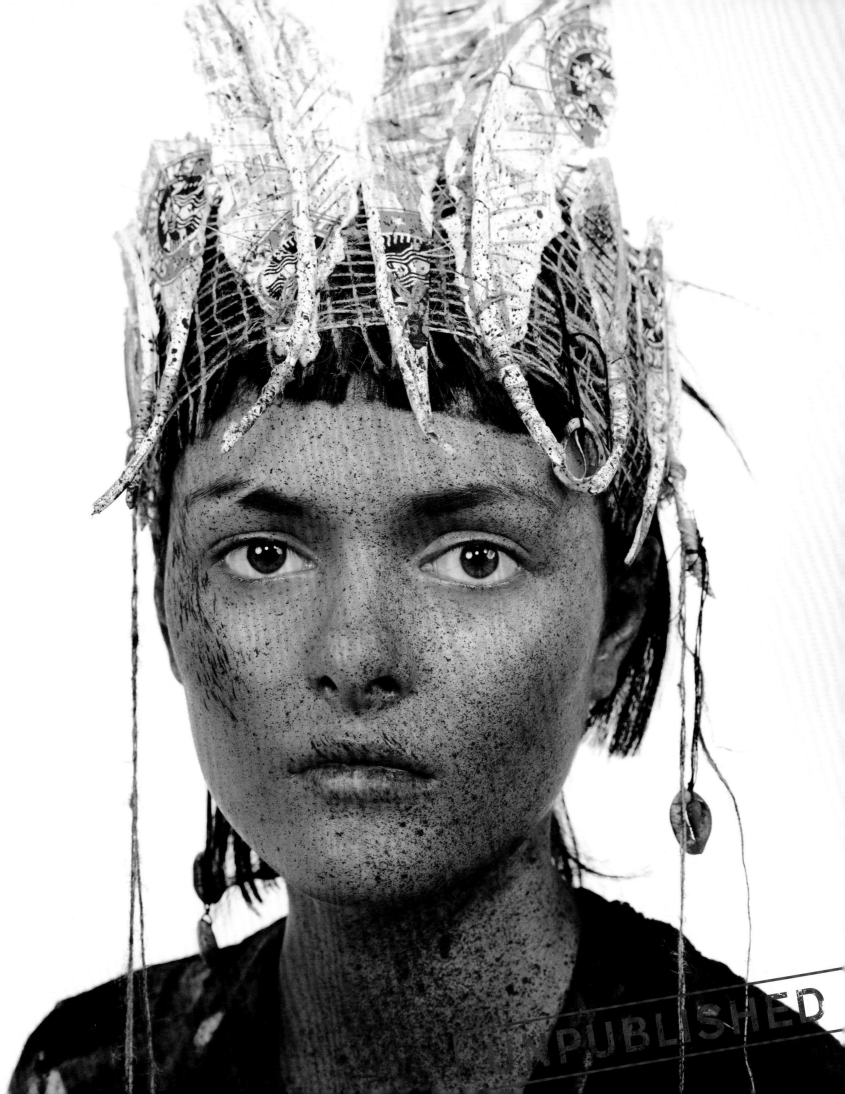

'GOOD KATE,

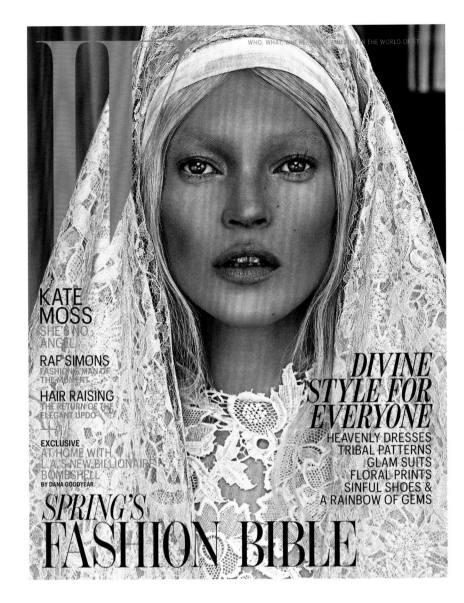

KATE
MOSS
SHE'S NO
ANGEL

RAF SIMONS
FASHION'S MAN OF
THE MOMENT

HAIR RAISING
THE RETURN OF THE
ELEGANT UPDO

EXCLUSIVE
AT HOME WITH
L.A.'S NEW BILLIONAIRE
BOMBSHELL
BY DANA GOODYEAR

SPRING'S
FASHION BIBLE

DIVINE
STYLE FOR
EVERYONE
HEAVENLY DRESSES
TRIBAL PATTERNS
GLAM SUITS
FLORAL PRINTS
SINFUL SHOES &
A RAINBOW OF GEMS

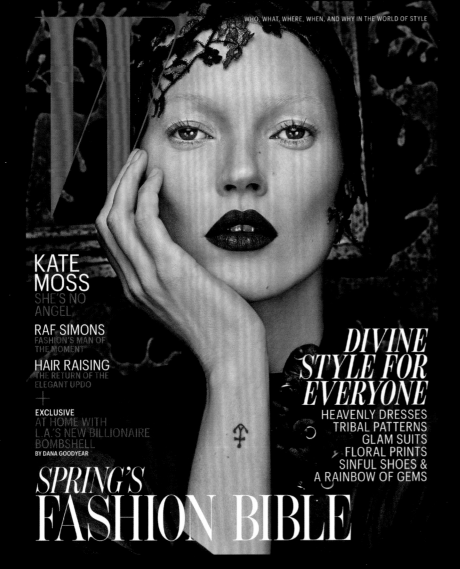

BAD KATE.'

'This was one of those stories that people look at and think it was so loaded. It was just like, I love Kate, I love Kate while she's good, I love Kate when she's being naughty. So we did this story of angelic Kate and dark Kate and Val just got it. She just got it. And all I remember was Kate being so focused and Val and I being quite naughty and laughing

W MAGAZINE NOVEMBER 2012; PHOTOGRAPHY STEVEN KLEIN; FASHION EDITOR EDWARD ENNINFUL; HAIR LUIGI MURENU; MANICURIST BERNADETTE THOMPSON; MODEL KEIRA KNIGHTLEY.

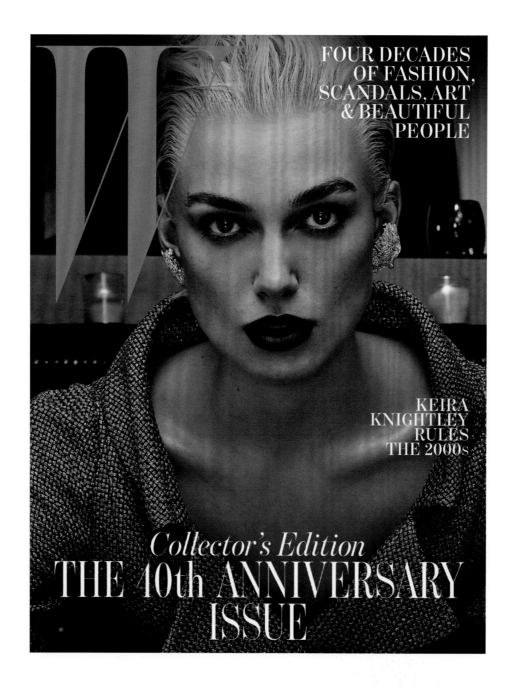

This was one of a series of covers I did with Steven. We had different actresses on the shoot, like Scarlett Johansson, Rooney Mara and Mia Wasikowska, and Steven wanted to make each woman into a character. Keira, who I had worked with a number of times, was amazing and said, 'OK Val, you can do whatever you like, but you are not bleaching my eyebrows'. And so really what I've done here is quite normal, beautiful makeup, but what's raw about it is Keira's attitude, and Steven's incredible light.

'OK VAL,
YOU CAN DO
WHATEVER
YOU LIKE,
BUT
YOU ARE NOT
BLEACHING
MY EYEBROWS.'

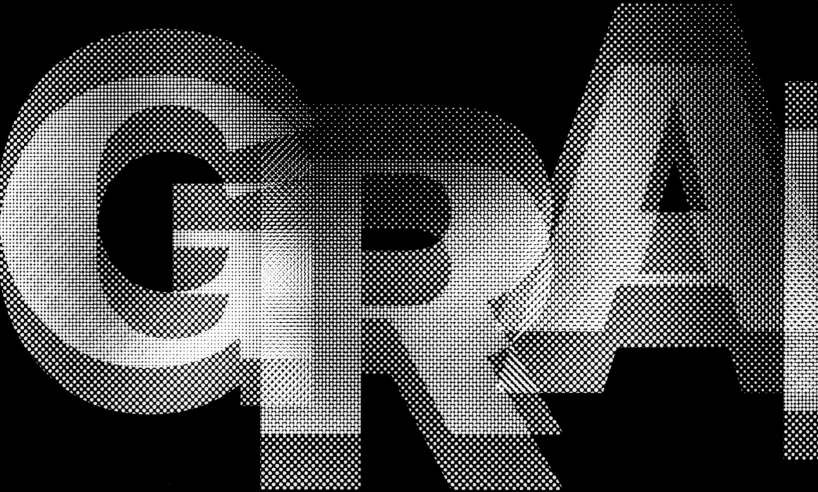

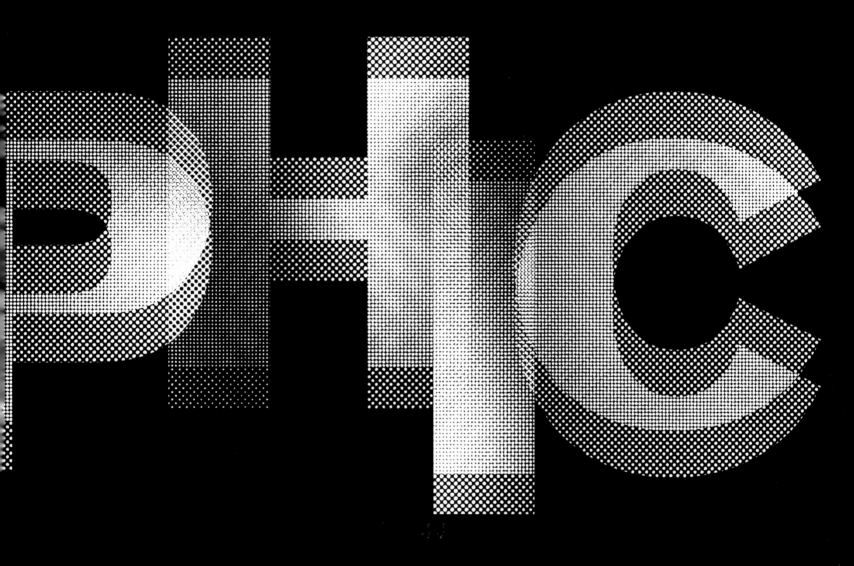

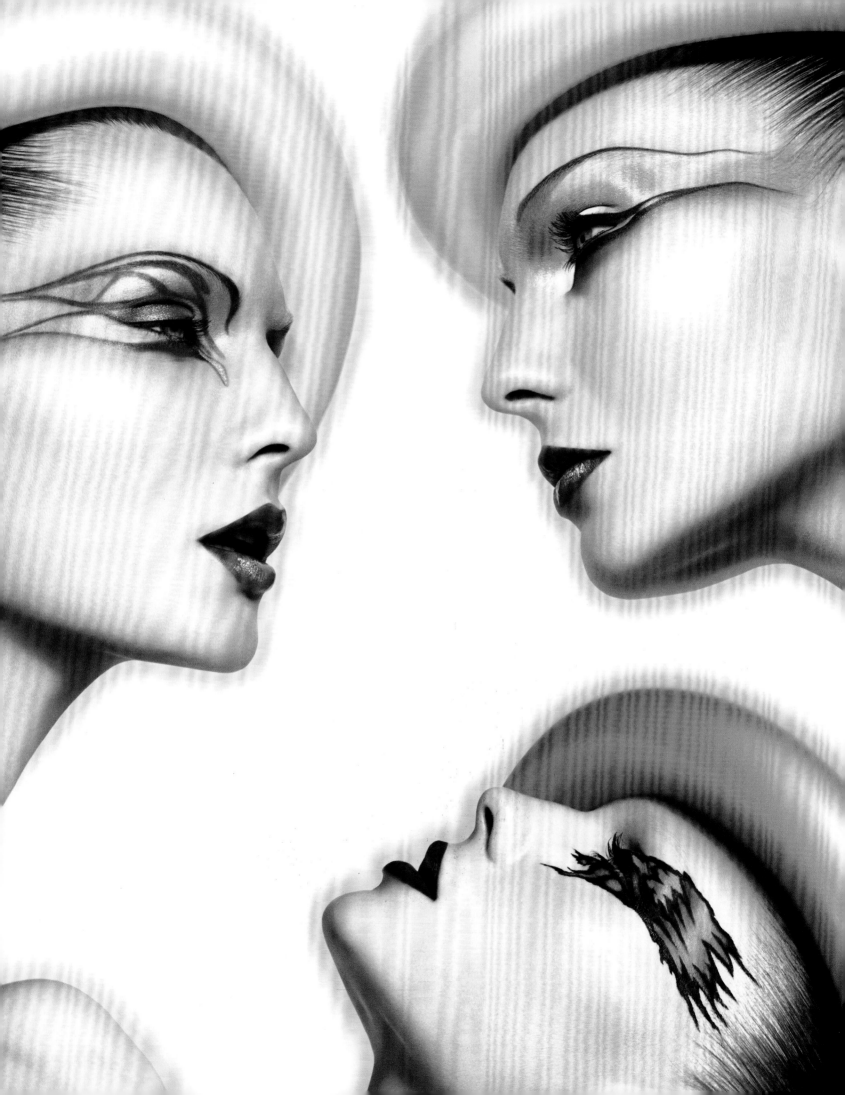

CROSSING THE LINE

Val's graphic work hits you like an adrenaline shot, then stares you down, snarling 'Look at me, but don't get too close'. This is powerful, dynamic, dramatic makeup – often about the simplicity of a single, bold gesture – that elongates eyes to create a menacing allure, pronounces mouths to render them too dangerous to kiss, and sharpens cheekbones to a point of peril.

Val's graphic makeup has its roots in punk. It is essentially about attention, power and drama. The punks of the seventies utilized makeup graphically to demand attention, via a feline eye or a vampire lip. And punk gave us possibly the most graphic beauty statement ever – taking an image of the Queen and piercing her stiff upper lip with a safety pin in protest against hypocrisy in the British establishment.

This chapter is about pure makeup drama. But dramatic gestures in makeup are Val's forté, like creating the face of a broken clown – as full-on as Pavarotti in *Pagliacci* – then wiping away the greasepaint, leaving only the graphic outline of the makeup in order to (in Val's words) 'let your imagination fill in the spaces'.

As with much of Val's work, there is an influence – albeit abstract – of art and artists. So in her graphic work we can see the influence of eighties Athena posters and album covers; the elongated, sweeping flamboyance of American illustrator Antonio Lopez; and the club-kid-gone-couture, almost geisha-like work of French photographer Serge Lutens. All have influenced Val with their caffeine kick of daring artistry – and none more than her muse, the sixties supermodel Veruschka, who was much appreciated by graphic, tribal body-paint artists, as seen in the radical art book *Trans-figurations* by photographer Holger Trülzsch.

And so it was a post-punk, anarchically inclined Val who entered the world of fashion in the nineties, at a time when 'graphic' was exploding on all levels. It was an era that witnessed the birth of Adobe Photoshop and saw the rise of graphic designers like Neville Brody and Phil Bicker of *The Face*, Peter Saville, the creative Svengali of Factory Records, and the American graphic design legend David Carson of *Ray Gun* – figures who were all so achingly cool it hurt. None of this was lost on the fledgling Val as she took to makeup with her own ideas on what was cool. With a graphic swipe at the 'no makeup' mantra of grunge, she began working on and creating more conceptually orientated shoots for magazines like *Dazed & Confused* – her way of ignoring what was otherwise a rather dull party.

V MAGAZINE; PHOTOGRAPHY MIGUEL REVERIEGO; HAIR PETER GRAY; MODEL KAROLIN WOLTER.

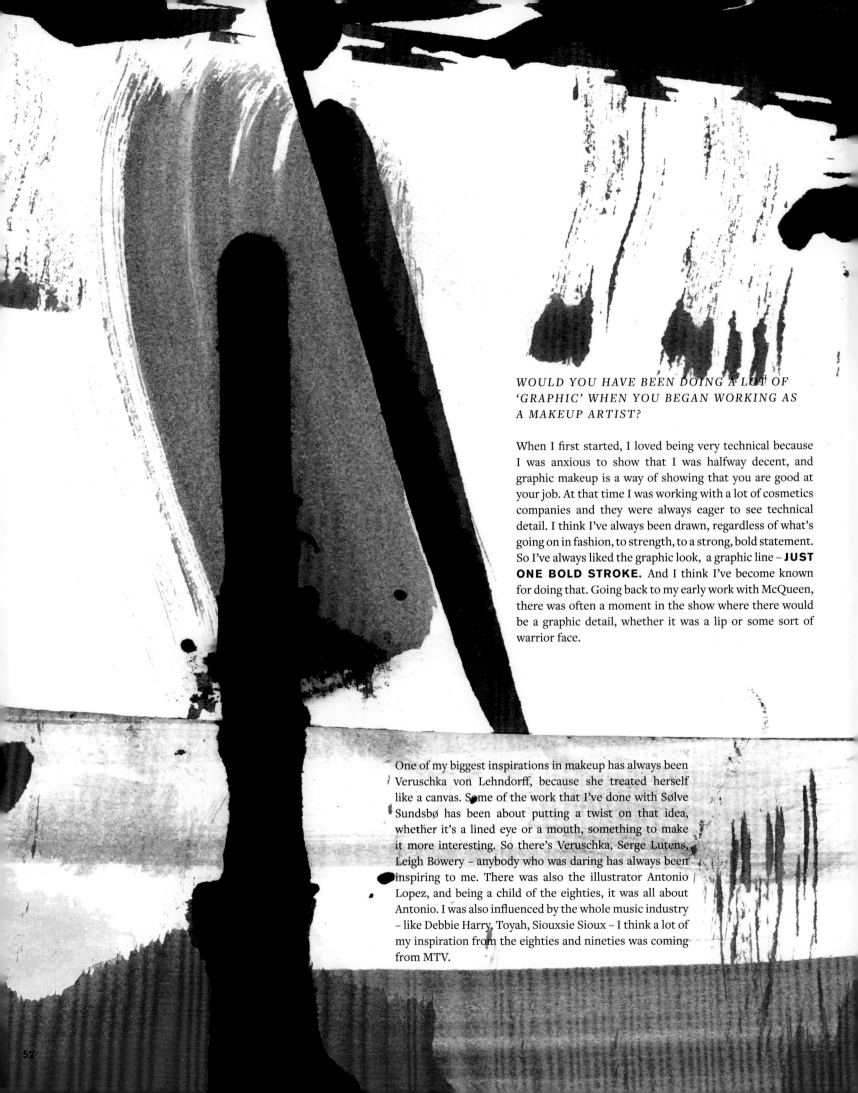

WOULD YOU HAVE BEEN DOING A LOT OF 'GRAPHIC' WHEN YOU BEGAN WORKING AS A MAKEUP ARTIST?

When I first started, I loved being very technical because I was anxious to show that I was halfway decent, and graphic makeup is a way of showing that you are good at your job. At that time I was working with a lot of cosmetics companies and they were always eager to see technical detail. I think I've always been drawn, regardless of what's going on in fashion, to strength, to a strong, bold statement. So I've always liked the graphic look, a graphic line – **JUST ONE BOLD STROKE.** And I think I've become known for doing that. Going back to my early work with McQueen, there was often a moment in the show where there would be a graphic detail, whether it was a lip or some sort of warrior face.

One of my biggest inspirations in makeup has always been Veruschka von Lehndorff, because she treated herself like a canvas. Some of the work that I've done with Sølve Sundsbø has been about putting a twist on that idea, whether it's a lined eye or a mouth, something to make it more interesting. So there's Veruschka, Serge Lutens, Leigh Bowery – anybody who was daring has always been inspiring to me. There was also the illustrator Antonio Lopez, and being a child of the eighties, it was all about Antonio. I was also influenced by the whole music industry – like Debbie Harry, Toyah, Siouxsie Sioux – I think a lot of my inspiration from the eighties and nineties was coming from MTV.

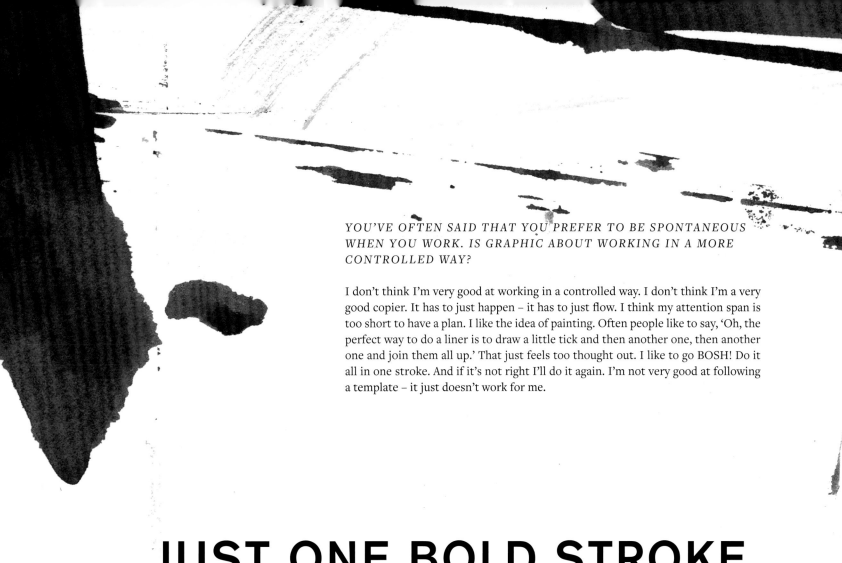

YOU'VE OFTEN SAID THAT YOU PREFER TO BE SPONTANEOUS
WHEN YOU WORK. IS GRAPHIC ABOUT WORKING IN A MORE
CONTROLLED WAY?

I don't think I'm very good at working in a controlled way. I don't think I'm a very
good copier. It has to just happen – it has to just flow. I think my attention span is
too short to have a plan. I like the idea of painting. Often people like to say, 'Oh, the
perfect way to do a liner is to draw a little tick and then another one, then another
one and join them all up.' That just feels too thought out. I like to go BOSH! Do it
all in one stroke. And if it's not right I'll do it again. I'm not very good at following
a template – it just doesn't work for me.

JUST ONE BOLD STROKE.

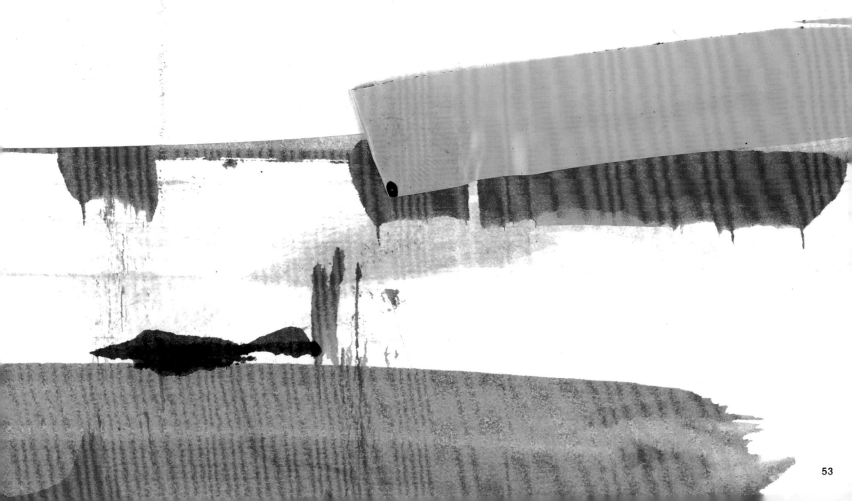

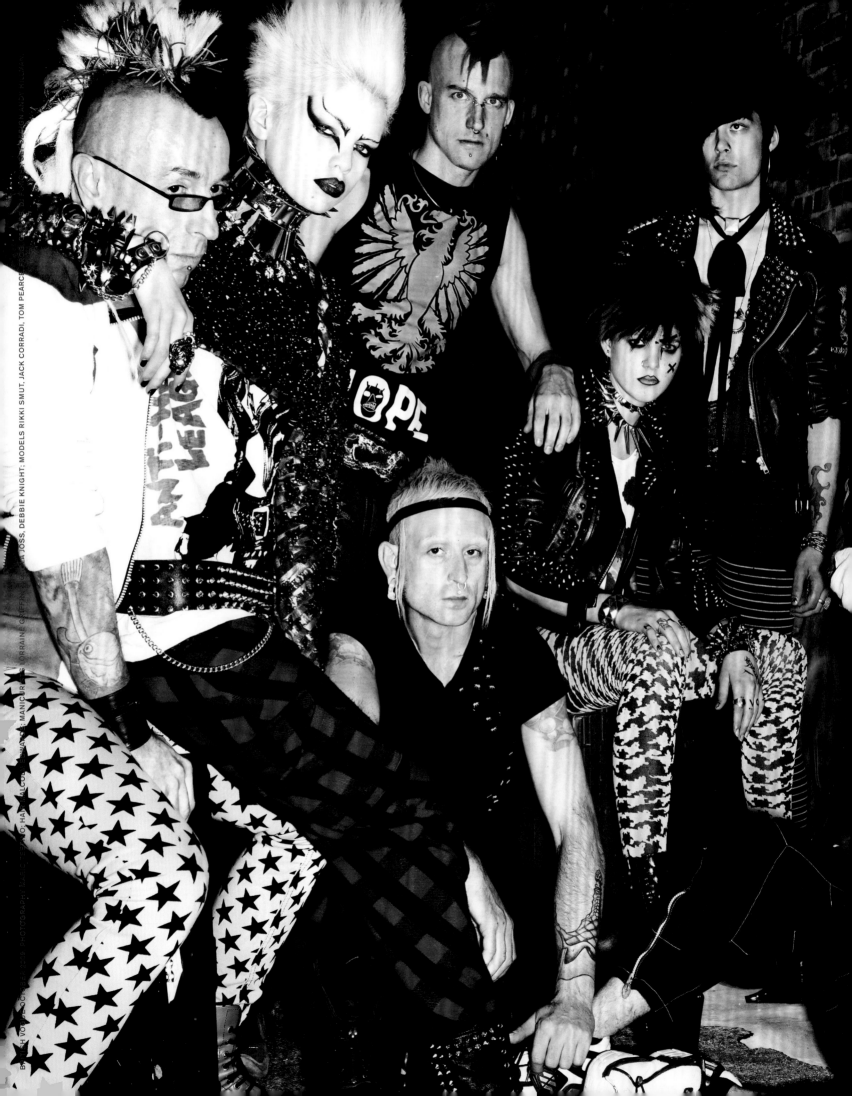

BRITISH VOGUE NOVEMBER 2009 PHOTOGRAPHY MARC LEBON; HAIR MALCOLM EDWARDS; MANICURE LORRAINE GRIFFIN JESSICA JOSS, DEBBIE KNIGHT; MODELS RIKKI SMUT, JACK CORRADI, TOM PEARCE

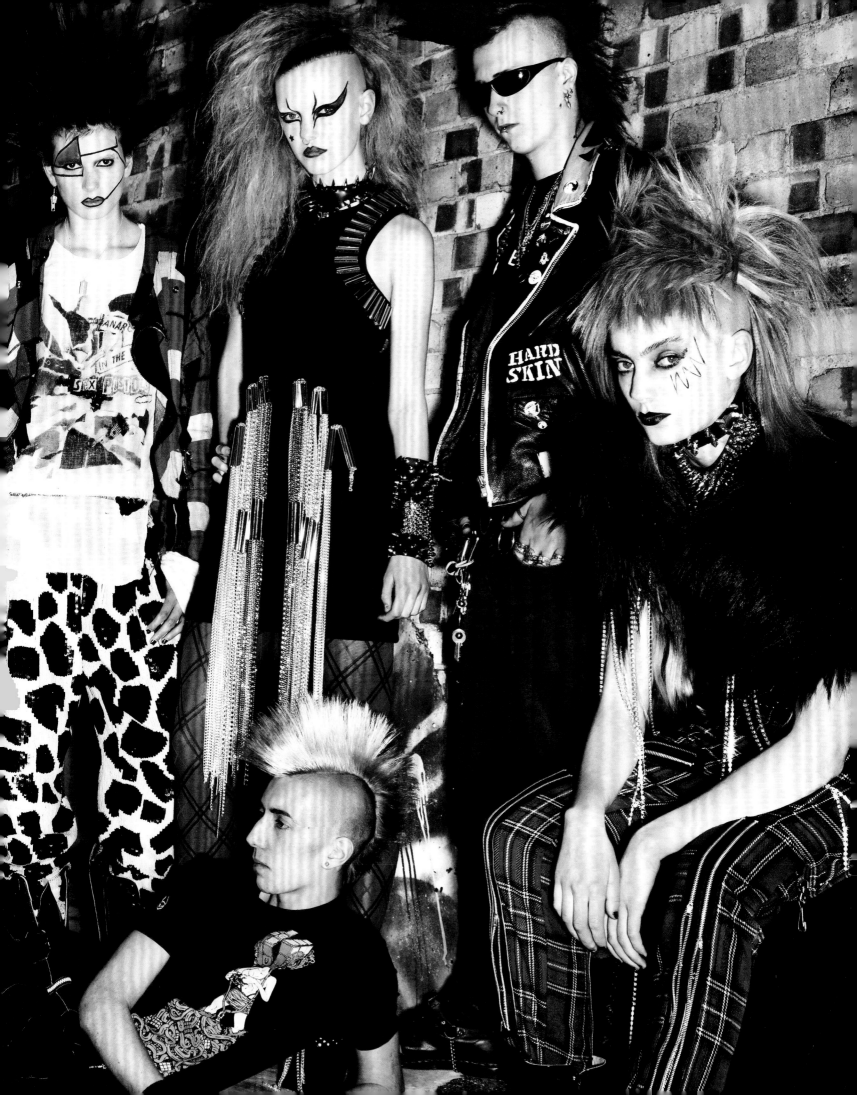

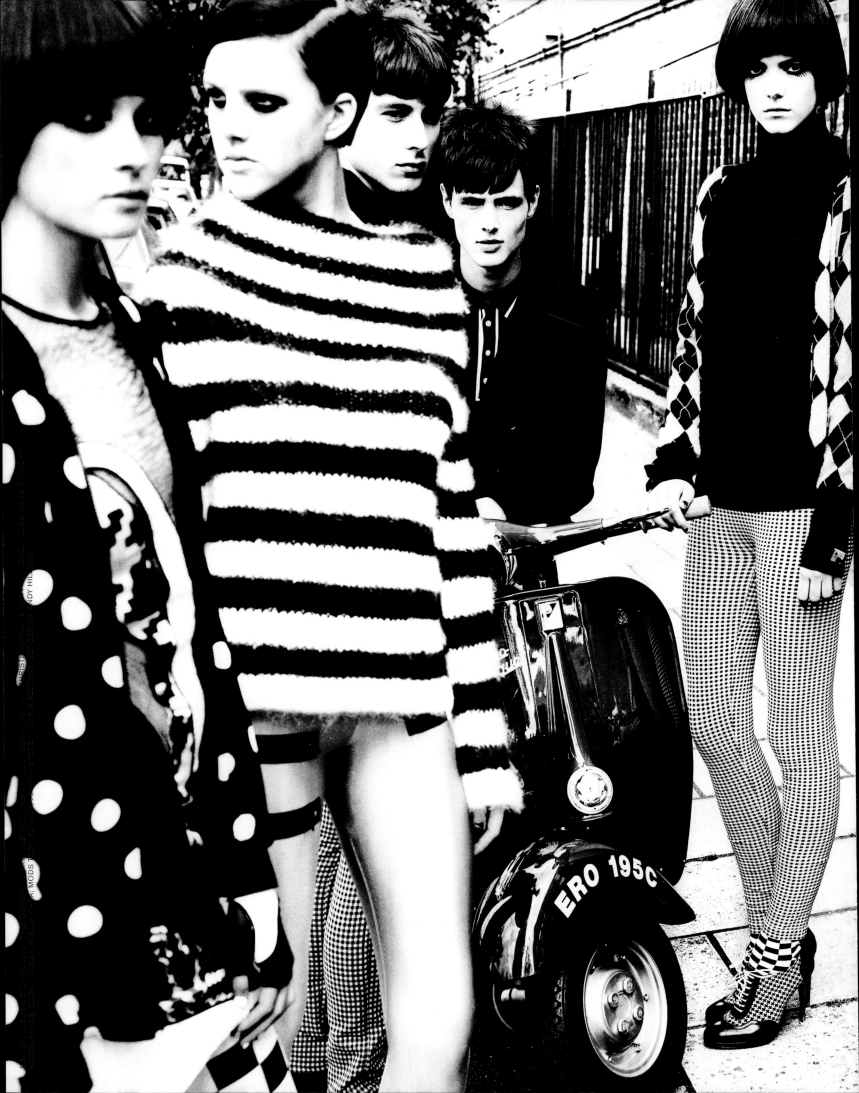

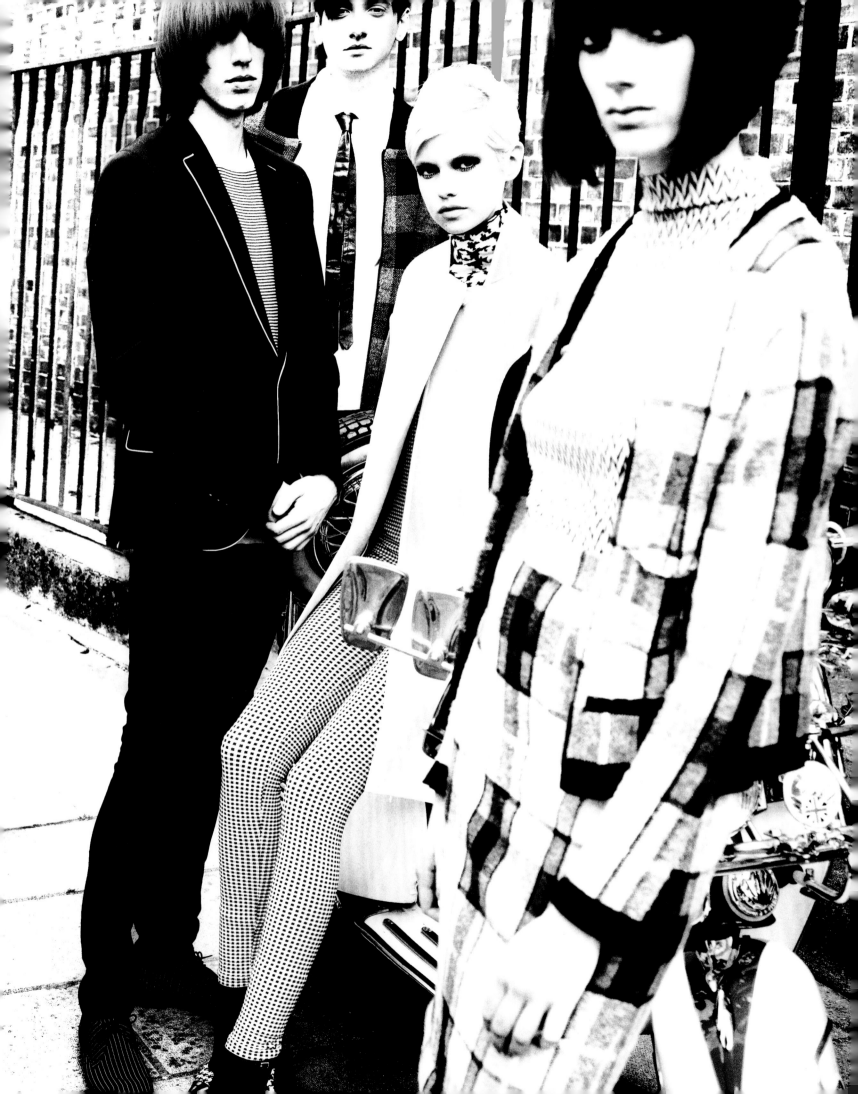

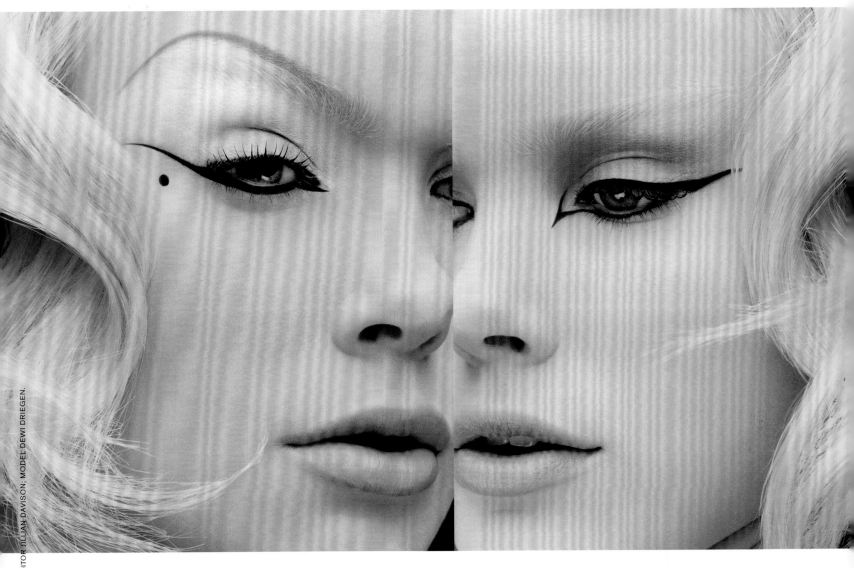

LET'S JUST *PUSH*

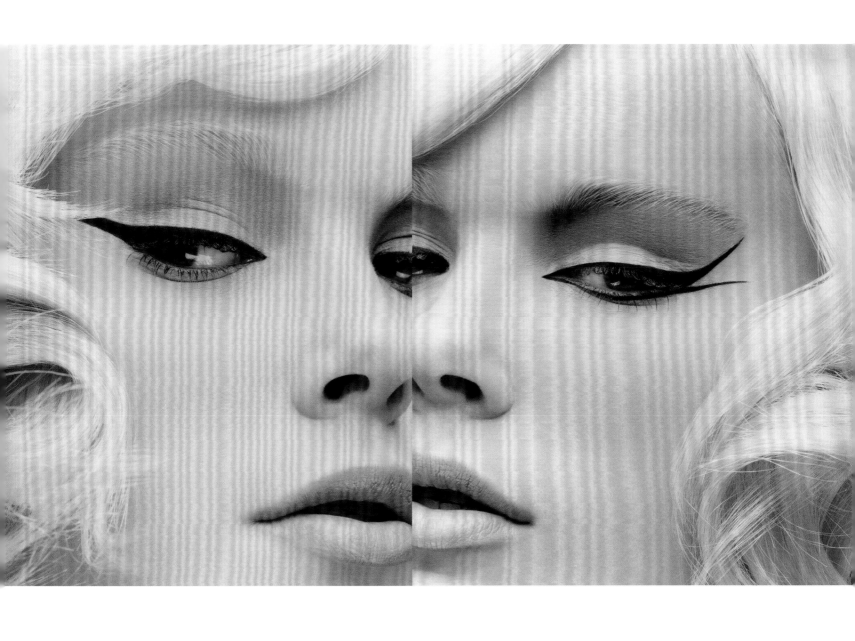

IT A LITTLE BIT

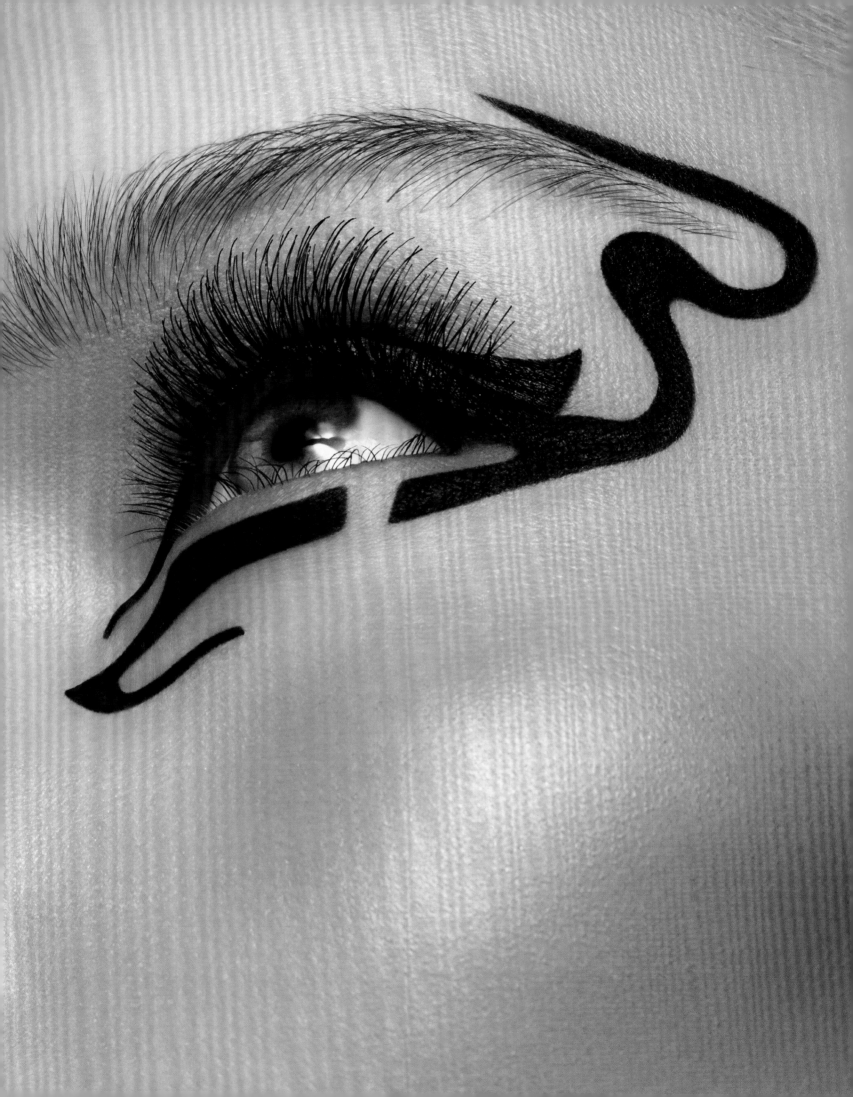

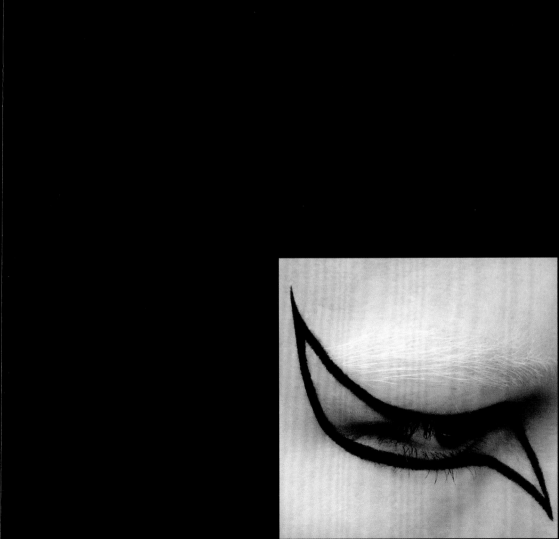

My first experience of Val, she kind of insisted on trying to shave off my eyebrows ... We really like to push Val because it kind of feels like she pushes us as well. She's got a very finite amount of time to do what she needs to do and I understand that need for focus.'

GARETH PUGH

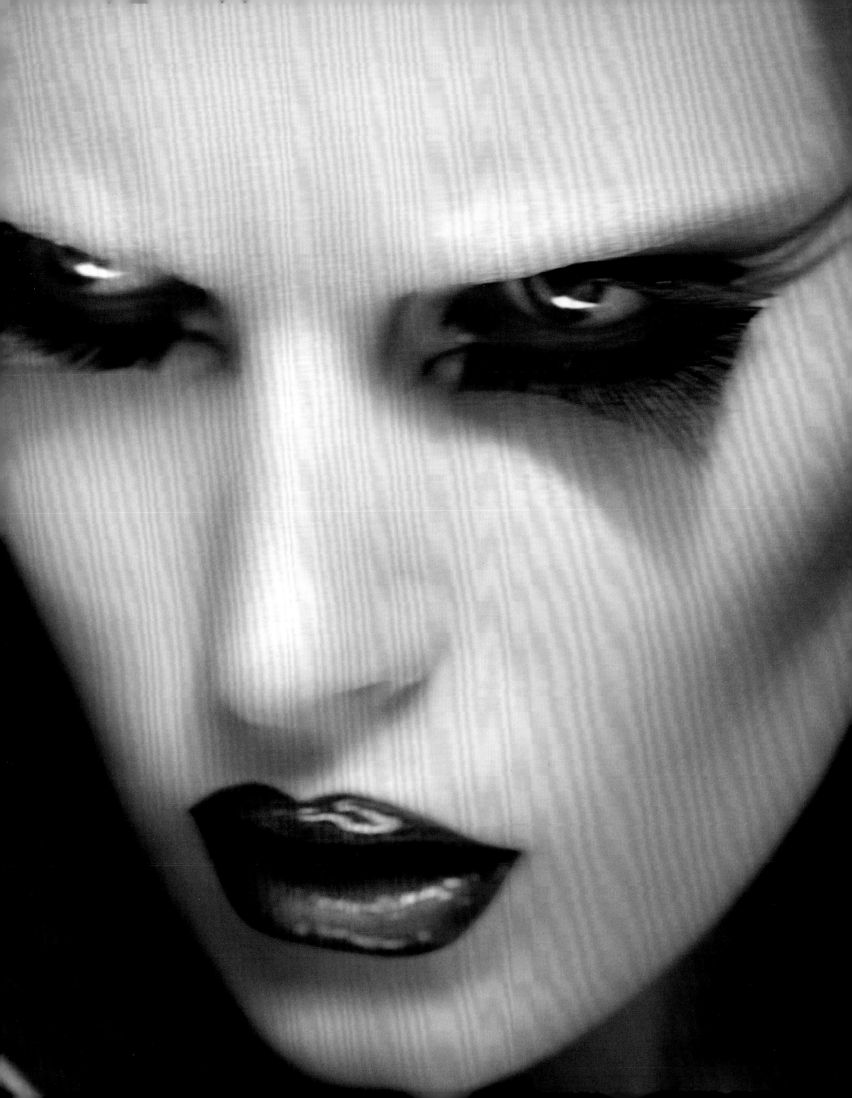

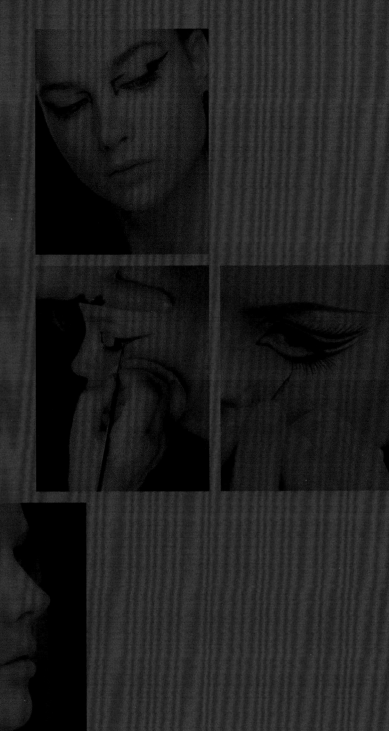

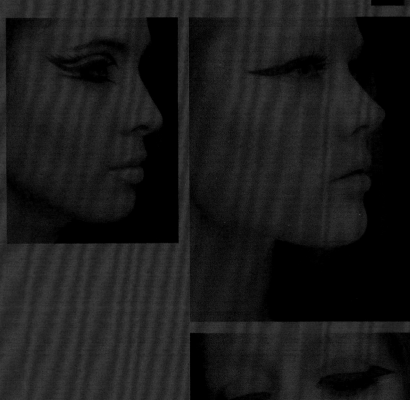

PHOTOGRAPHY LUCA CANNONIERI.
THE FACE 2001. PHOTOGRAPHY LIZ COLLINS; FASHION EDITOR KATIE GRAND; MODEL DEVON AOKI.

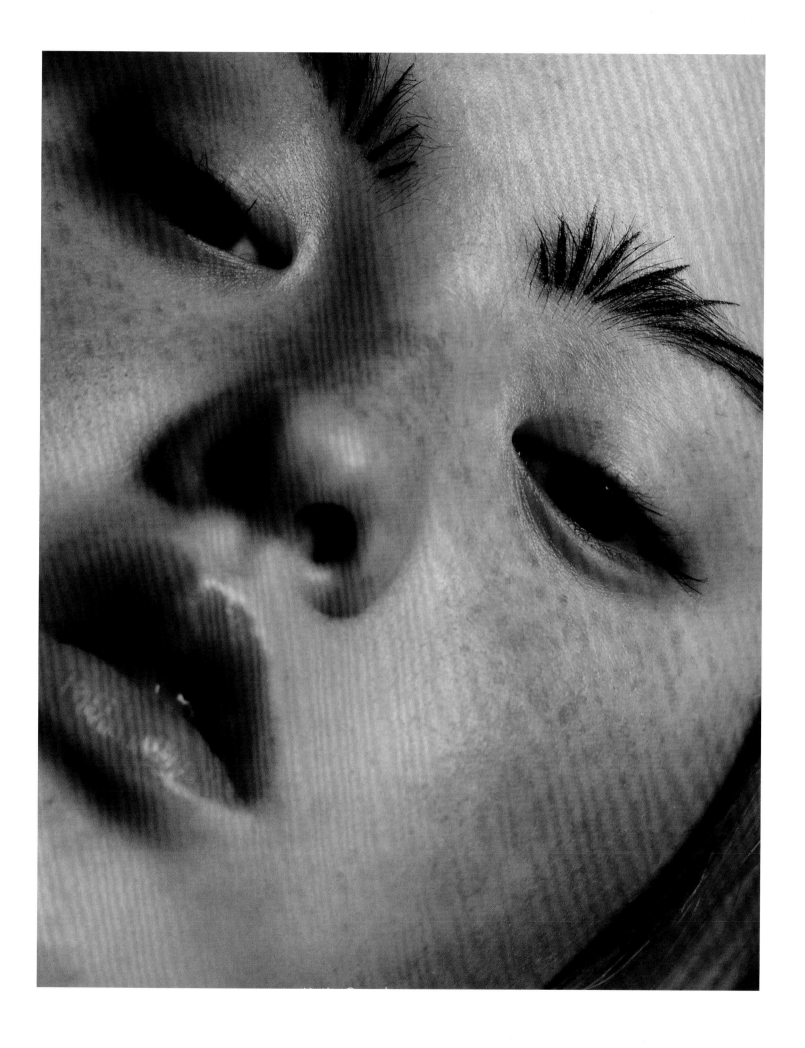

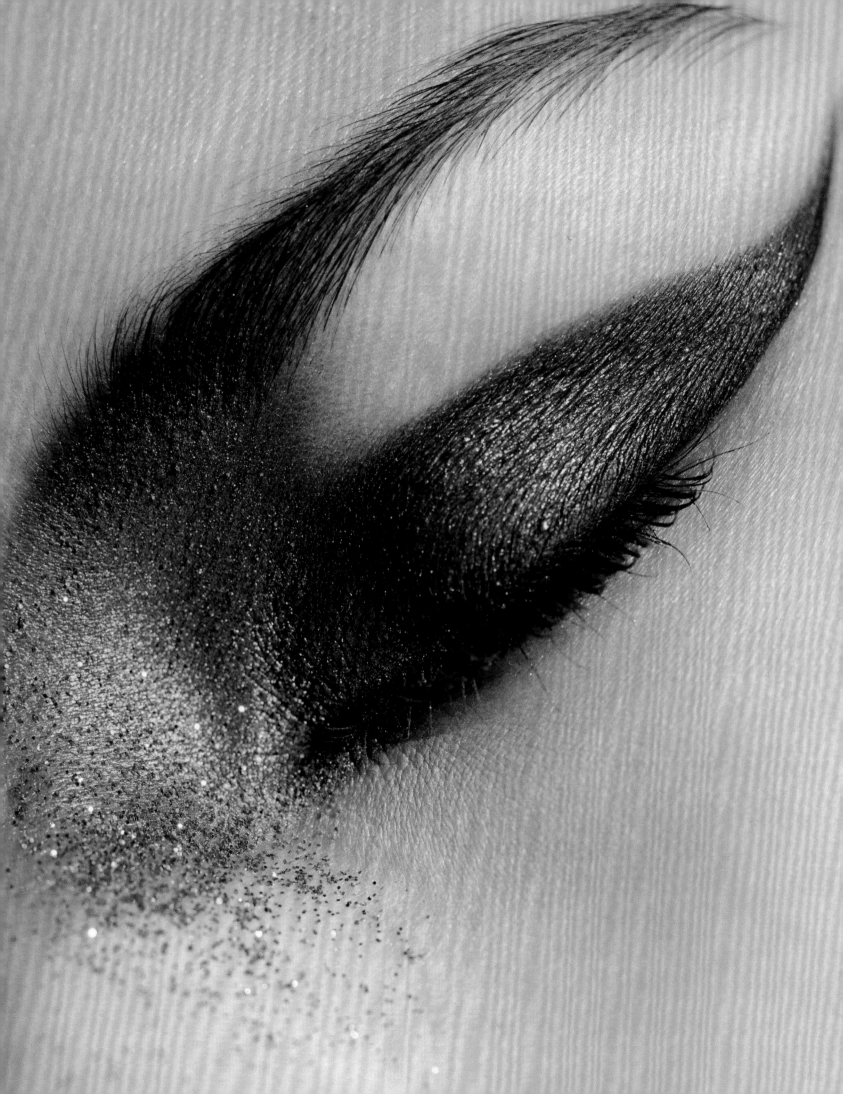

I just like the simplicity of a single gesture, whether that be in colour, carbon or glitter. I often think that sometimes that's all you need to make it look fresh.

VOGUE NIPPON APRIL 2003: PHOTOGRAPHY RICHARD BUSH.
FOLLOWING PAGES: NUMÉRO 57, OCTOBER 2004; PHOTOGRAPHY RICHARD BUSH; MODEL POLINA KUKLINA.

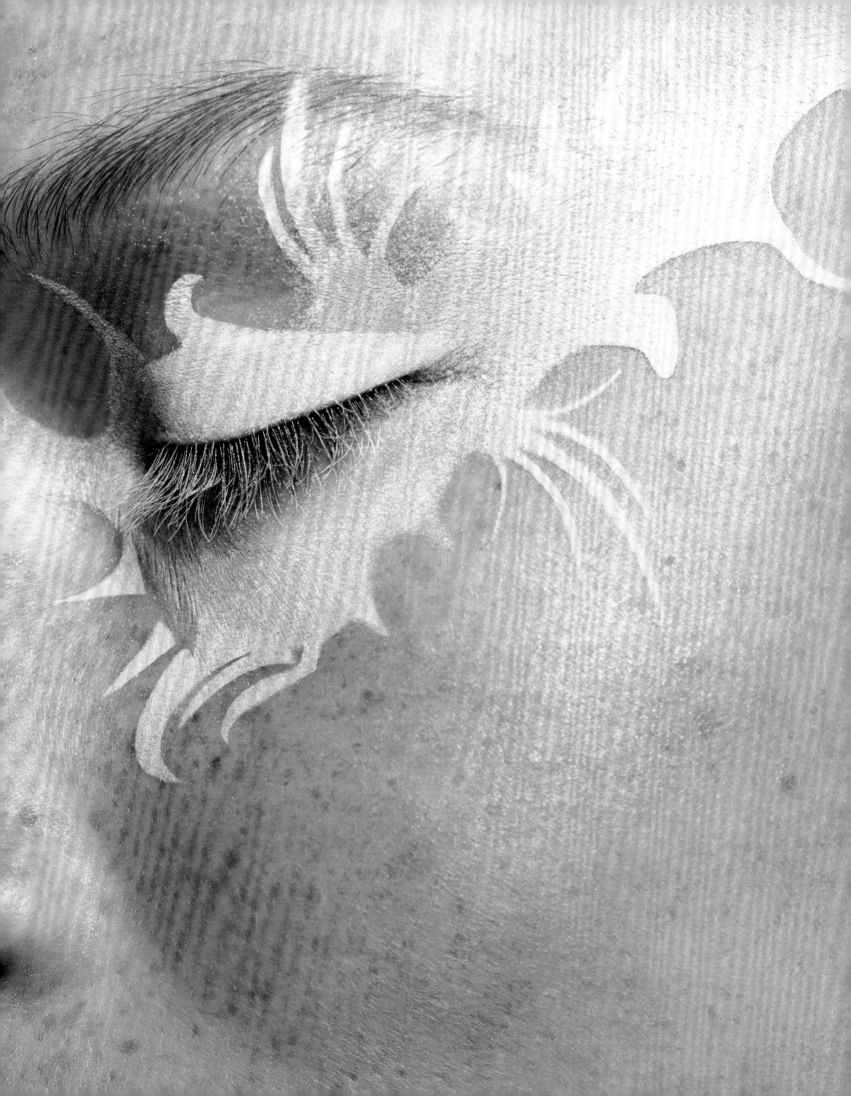

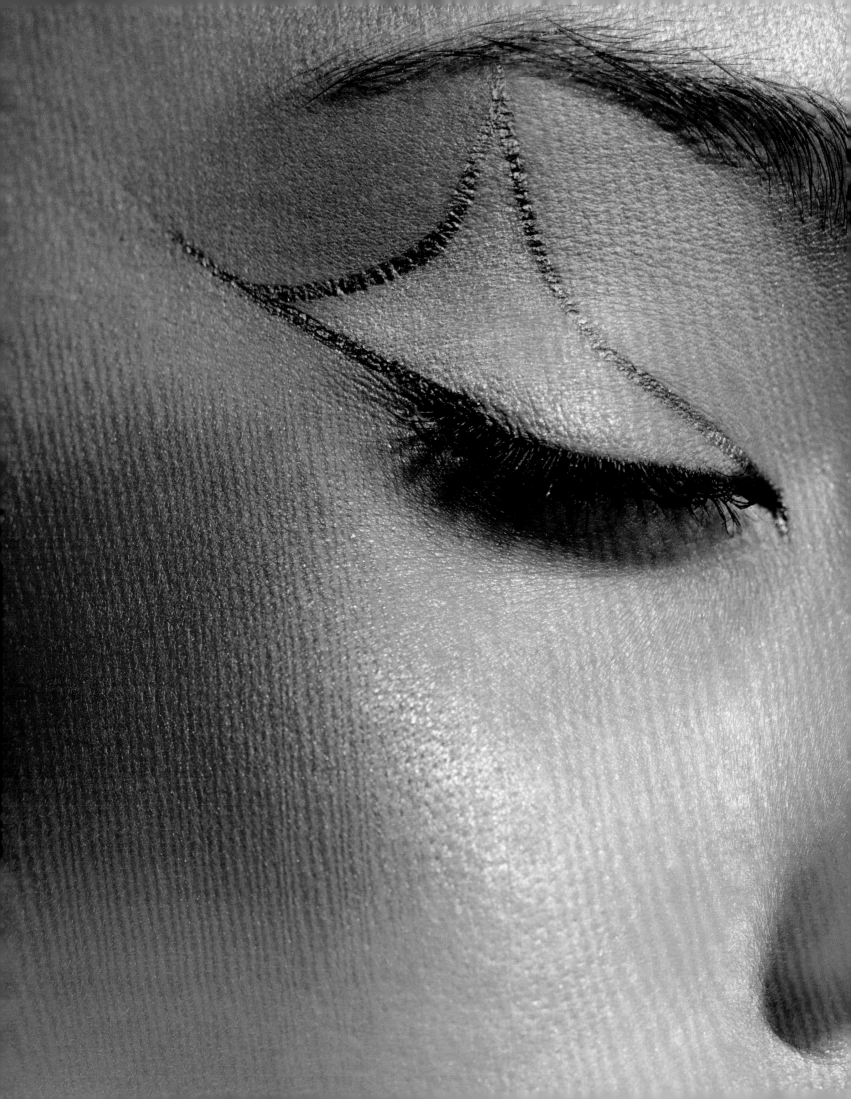

ESSENTIALLY, YOU'RE

PAINTING

A

NUMÉRO 108, NOVEMBER 2009; PHOTOGRAPHY MIGUEL REVERIEGO; HAIR KEN O'ROURKE; MODEL ANJA RUBIK.

IF I THINK OF A GRAPHIC EYE I THINK OF AMY WINEHOUSE, AND THIS IMAGE IS LIKE A COLOURFUL VERSION OF HER MAKEUP.

This was a story about eight completely different make-ups on Anja. I wanted to do something that was a bit **'IN YOUR FACE'** graphic, sort of punky, but I didn't want to use black because we do that so much already. So I thought, 'OK, why don't we take an odd-coloured lipstick, like a lavender, and do a navy brow and a yellow eye?'

I DON'T INSTANTLY RECOGNIZE ANJA IN THIS IMAGE, SO WOULD YOU SAY GRAPHIC MAKEUP IS PARTICULARLY TRANSFORMATIVE?

Yes, because you're painting, essentially, you're painting a picture. It's empowering. I think makeup can make you feel more confident, more powerful. I like the feline aloofness of a graphic eye that says, 'Fuck you. This is me.'

PICTURE

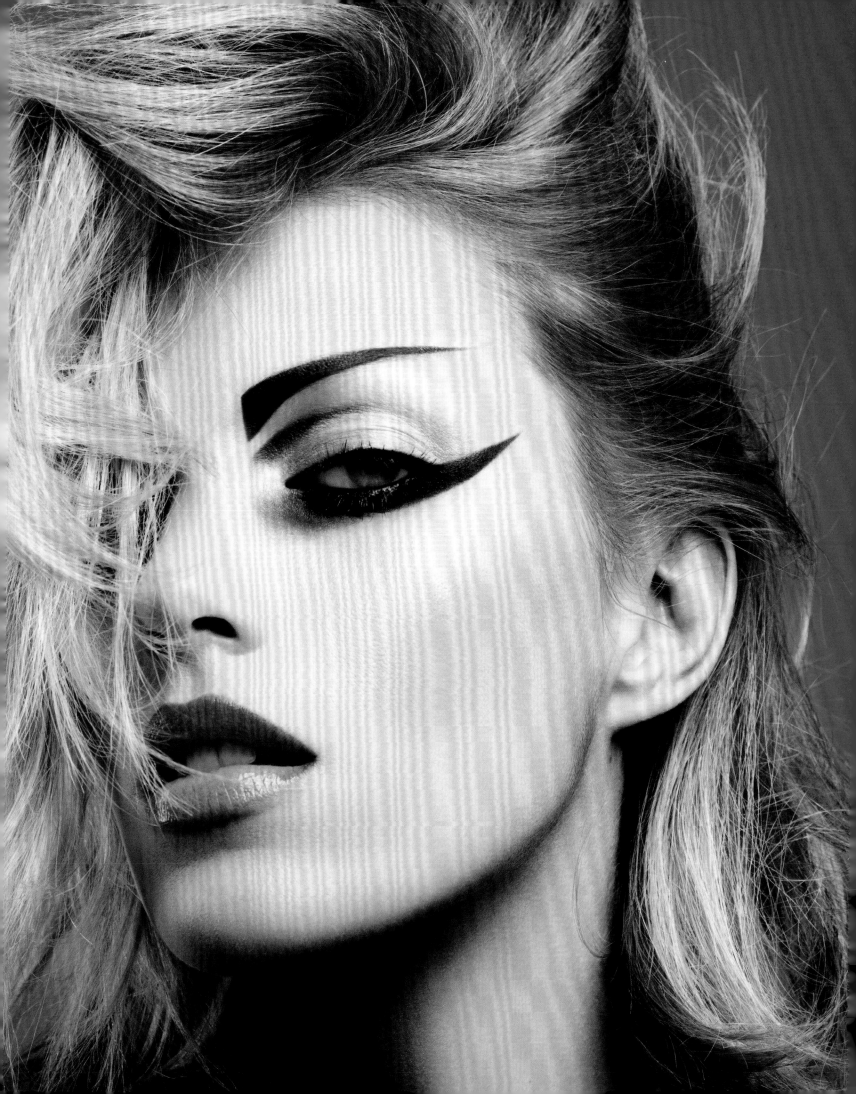

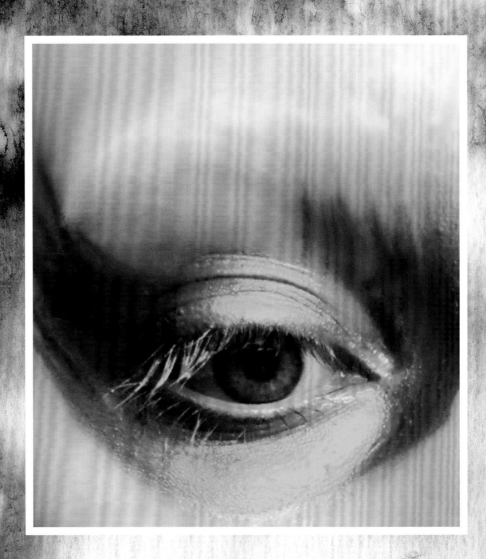

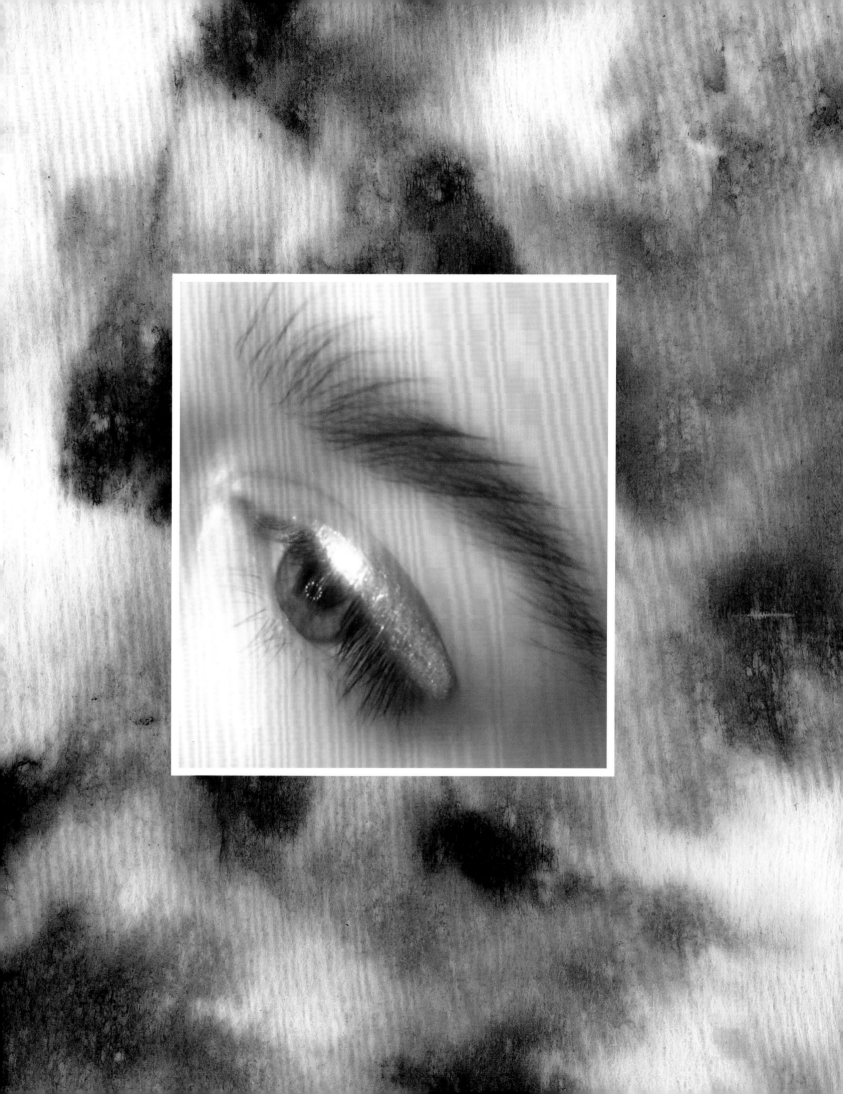

BRITISH VOGUE NOVEMBER 2010; PHOTOGRAPHY NICK KNIGHT; FASHION EDITOR LUCINDA CHAMBERS; HAIR SAM MCKNIGHT; MANICURIST MARIAN NEWMAN; MODEL RAQUEL ZIMMERMANN.

This shoot was with Nick, Lucinda, Sam and Marian. I remember Lucinda said it was going to be blacks and whites with creams, and Nick was going to desaturate the tones in the pictures. It was either going to be low colour or black-and-white shots. I didn't want to do a Peggy Moffitt or a Twiggy; I wanted to do it so that it felt more 'now' than a copy of the sixties or seventies. So it was all about this black on the eye, very graphic. I was referencing the photographer Irina Ionesco. So I started there and just went off on a tangent. But what's nice about this shoot is that it looks like a sitting: like a Cecil Beaton gone Mad Max.

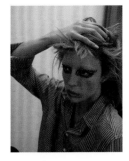

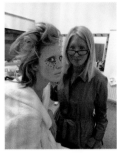

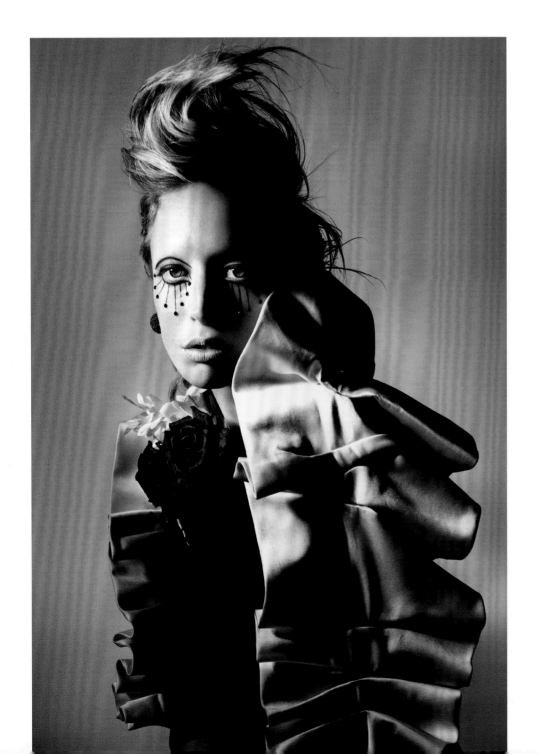

LIKE
A
CECIL
BEATON
GONE
MAD
MAX

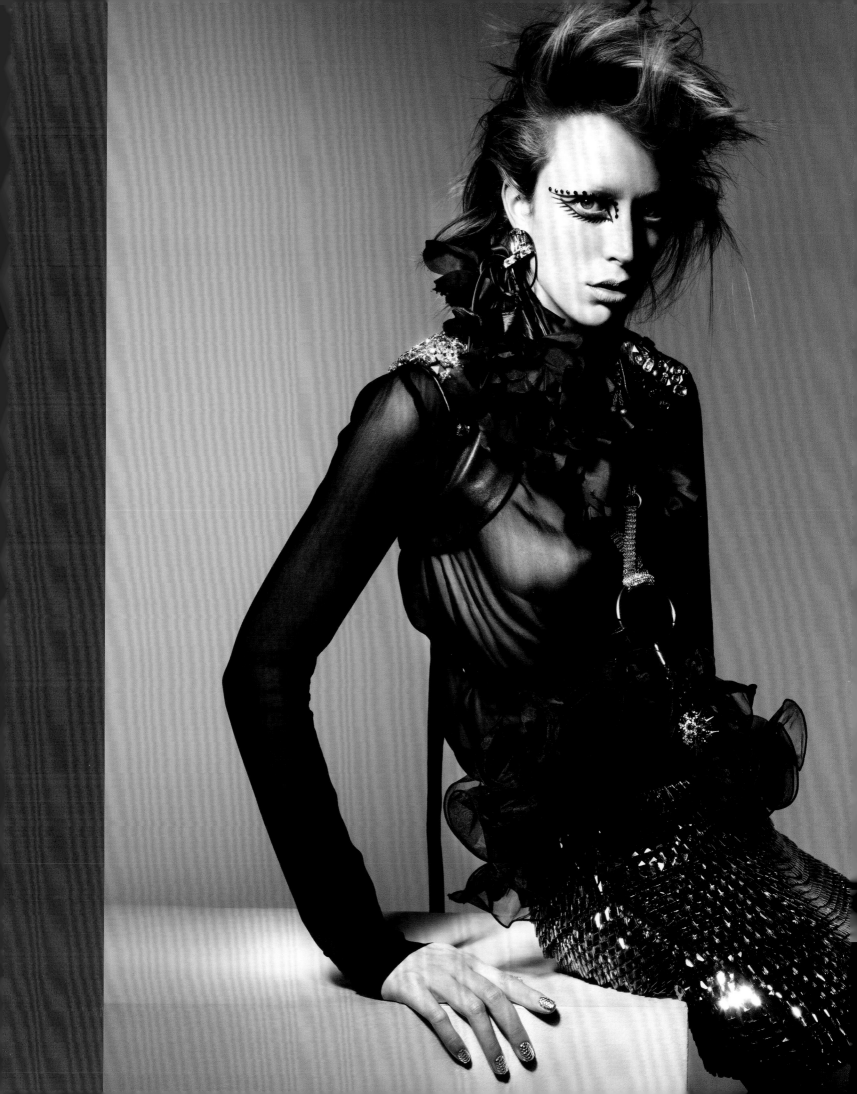

VOGUE ITALIA JUNE 2009: PHOTOGRAPHY MICHELANGELO DI BATTISTA; FASHION EDITOR ALICE GENTILUCCI; HAIR: STÉPHANE LANCIEN; MODEL: ALEK ALEXEYEVA.

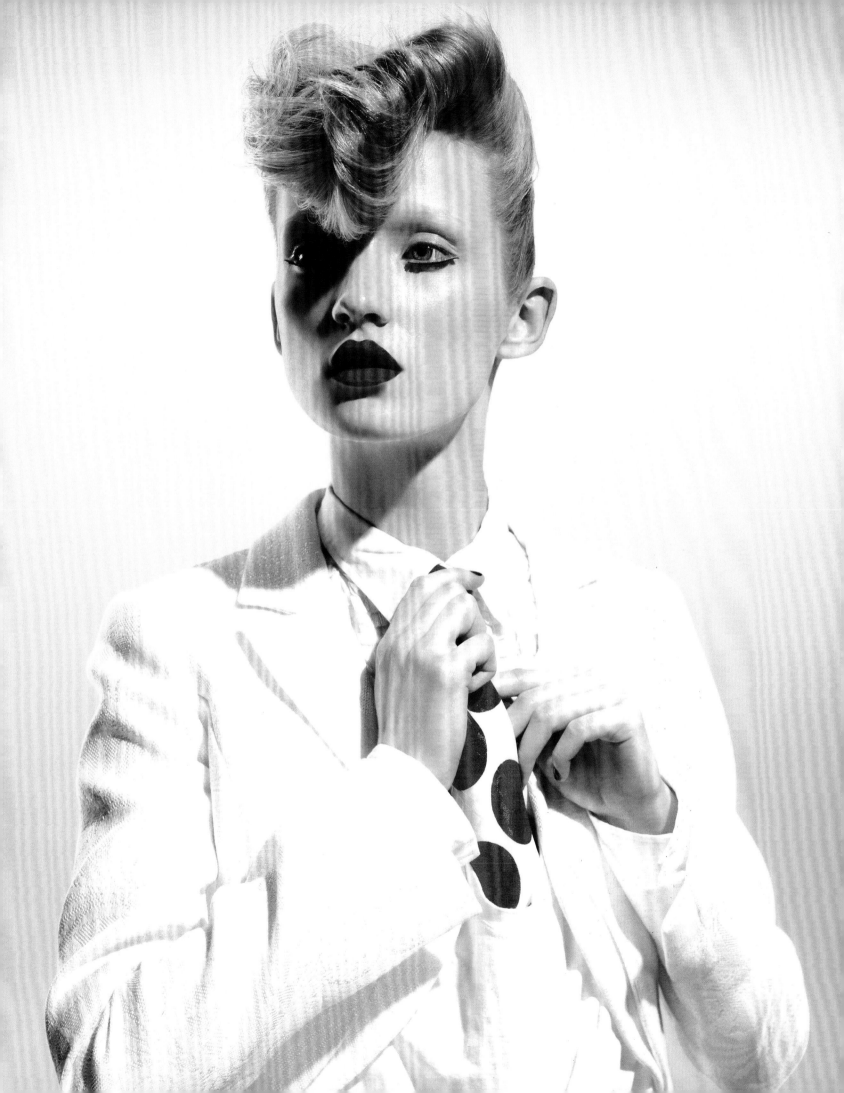

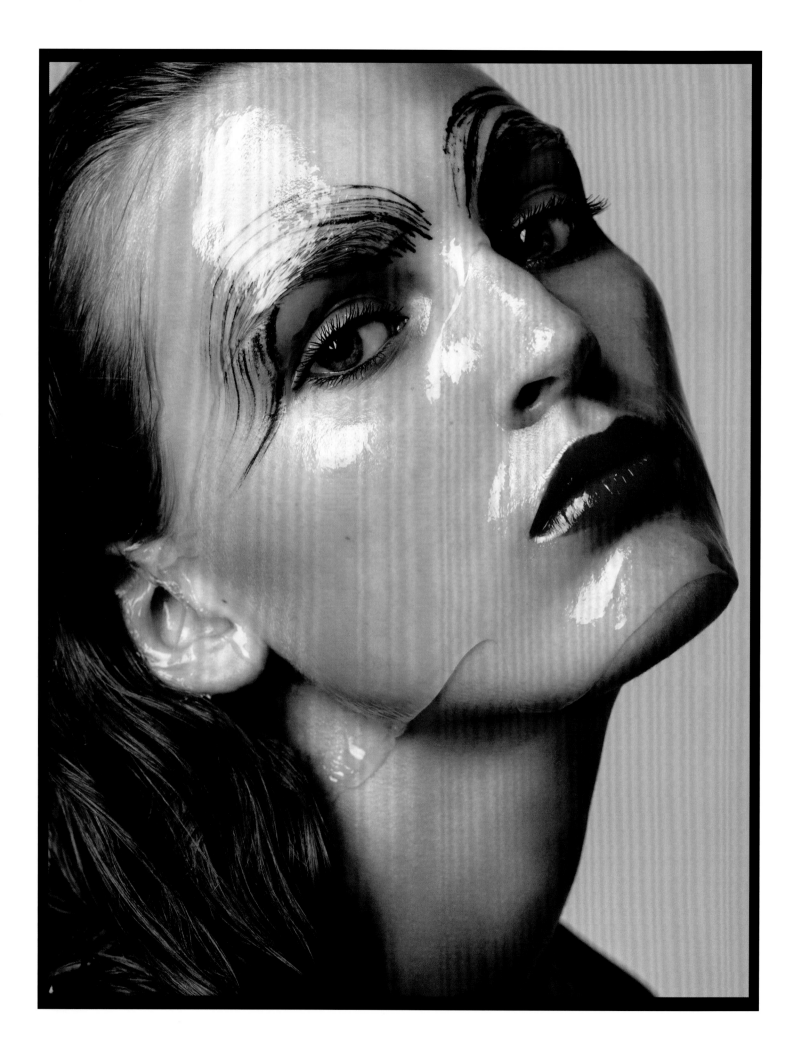

IT'S HONEY, ACTUALLY.

It's from a shoot I did for *10* magazine. I like beauty in the extreme and I get worried people will get bored if I do a nice, lovely beauty story, so I always have to fuck it up in some way. But retain the beauty. So for this I thought, 'OK, let's do a graphic eyebrow, but not as you know it'. I wanted to do something very linear. So I bleached Ali's eyebrows, painted on these black lines, added a bit of colour to the lip and then said, 'OK, now let's pour honey on her.'

I took a massive risk by pouring honey over this already graphic makeup. If you don't get the shot in a situation like this you've got to take the whole thing off and do it again. And will I get that same, spontaneous roundness of the brow? No, probably not. So sometimes I make it very difficult for myself, but then I just love those kind of 'Will we, won't we? Is it going to happen?' moments.

I LIKE THAT IT'S A MOMENT AND WHEN THE MOMENT'S GONE, IT'S GONE.

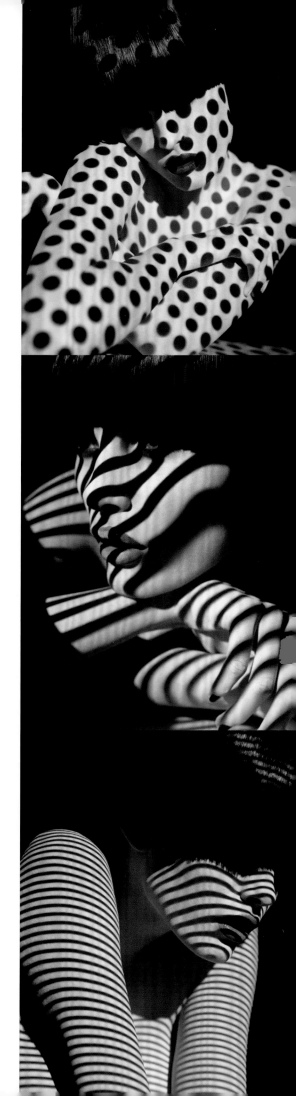

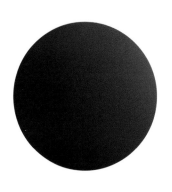

Lip Service

NUMÉRO 93, MAY 2008; PHOTOGRAPHY SØLVE SUNDSBØ; HAIR MALCOLM EDWARDS; MANICURIST SOPHY ROBSON; MODEL EDITA VILKEVICIUTE.

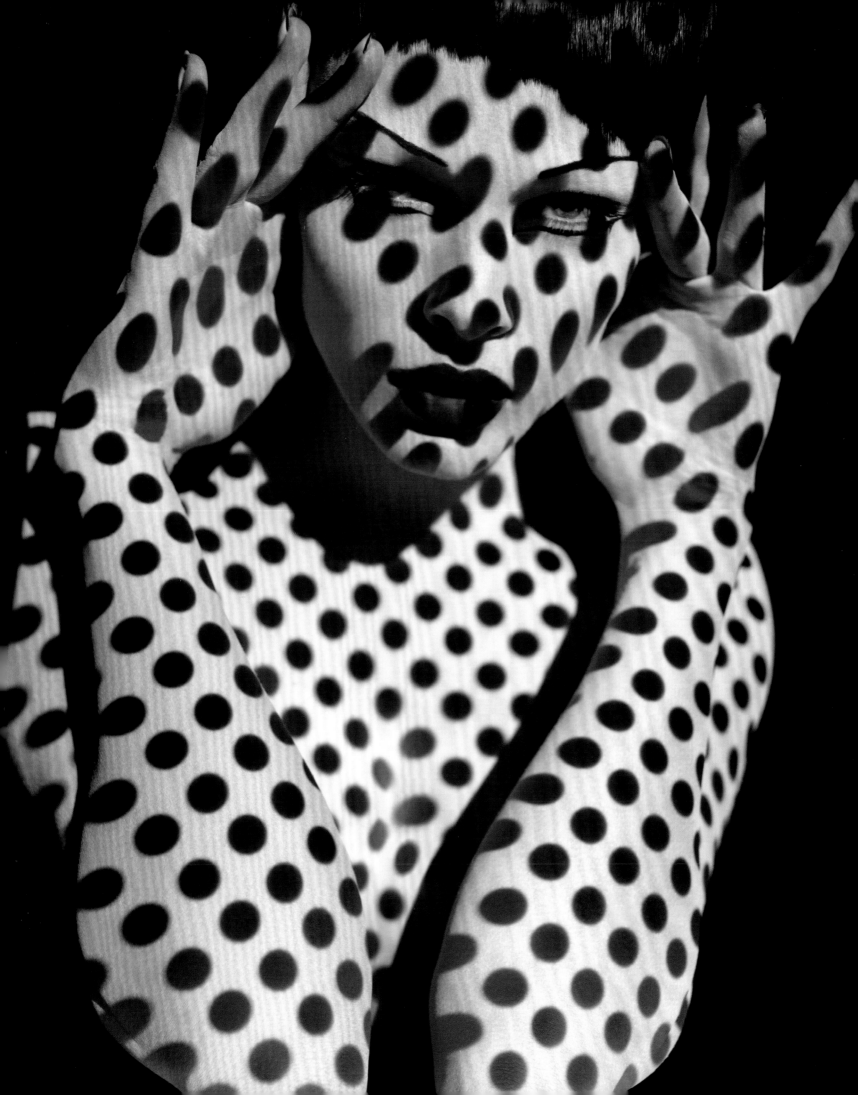

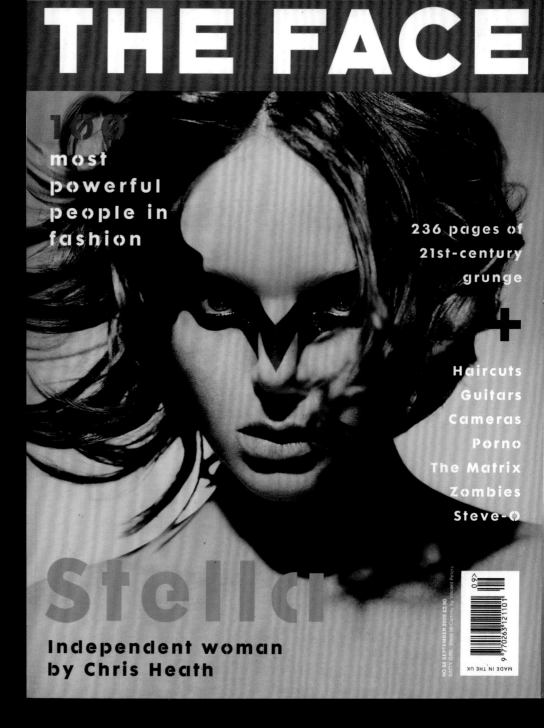

THE FACE

100 most powerful people in fashion

236 pages of 21st-century grunge

+

Haircuts
Guitars
Cameras
Porno
The Matrix
Zombies
Steve-O

Stella

NO 68 SEPTEMBER 2002 £2.90
BATTY GIRL: Stella McCartney by Vincent Peters

MADE IN THE UK

Independent woman
by Chris Heath

When I did these covers for *the Face* I think Stella had just begun her label and it was an iconic time for women in fashion. We wanted to pull them all together – it was something like three or four different covers, with an iconic woman on each one – so we decided, let's give them all masks, but let's do a different mask on each woman. So Phoebe Philo, for example, was a sort of highway woman, and Stella was a bit more superwoman/tribal. But it was all about some kind of black around the eyes. In the nineties

THE FACE

**100
most
powerful
people in
fashion**

236 pages of
21st-century
grunge

Haircuts
Guitars
Cameras
Porno
The Matrix
Zombies
Steve-O

Phoebe

Princess purr-fect!
by Chris Heath

NO 68 SEPTEMBER 2002 £2.90
MISS KITTEN: Phoebe Philo by Vincent Peters
MADE IN THE UK

WHY SHOULD MAKEUP STOP AT THE EYES AND LIPS?

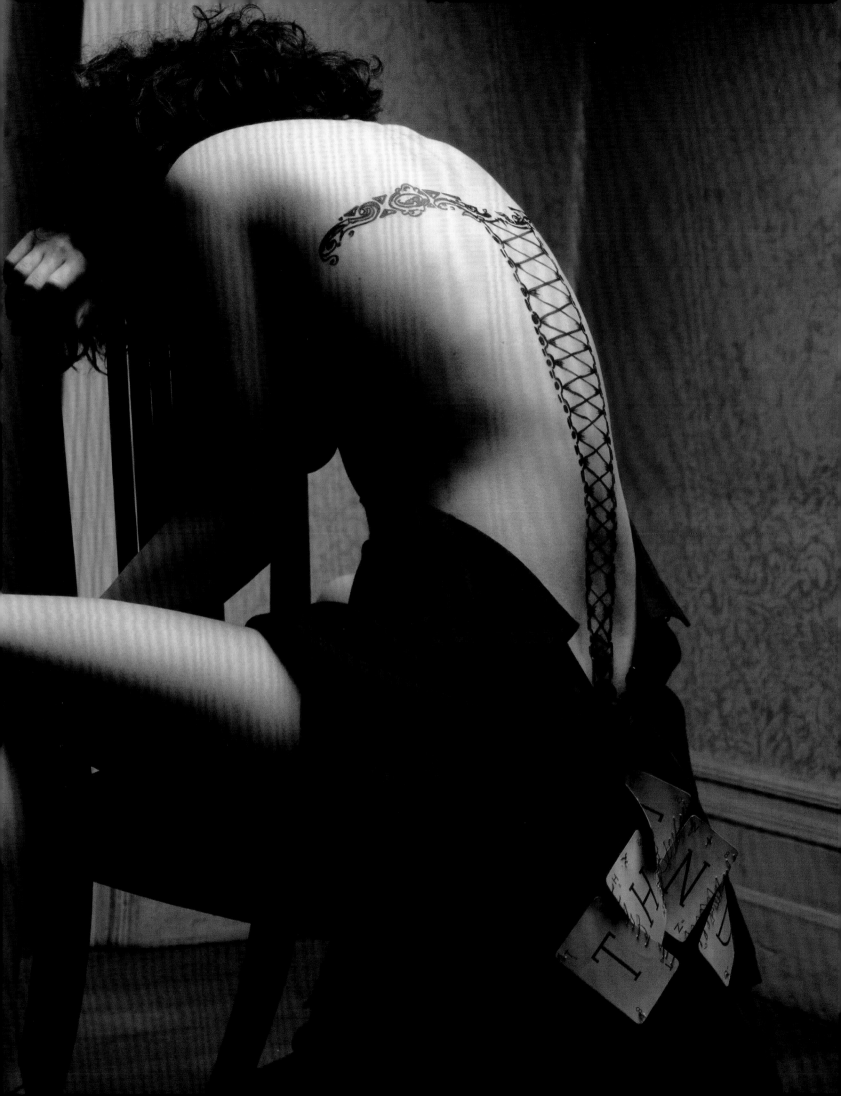

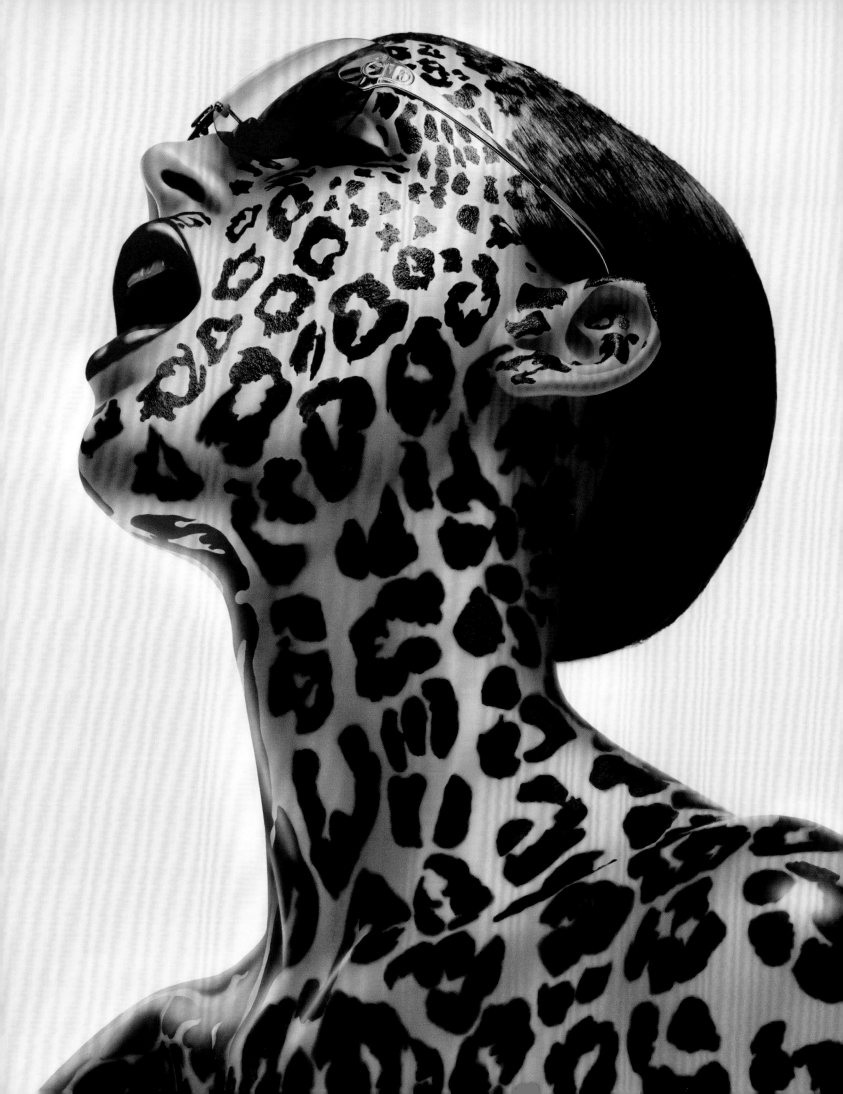

'I LOVE MAKEUP WHEN IT'S TRANSFORMATIVE.

I DON'T HAVE A STRONG OPINION ON THE COLOUR OF RED, OR THE LENGTH OF THE LASHES, OR THE COLOUR OF THE BLUSH. BUT I LOVE IT WHEN IT'S TRANSFORMATIVE. I LOVE WORKING WITH VAL BECAUSE SHE'S CAPABLE OF DOING IT, WHICH VERY FEW PEOPLE ARE. AND SHE LOVES DOING IT. SHE LOVES THAT TRANSFORMATIVE PROCESS. BUT SHE'S WILLING TO GO MUCH FURTHER.'

SØLVE SUNDSBØ

FASHION IMAGES DE MODE NO. 6, 2002 COVER; PHOTOGRAPHY SØLVE SUNDSBØ; MODEL LIBERTY ROSS.

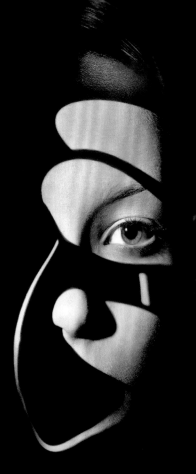
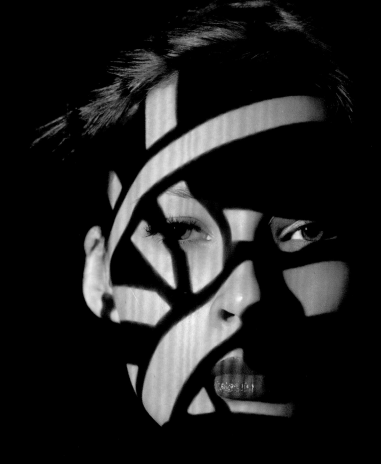

NUMÉRO 57, OCTOBER 2004; PHOTOGRAPHY RICHARD BUSH; HAIR PETER GRAY; MODEL TIIUK KUIK.

LIGHTING PLAYS A BIG PART IN YOUR WORK, THE TECHNIQUES USED SEEM SO VARIED.

Here, Richard was using projections onto the face. The makeup was in fact relatively simple; it was the way it reacted with the projection that made it quite a cool beauty story. Because it's not always about the makeup: it's about, would you want to look at it again? The relationship between photographer and makeup artist determines how it looks. You can do the most incredible makeup and if it's not lit right, you can't see it. When I go into a shoot or show, the first thing I need to know is what the lighting is going to be like.

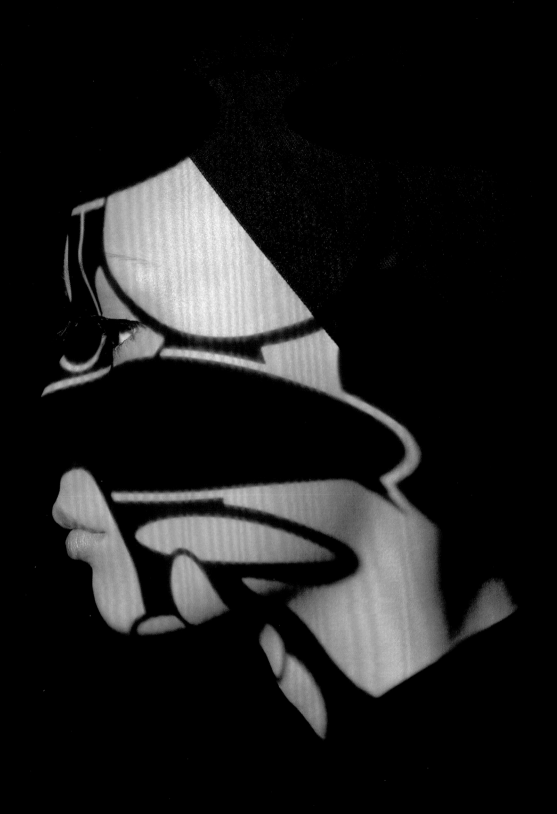

IT'S NOT ALWAYS ABOUT THE MAKEUP

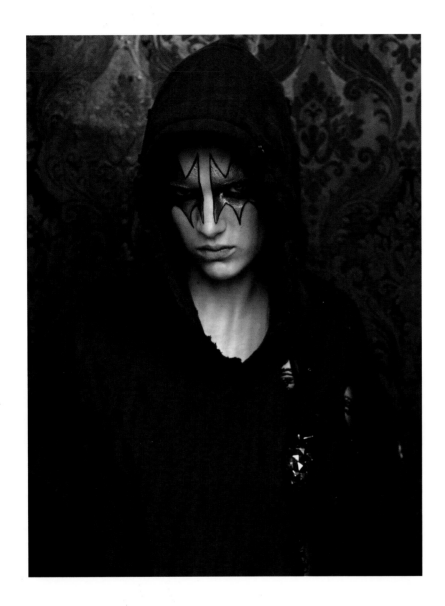

This was a shoot for British *Vogue* (opposite). Many times when I've worked with Alasdair he's wanted the makeup to be real and natural, but this time he and Kate were thinking The Human League so I'm like 'What, really? Bright blue eyeshadow and red lips!?' I finished doing Anna's makeup and I thought, with the pink blusher he's probably going to think I've gone too far ... But phew! I got away with it.

SELF SERVICE SS 2014.; PHOTOGRAPHY ALASDAIR MCLELLAN; FASHION EDITOR JANE HOW; HAIR ANTHONY TURNER; MODEL ASHLEIGH GOOD. BRITISH VOGUE SEPTEMBER 2014; PHOTOGRAPHY ALASDAIR MCLELLAN; FASHION EDITOR KATE PHELAN; HAIR DUFFY; MODEL ANNA EWERS.

For this picture of Ashleigh (above) we were shooting in the Camden Palace nightclub in London. They wanted natural makeup, they wanted to keep it real. Then, out of nowhere, they suddenly said, 'Oh, can you do something interesting? Actually, why don't you do Kiss makeup?' And so I did. It was touch and go as to whether it was going to make it into the magazine because it was the only shot with makeup in the whole story. But actually it feels quite fitting in there. But with Alasdair there's often going to be a point where he says, 'Go and do something out of the ordinary'.

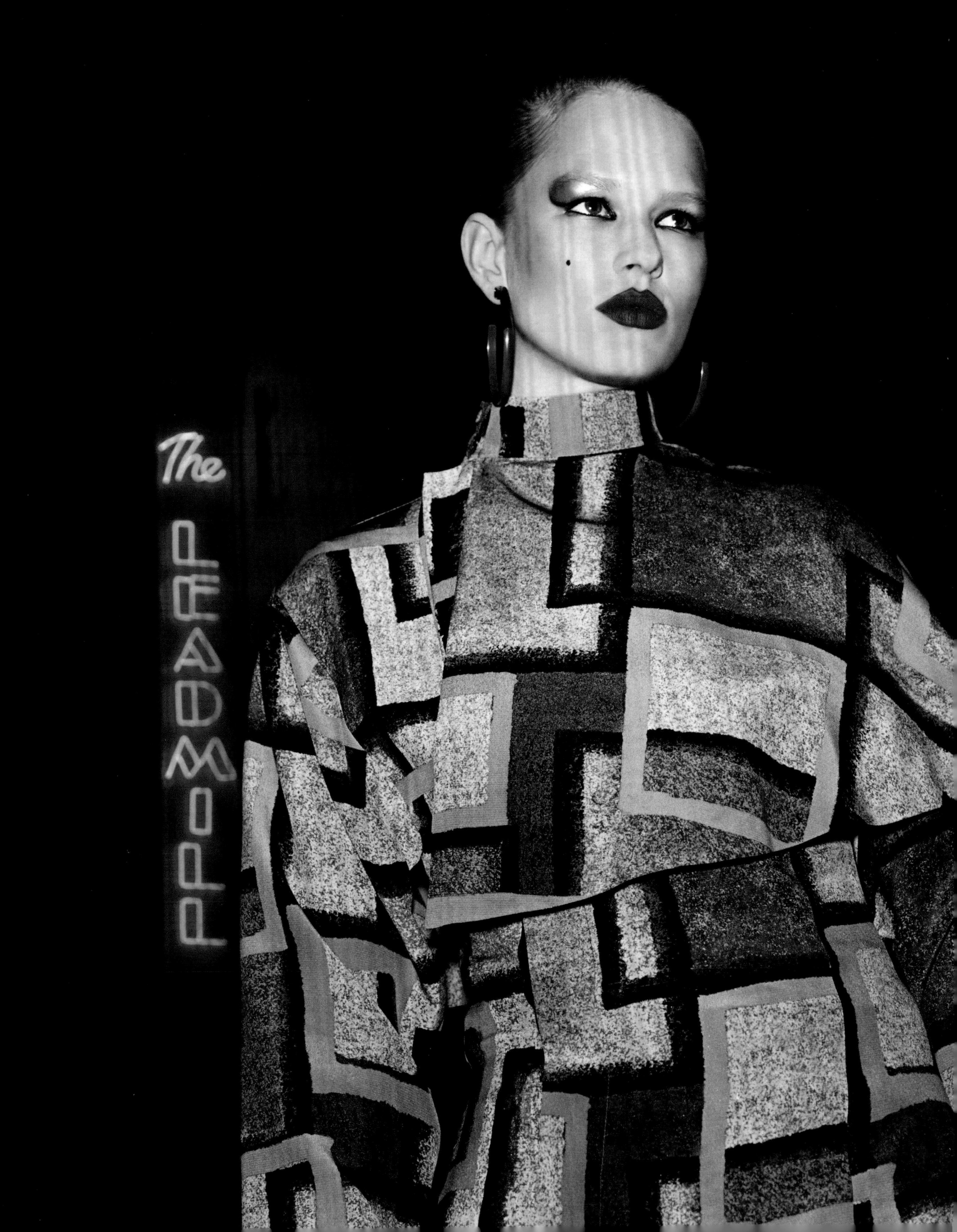
The
LEADMILL

VIVIENNE WESTWOOD RED LABEL SS15; PHOTOGRAPHY LUCA CANNONIERI; MODELS NYKHOR, MARTA ORTIZ, CHEN LI, ALEKSANDRA T, STINA OLSSON.

'I think that Val is as good at makeup as I am at designing clothes. And I'm good at makeup as well, but that's not been my full-time job. I might be as good as Val if it had been ...'

VIVIENNE WESTWOOD

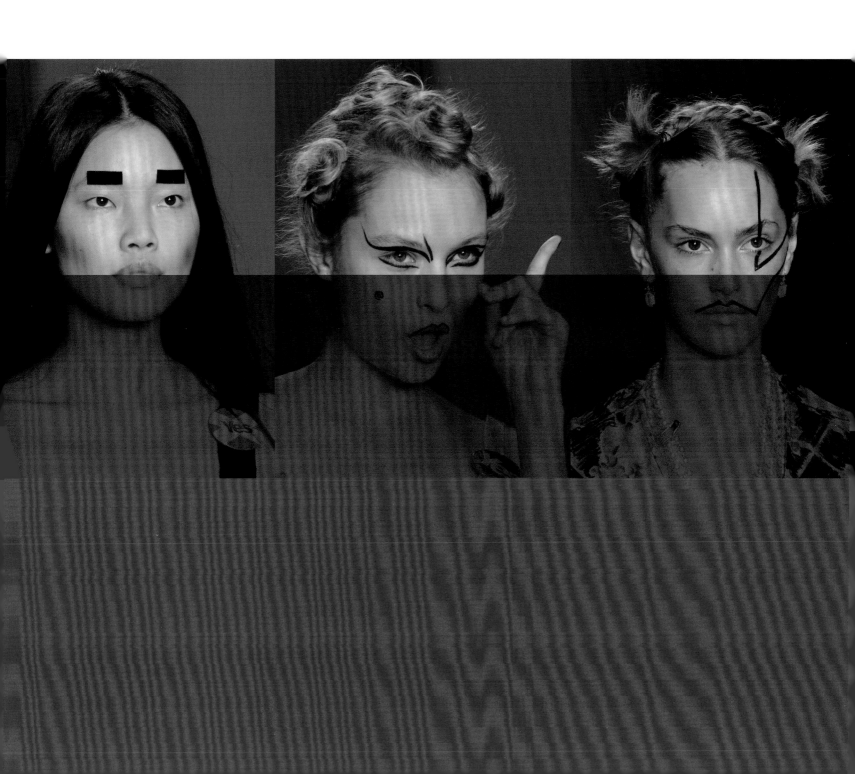

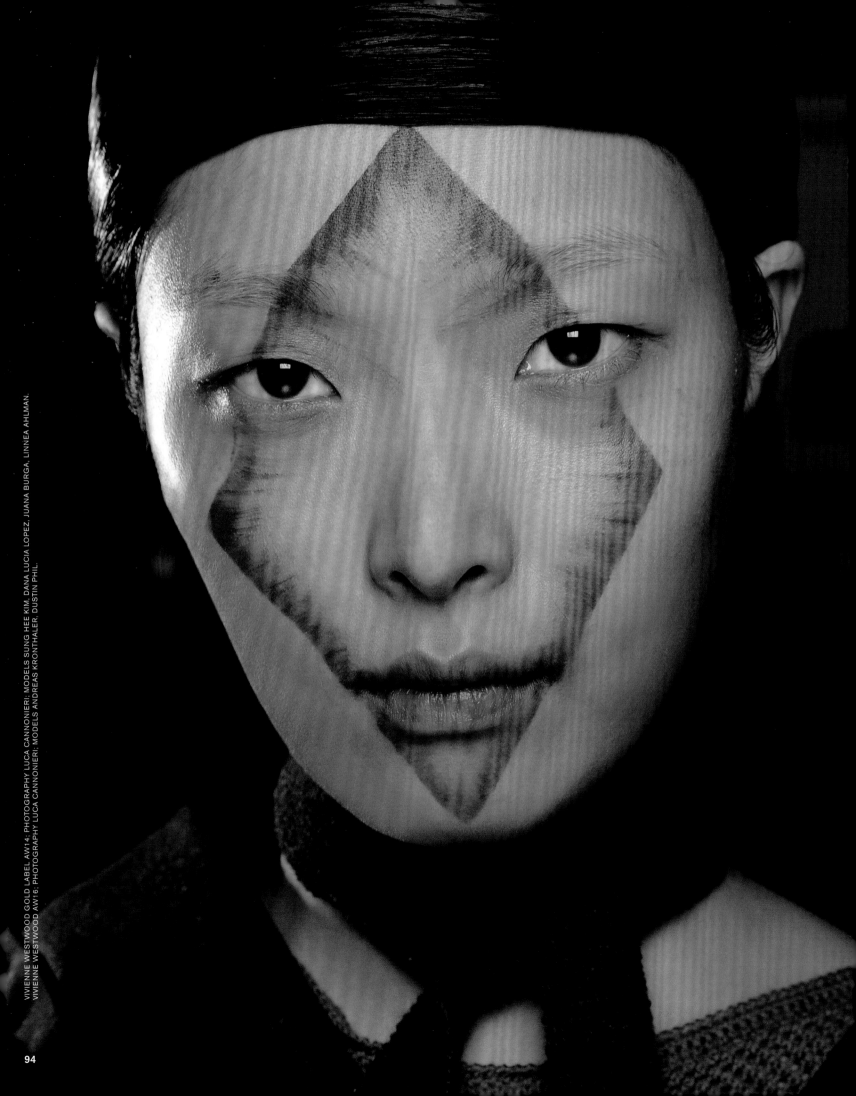

VIVIENNE WESTWOOD GOLD LABEL AW14: PHOTOGRAPHY LUCA CANNONIERI; MODELS SUNG HEE KIM, DANA LUCIA LOPEZ, JUANA BURGA, LINNEA AHLMAN.
VIVIENNE WESTWOOD AW16: PHOTOGRAPHY LUCA CANNONIERI; MODELS ANDREAS KRONTHALER, DUSTIN PHIL.

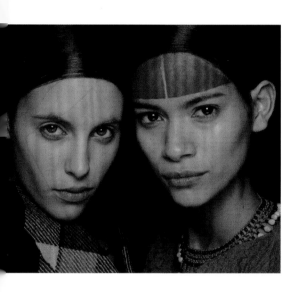
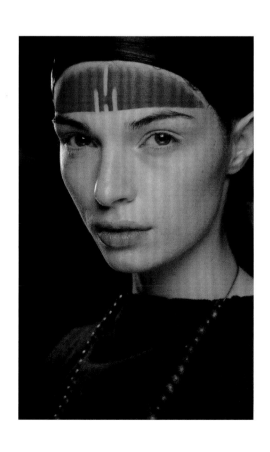
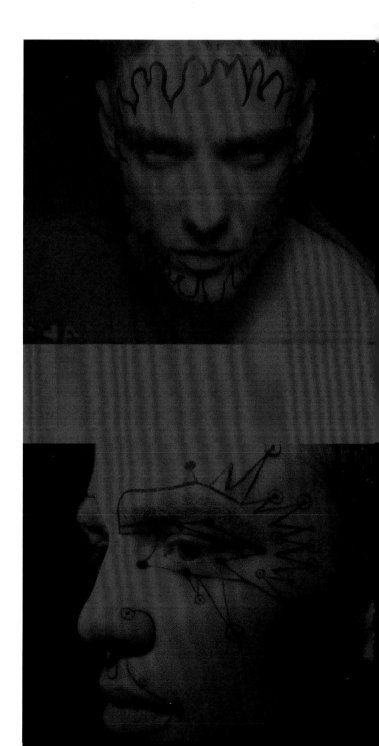

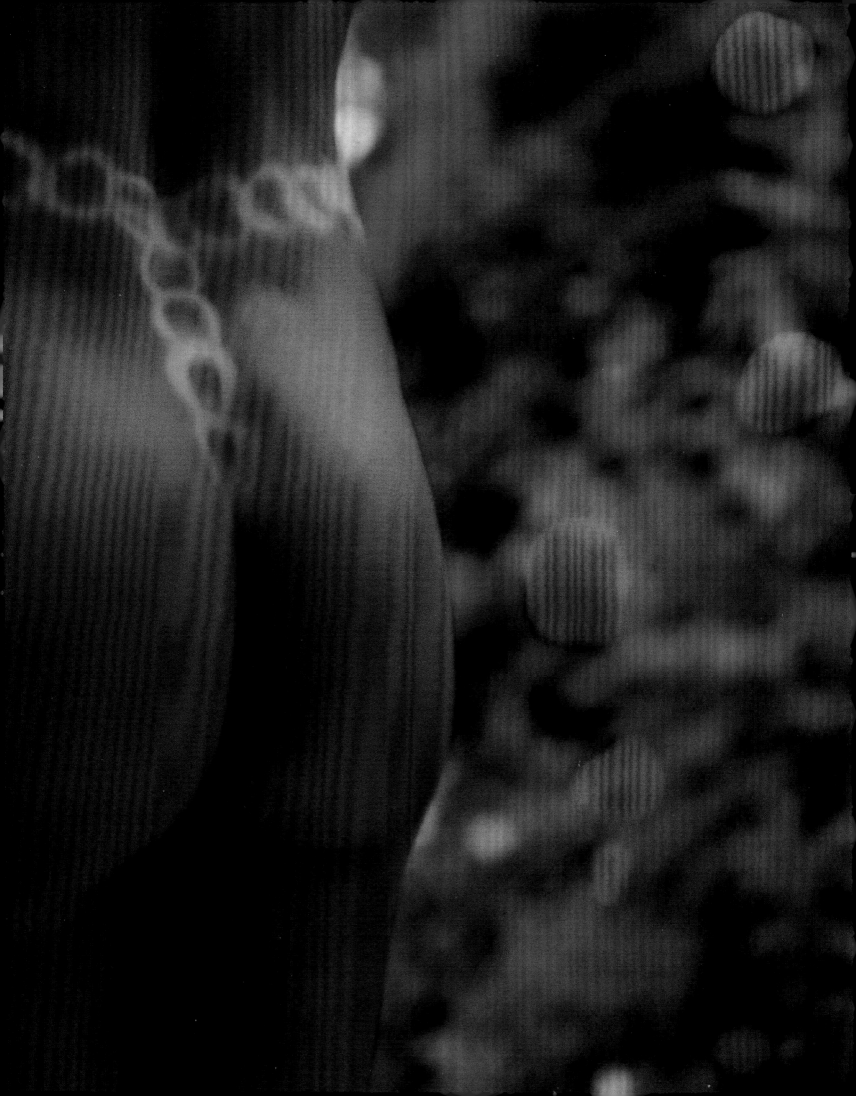

OH, MY GOD.

Well, in those days we didn't really have any money for models!

KATY ENGLAND

I THINK GRAPHIC IS OFTEN SEEN AS A MORE SERIOUS STYLE OF MAKEUP, BUT ARE THERE ANY HUMOROUS MOMENTS?

Well, there was the time we photographed Katy England's bottom. It's a shoot about tan lines that I did for *Dazed & Confused* with Katy. Basically, we were on very tight budgets at the time, so this was a case of, 'You've got a nice garden, Val, why don't we shoot it there?' I remember I was a bit obsessed with my roses. Katy put on a chain-mail G-string by Gucci, I fake-tanned her, and then we just carefully took it off. It was all about this absence of clothing. We were all about a concept then, and really, really serious. And this is how Katy's bottom appeared in a fashion shoot.

DAZED & CONFUSED, AUGUST 1996; PHOTOGRAPHY PHIL POYNTER; FASHION EDITOR KATY ENGLAND; HAIR ADAM BRYANT; MODEL KATY ENGLAND.

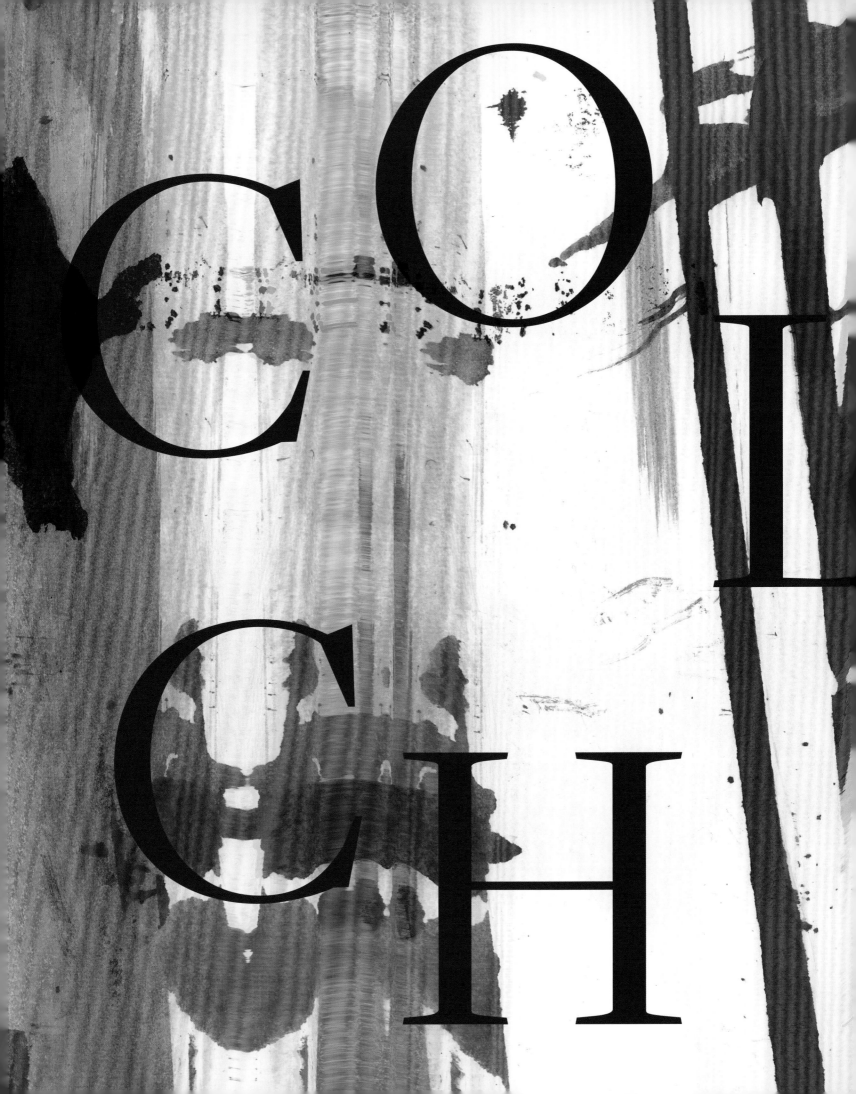

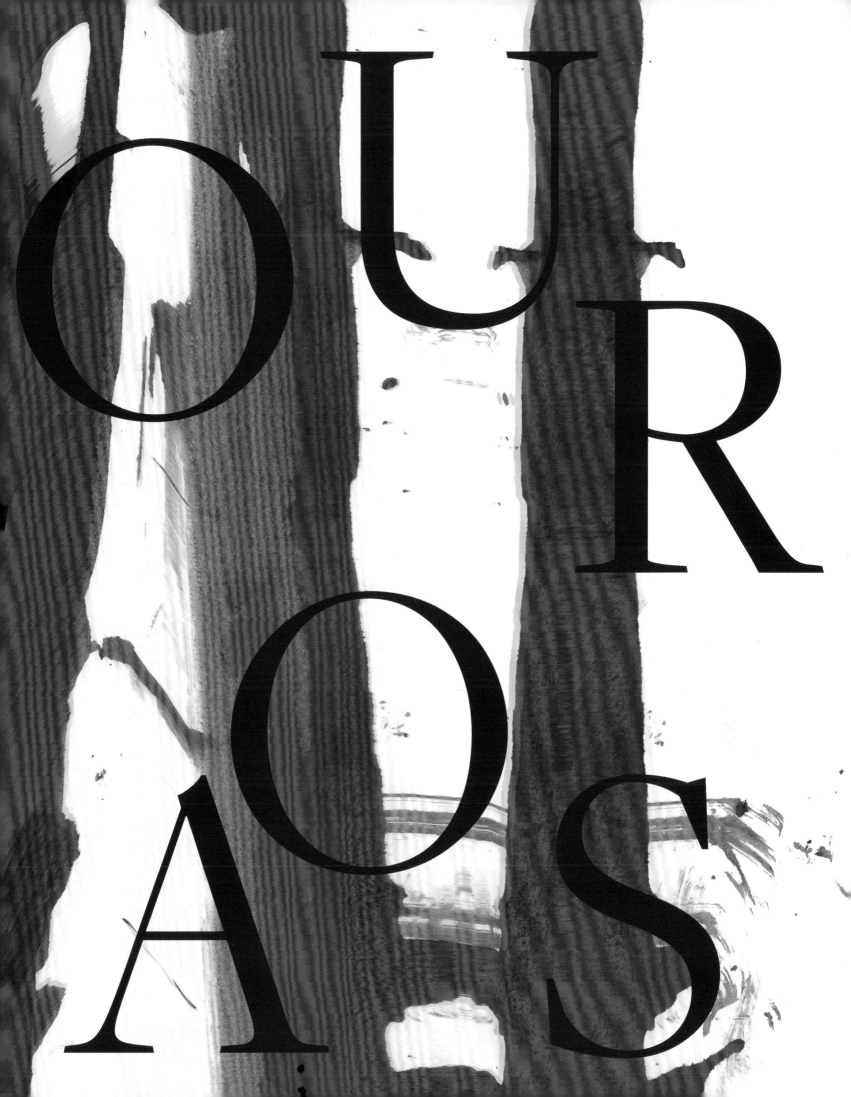

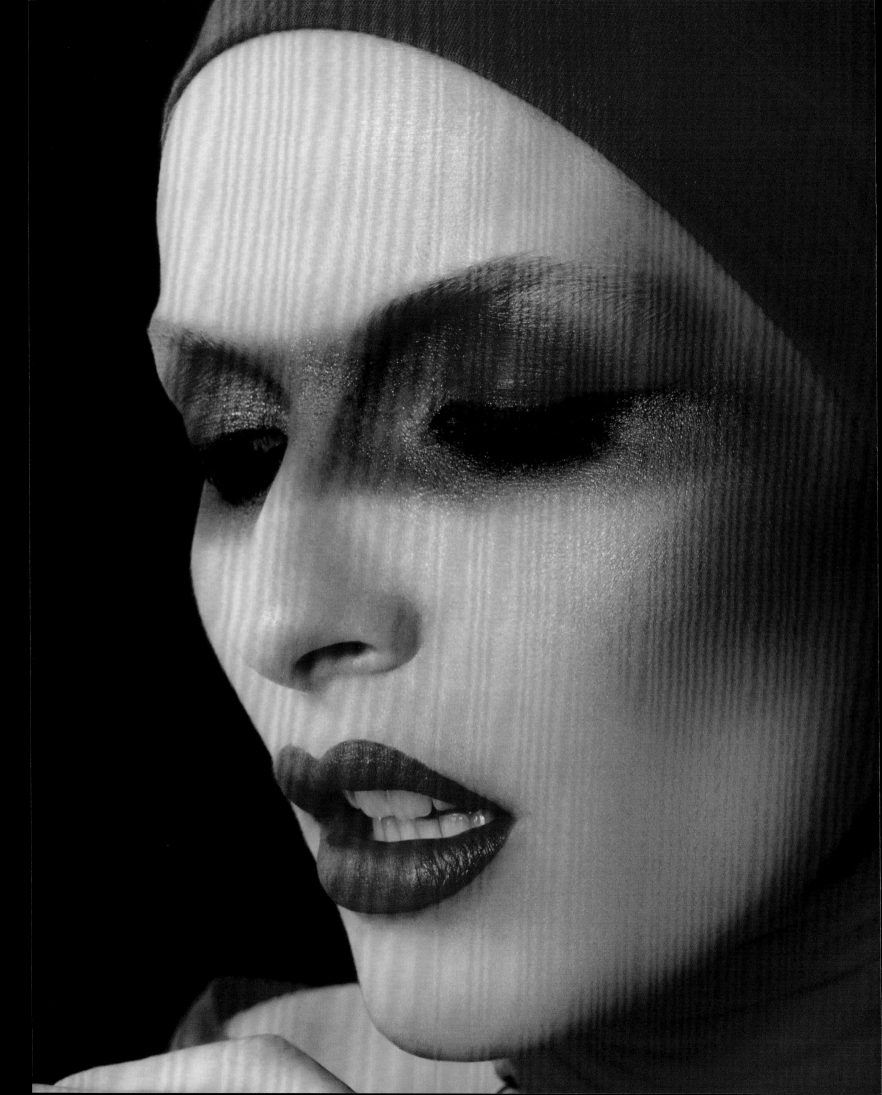

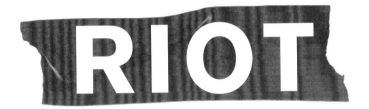

IN A PAINTBOX

When the experimental psychologist Timothy Leary wrote *The Psychedelic Experience* he wasn't thinking about makeup but he was considering mind-expanding colour. In this chapter, Val takes us on her own, at times hallucinatory, trip through the infinite spectrum of beauty.

When asked to define her more colour-orientated work, Val often uses the term 'colour chaos'. This description is true to a point, as in fact much of her work here has been applied with the free-form, almost stream-of-consciousness style that is her trademark. However, what is also clear is how much Val elevates colour in her work, bringing it to a heightened level of artistry. This is not makeup intended to inspire an Instagram response of flowers and unicorn emojis.

Colour in art can suggest the life force in nature, or our anxiety towards a frightening modern world, and Val's use of colour in her makeup art provides a direct insight into her own emotions and moods. Think of Jackson Pollock's feverish drip paintings, the spray-painted art pieces of Marco Rea and the dreamy darkness of Instagram artist Unskilled Worker: anyone who sniffs at the idea that makeup can be considered a true art form should take note. In many of the images here, Val is not selling us anything – she is, like many true artists, being unbridled and expressionistic for the sake of creating a great image, and clearly her work can hold its own.
As Vivienne Westwood once said, 'Val is hyper-artistic'. And she should know.

Much of Val's colour world is a psychedelic one, and her influences in this chapter shift like the glittering particles of a kaleidoscope: imagine an eighteenth-century powdered and rouged courtesan who has time-travelled to the set of eighties punk movie *Liquid Sky* via a sixties commune of flower children and you get the drift.

One would like to imagine that by sometimes detaching line from colour, Val is perhaps showing an almost nebulous move towards a new creative renaissance in beauty – leading us away from the grey, linear and increasingly Orwellian world in which we presently live. And while we would expect nothing less of Val, it should be noted that in the self-conscious, ever commercialized worlds of fashion and beauty, daring ventures into colour are only travelled by the brave. So here, Val reveals a portal to a world of colour and beauty that we would never have imagined, had she not opened up the doors of our perceptions.

VOGUE ITALIA 2003; PHOTOGRAPHY NORBERT SCHOERNER; MODEL RIE RASMUSSEN.

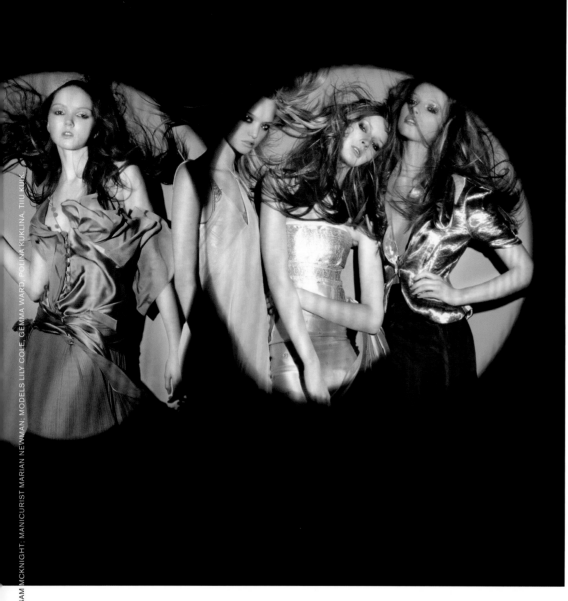

BRITISH VOGUE APRIL 2004; PHOTOGRAPHY NICK KNIGHT; FASHION EDITOR KATE PHELAN; HAIR SAM MCKNIGHT; MANICURIST MARIAN NEWMAN; MODELS LILY COLE, GEMMA WARD, POLINA KUKLINA, TIIU KUIK

WOULD YOU SAY THAT WORKING WITH COLOUR IS WHEN YOU'RE PARTICULARLY INTERPRETIVE WITH YOUR MAKEUP?

I think so. Sometimes when I look at a face I think about how the light would hit it. Like if she was in a nightclub and there was psychedelic lighting, but she's living it. Glam rock is something I reference a lot, and I think there are a lot of glam rock, New Romantic and punk elements that cross over. And they always say that you do the things that were part of your youth. I think that's quite apparent in my work.

I love the whole psychedelia thing. I think you draw on your past to inspire you, whether that's the theatre, music, a movie or a great club or party that you were at.

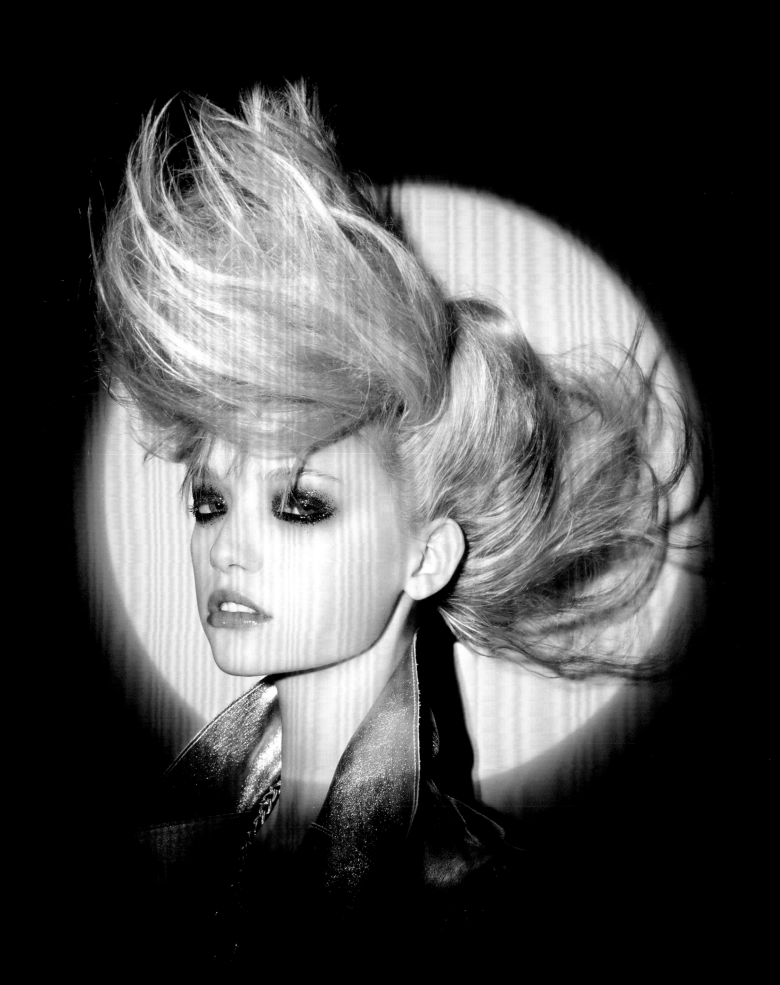

V MAGAZINE 47, SUMMER 2007; PHOTOGRAPHY MARIO TESTINO; ART DIRECTION STEPHEN GAN; FASHION EDITOR BEAT BOLLIGER; HAIR MARC LOPEZ; MANICURIST LORRAINE GRIFFIN; MODEL CATHERINE MCNEIL.

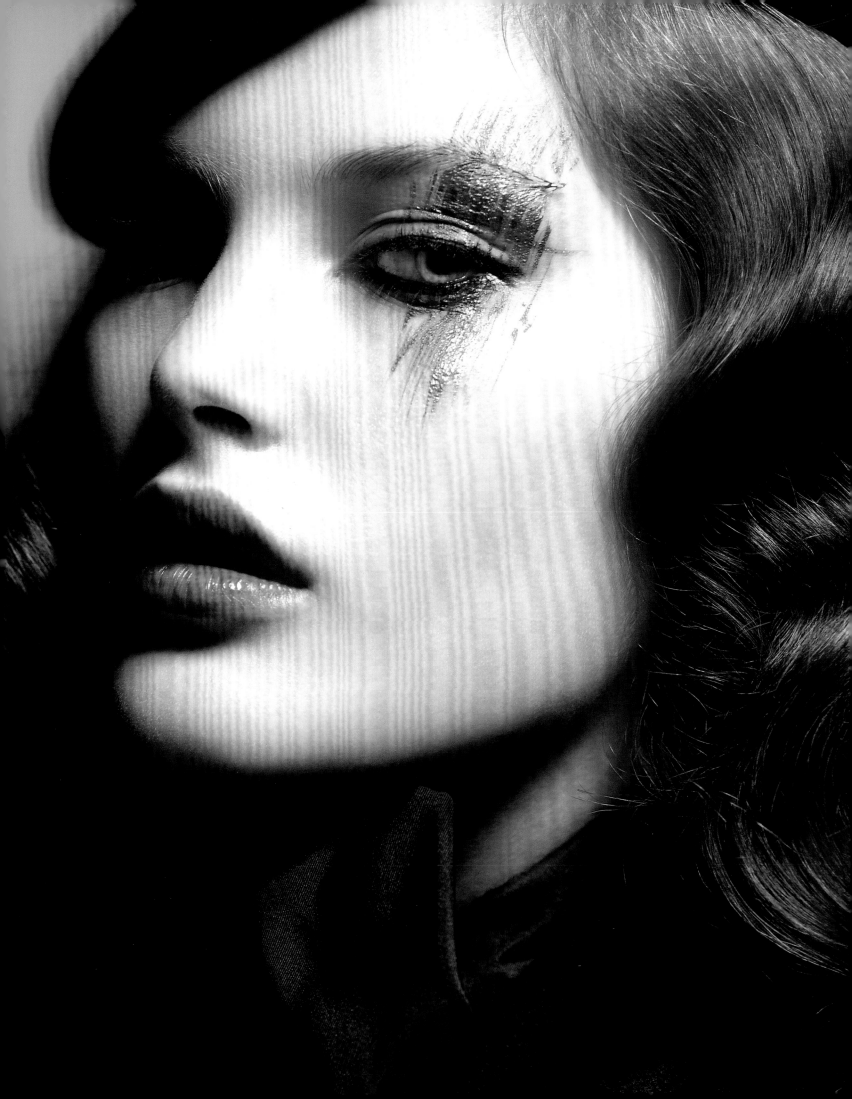

'If you show Val just kind of pretty stuff that's very beautiful, she's less excited than if you show her stuff which is

DANGEROUS
OR IMMORAL
OR DEGENERATE

or all those sort of words that people pile on this stuff. Because, it feels like it's being subversive. It feels like you're not just conforming, you're actually showing beauty where perhaps you see it and other people don't. When we first started SHOWstudio there was no Facebook, there was no YouTube, there was no light broadcasting. I nevertheless decided light broadcasting was a thing I wanted to do; it was a thrill actually saying "okay, this is us talking directly to our audience".

WE JUST DID STUFF
WE WANTED TO DO.

With the "Make it up" film Val decided the best thing to do was to line the girls up and she put rubber bands around them to make their limbs look more like Hans Bellmer in a way. And then she decided the best way to apply makeup, to apply colour, was with a pump-action water pistol. But she had this super soaker, and those water pistols are machine guns for paint.

SO YOU'VE GOT THIS FUNNY BLONDE WOMAN
SPRAYING THESE NEAR-NAKED GIRLS.

And they're laughing and Val was really, clearly enjoying herself, just being able to paint on these human forms. So, the performance part of it was the joy of doing it live.'

NICK KNIGHT

106

*THE FILM YOU MADE WITH NICK KNIGHT REMINDS ME OF THE
'COLOUR CHAOS' OF THE HOLI FESTIVAL IN INDIA.*

Nick had just launched SHOWstudio and he said, 'I want you to demonstrate makeup for me in a film, no one's ever done a makeup demonstration before online.' Nick's was the only online magazine at that time and I said, 'No, I don't want to do it because I think watching somebody do a makeup tutorial is really boring.' This was long before the whole YouTube thing. But Nick really wanted me to do it and he said, 'Look, we're going to come at it from a different angle'. I said, 'I want it to be arty. I don't want to just draw a winged eyeliner, or put on a perfect fuchsia lip.' Nick said, 'I'm going to give you a painting and I want you to take direction from that.'

He gave me a Picasso called *Les Demoiselles d'Avignon*. It's five girls and they're all na-ked, and it really inspired me. I said, 'I want a group of girls, all different body shapes, tall, short, voluptuous, not so voluptuous. I want lots of different body shapes to rep-resent all women, because, let's face it, we are not all a perfect size 10! So they're all going to be in this elastoplast-coloured underwear and I'm going to get fake bottoms and fake boobs, I'm going to strap them to the wrong parts of their bodies. So we're treating them like an art installation.' I also got elas-tic bands and nude tights because I wanted to tie up different parts of their limbs so that they became more Hans Bellmer-like. Some of them would also be wearing see-through masks. Then I was going to paint them like a paint-er would, as opposed to a makeup artist. I was think-ing of Jackson Pollock and Yves Klein.

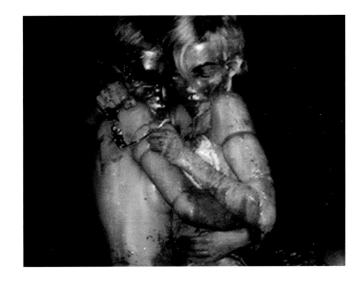

I had a big box of paint-brushes, household items, art brushes and these big water pistols that I was go-ing to fill with colour. I said to Nick, 'I'm just going to paint them. I don't know how it's going to turn out. I'm just going to do it.' And then Nick said, 'Well, we need to see you in the film. We need to know it's you.' I used to wear these car-mechanic boiler suits – I was obsessed by them – and Nick came along with white paint and painted 'VAL' on the back of the one I was wearing and said, 'OK. Off you go'. I think I had to do it all in three minutes.

So I painted all these girls, very quickly, into a collage and then finally I took the water guns and just blasted them with paint. What was great was the way Nick edited it and put it to music. It felt like he had really summed me up – chaotic and slightly mad.

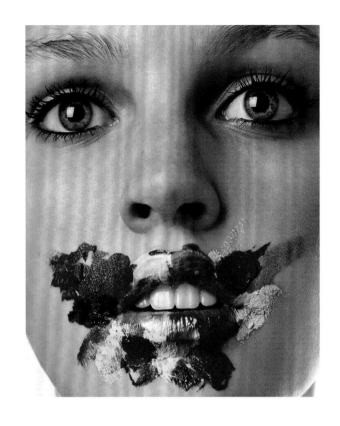

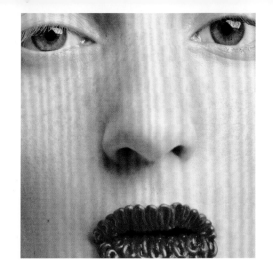

I was inspired by Irving Penn and the idea of

'LET'S EAT IT!
LET'S EAT ALL
THE COLOURS!'

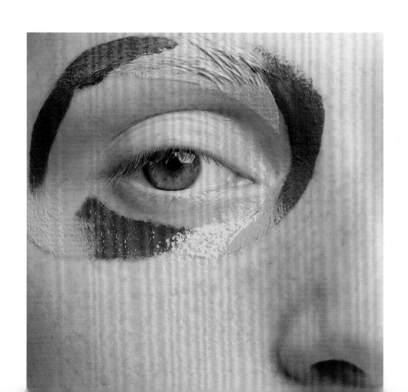

CRÈME MAGAZINE: PHOTOGRAPHY RICHARD BUSH.
10 MAGAZINE: PHOTOGRAPHY RICHARD BUSH; FASHION EDITOR SOPHIA NEOPHITOU; MODEL ALI STEPHENS.

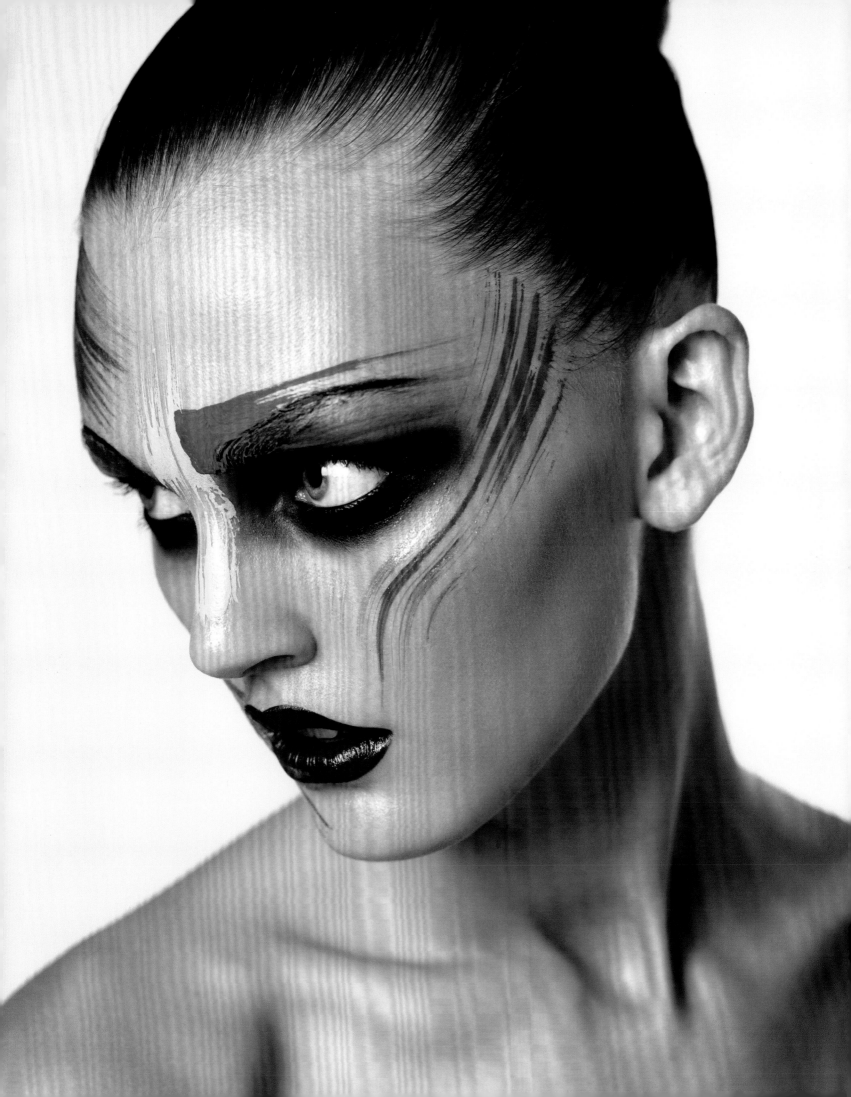

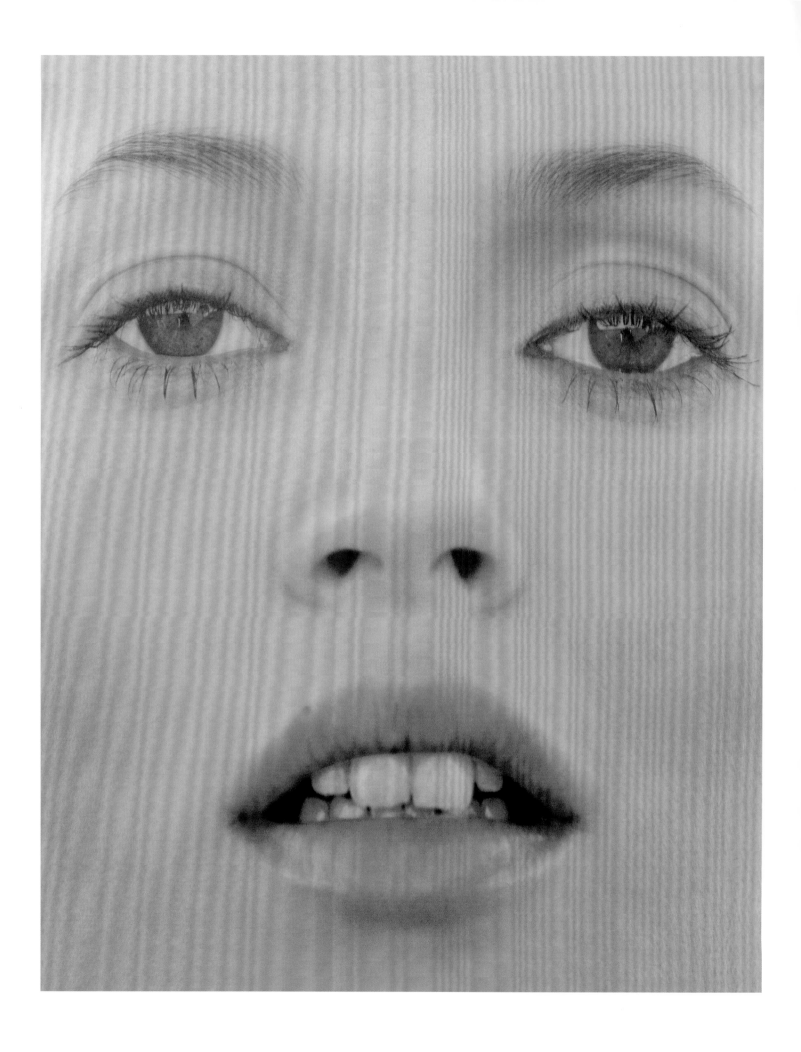

I was very excited to work with Corinne and we went to shoot what was a fashion-come-beauty story in a seventies-style house in Brighton. We moved to shoot on the beach and were in a Winnebago, and I was deciding what I was going to do for the next makeup. We were going to be shooting on the beach and everything I'd done so far had been like a little appliqué, like daisies or butterflies, so I thought, 'maybe I should do a little bit of proper makeup here. I'll do some rainbow eyes'. I started to do this lovely yellow into green into lilac into blue eye and Corinne came running up to the van yelling, 'I need Kate now! We're losing light. I've got to shoot her now. Come on, you've got to be finished!' And I lost my rag and said, 'It's a fucking beauty story!' But Corinne insisted on taking her, so I just said, 'OK, take her!' Neil said, 'But you've only done one eye.' And that's how this asymmetric makeup came about. We shot her like that and it was a beautiful picture. And then Corinne said, 'So, what are you going to do for the last two shots?' And I said, **'THERE'S NO MORE MAKEUP. THERE'S NO MORE LIGHT. THAT'S IT!'** And I think that was the first and last time I ever worked with Corinne.

BRITISH VOGUE FEBRUARY 2002; PHOTOGRAPHY CORINNE DAY; FASHION EDITOR LUCINDA CHAMBERS; HAIR NEIL MOODIE; MANICURIST GLENIS BAPTISTE; MODEL KATE MOSS.

'It's a genius picture isn't it? It's so Corinne. Corinne was probably the only person who could capture that.'

KATE MOSS

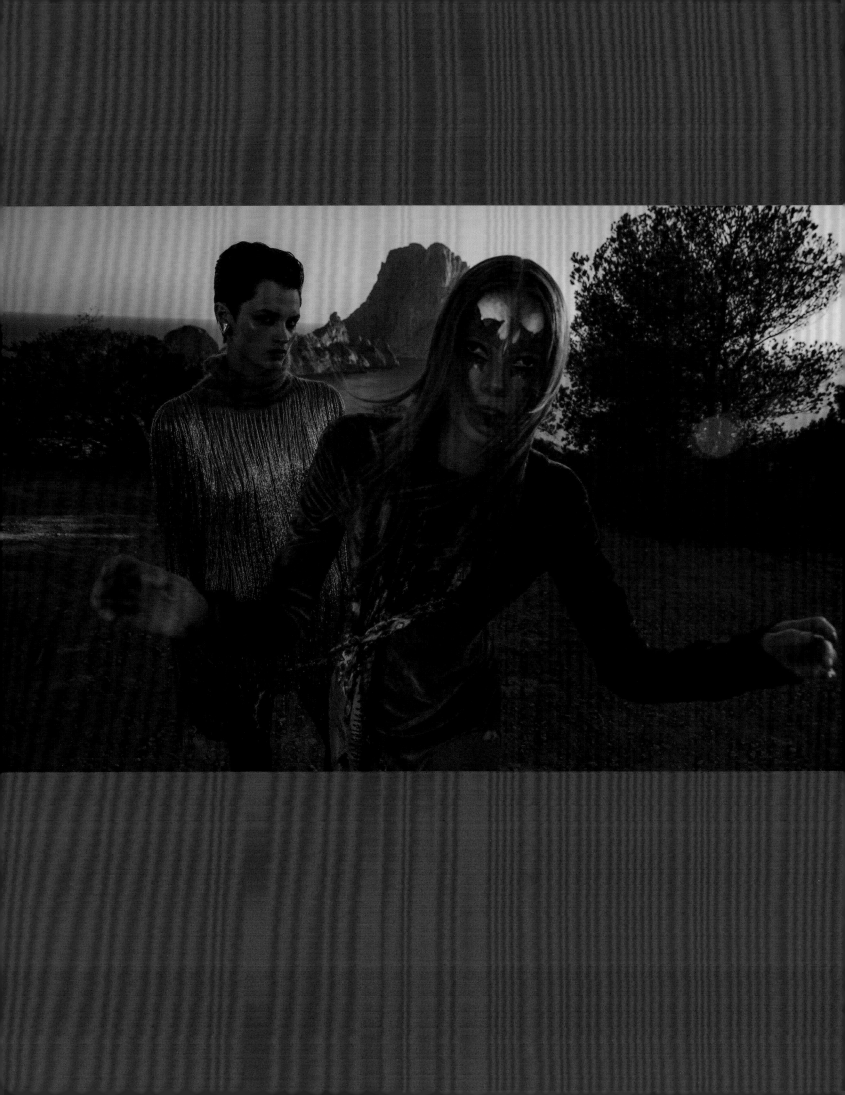

YOU'VE GOT TO FIND A WAY OF DOING IT

I WOULD SAY THAT COLOURFUL MAKEUP IS NOT EVERYBODY'S FIRST CHOICE?

I think you've got to understand what you're trying to achieve. The way I do colour best is to do it instinctively and quite free-form. I think that anything that looks like it's harking back to the sixties, seventies or eighties, that's when it just looks old. You've got to find a way of doing it and breaking it up, and then that's what makes it look fresh.

AND BREAKING IT UP

M MAGAZINE, LE MONDE 2017; PHOTOGRAPHY INEZ & VINOODH; FASHION EDITOR ALEKSANDRA WORONIECKA; HAIR WARD; MODELS JULIA HAFSTROM, ISABELLA EMMACK.

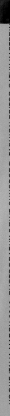
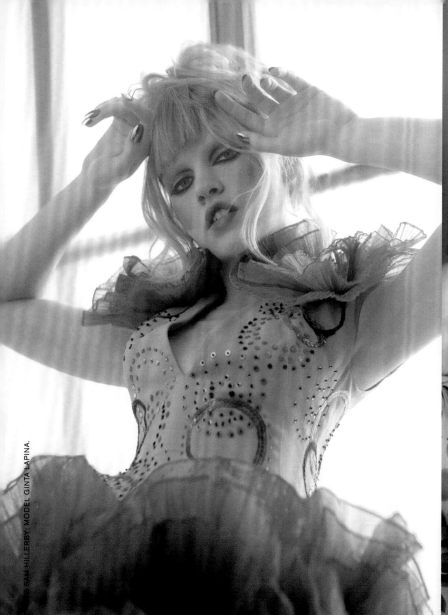
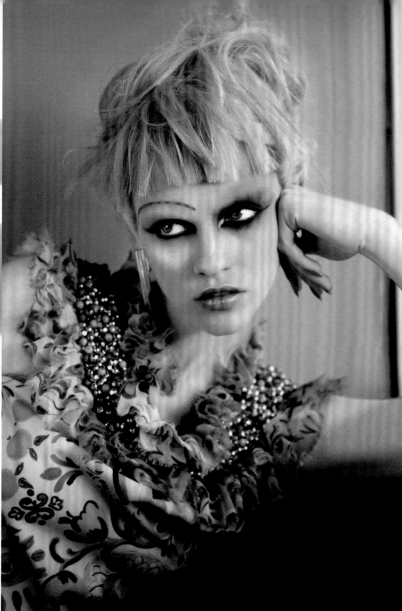

'WHAT I LOVE ABOUT THESE PICTURES, ESPECIALLY THE MAKEUP, IS THAT SHE'S NOT AN OBVIOUSLY ROMANTIC CHARACTER, SHE'S MORE NEW ROMANTIC, MORE PUNK. YOU TAKE SOMETHING FROM ONE WORLD AND PUT IT INTO ANOTHER.'

SØLVE SUNDSBØ

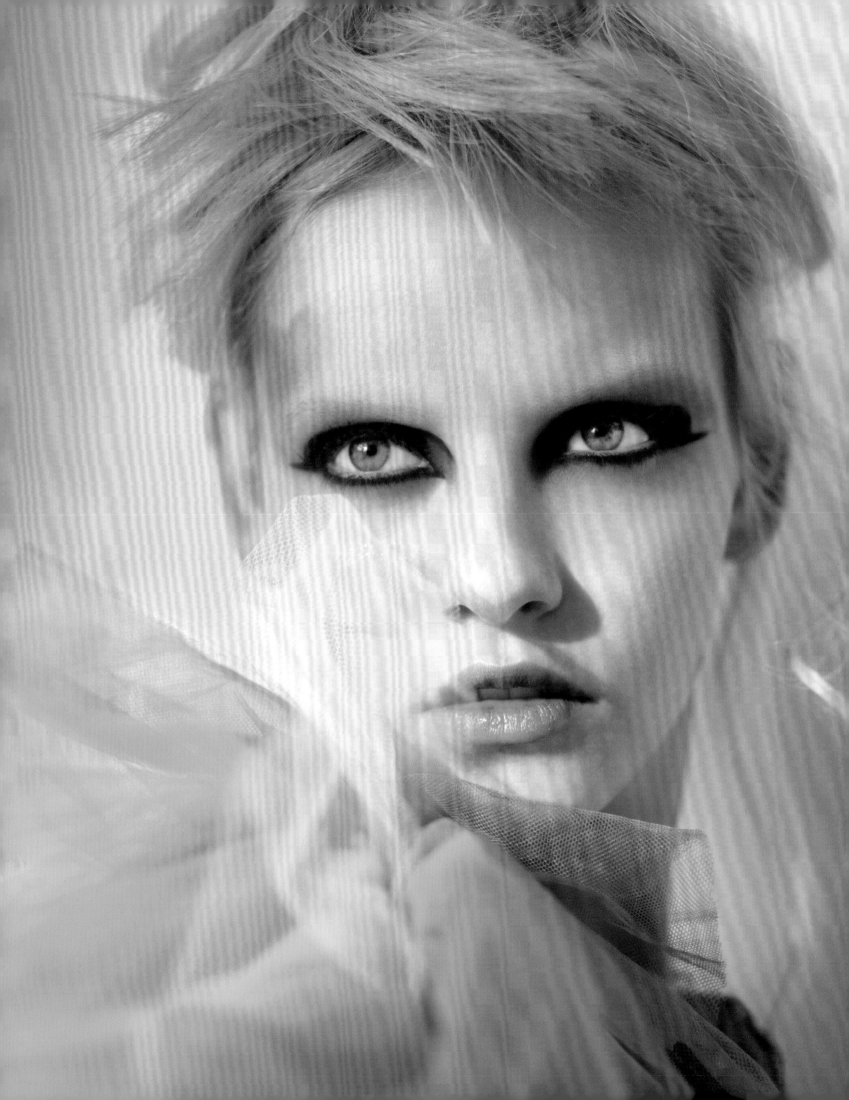

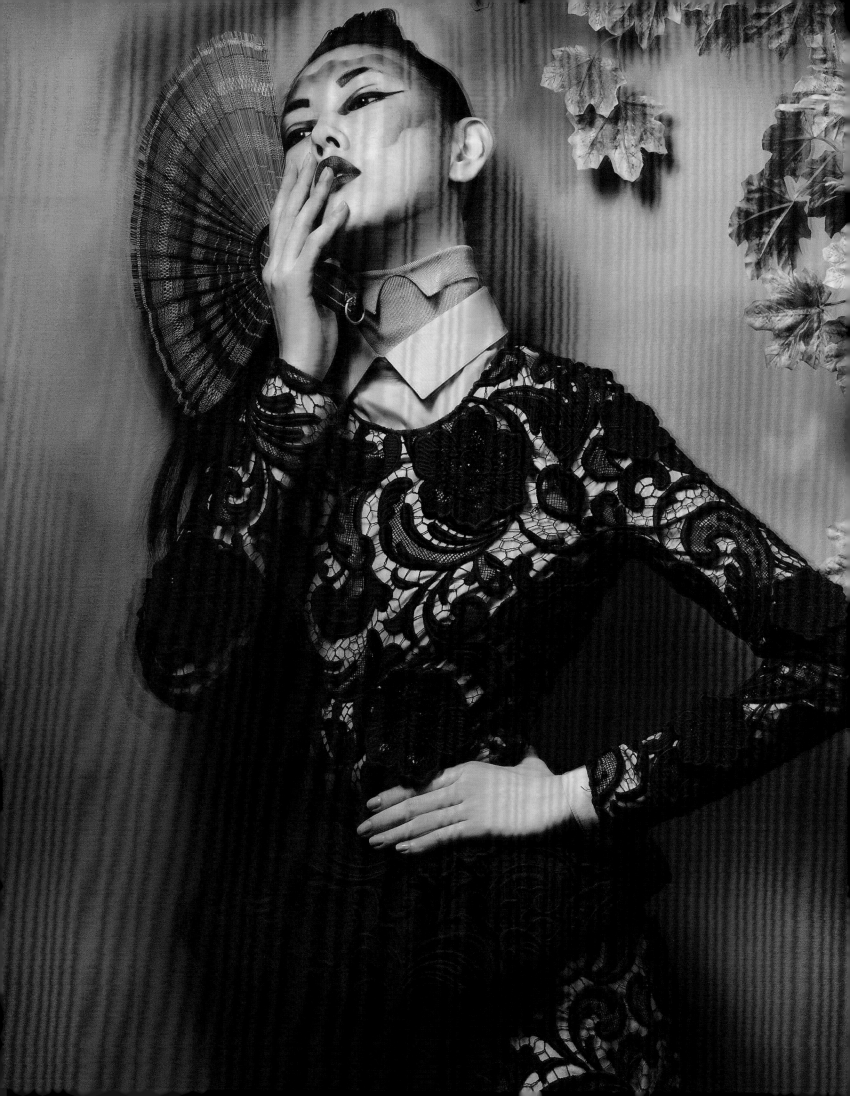

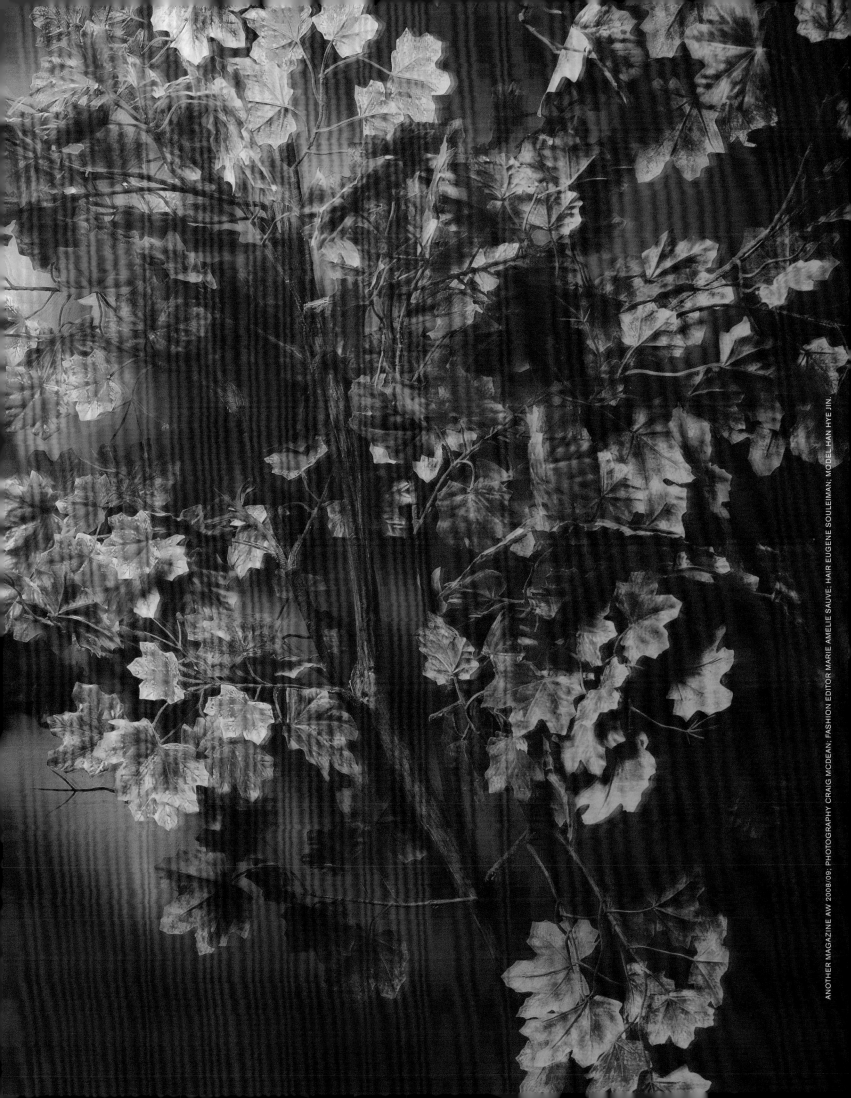

ANOTHER MAGAZINE AW 2008/09; PHOTOGRAPHY CRAIG MCDEAN; FASHION EDITOR MARIE AMELIE SAUVE; HAIR EUGENE SOULEMAN; MODEL HAN HYE JIN.

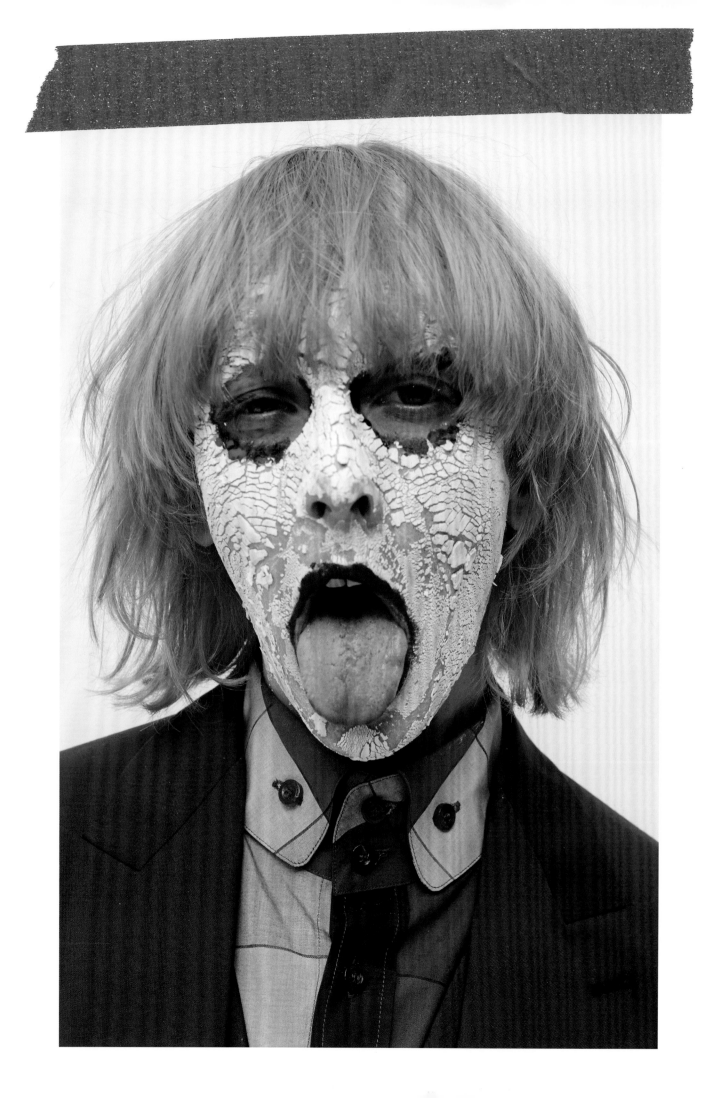

'IT LOOKED LIKE THE MAKEUP WAS UNDERNEATH, THE EYE MAKEUP WAS RINGED WITH BLUE SO THE BLUE WAS UNDERNEATH THE WHITE CRACKED THING AND THE LIPS WERE UNDERNEATH THE WHITE CRACKED SKIN AND IT LOOKED REALLY, REALLY GOOD. IT WAS VERY CLEVER HOW SHE DID AN ALTERNATIVE WHITE FACE AND MADE IT LOOK LIKE THAT.'

VIVIENNE WESTWOOD

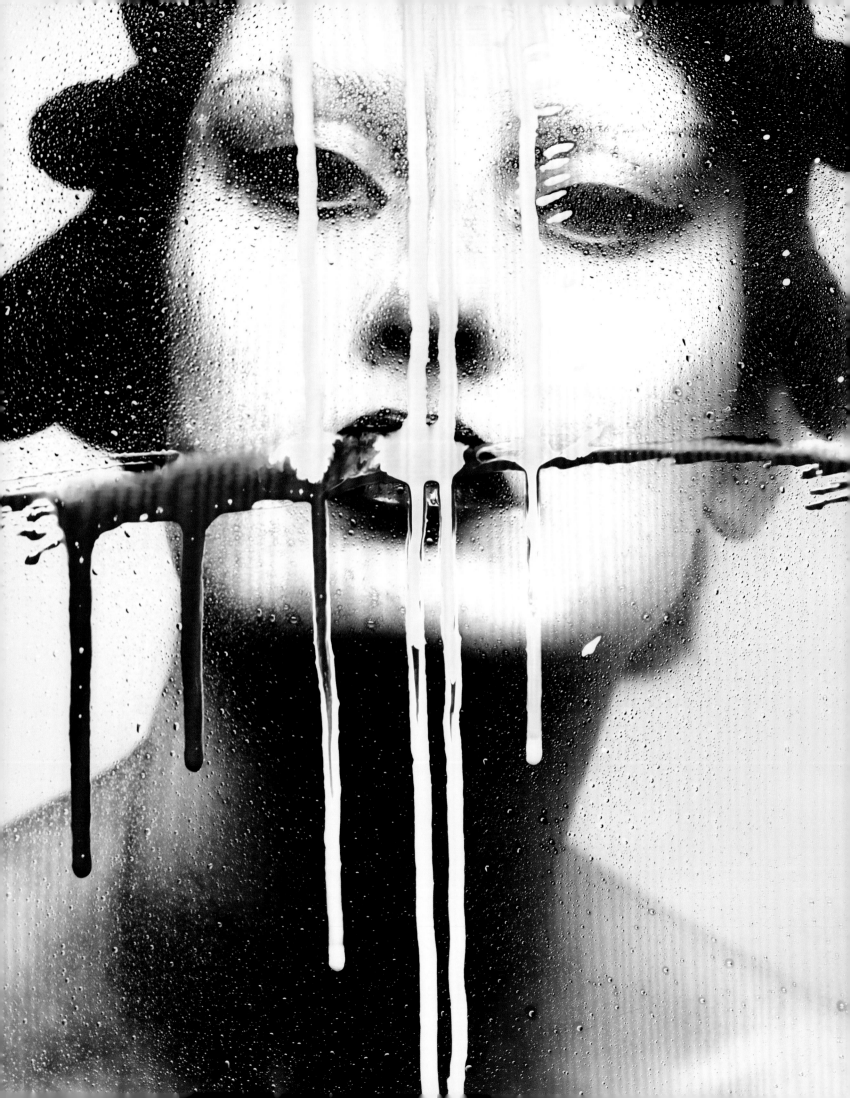

FOR THIS SHOOT, MY FIRST THOUGHT WAS ERIN O'CONNOR.
I RANG HER AND SAID, 'LOOK, I'M GOING TO THROW PAINT AT YOU.
I WANT TO TREAT YOU LIKE A SCULPTURE.

ARE YOU UP FOR IT?'

ERIN SAID, 'LOOK DARLING, WHY NOT?
YOU'VE ALREADY BARED MY TITS AND
SHOVED A BIG FAKE NOSE ON ME AND
CALLED THAT BEAUTY!'

'MARCO REA HAD TAKEN FASHION MAGAZINES AND TURNED
THEM INTO ART. SO WHY DON'T WE JUST TAKE A PHOTOGRAPH
AND TURN IT INTO A PAINTING?'

SØLVE SUNDSBØ

OPPOSITE AND FOLLOWING PAGES: MISSION MAGAZINE 2017; PHOTOGRAPHY SØLVE SUNDSBØ; HAIR SCOTT ADE; MANICURIST MARIAN NEWMAN; MODEL ERIN O'CONNOR.

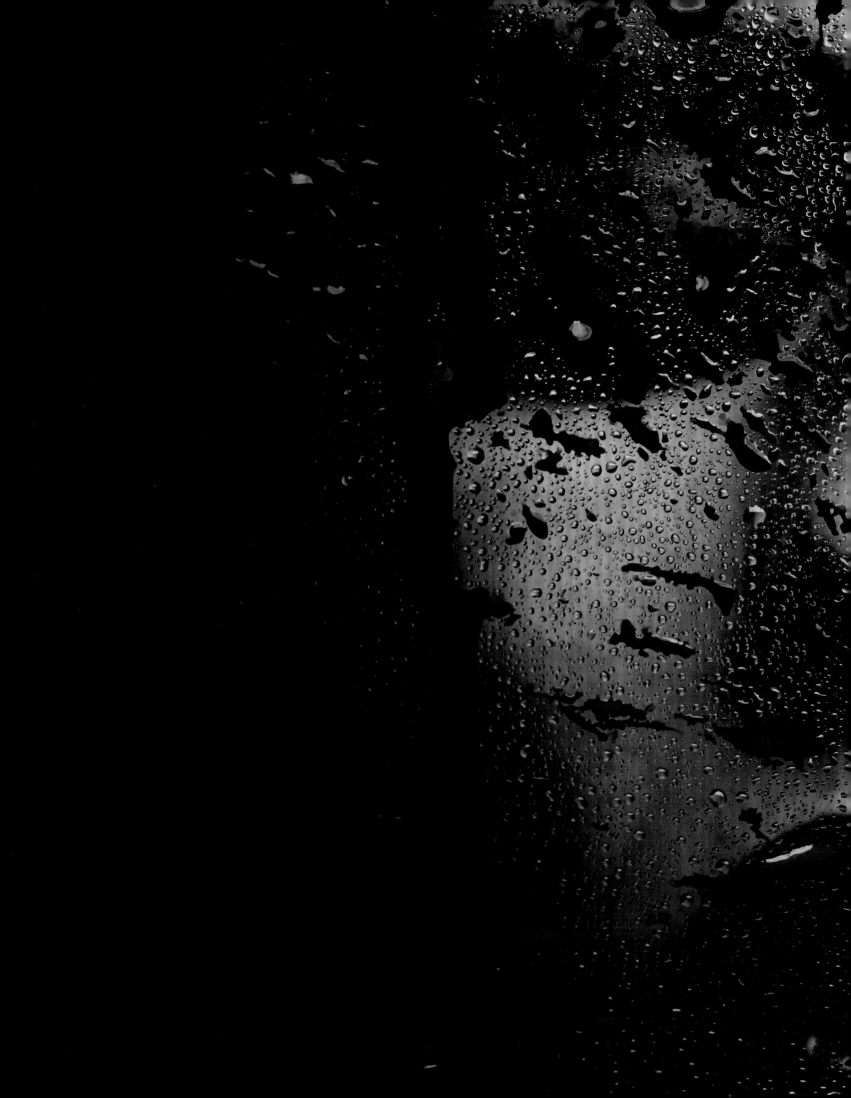

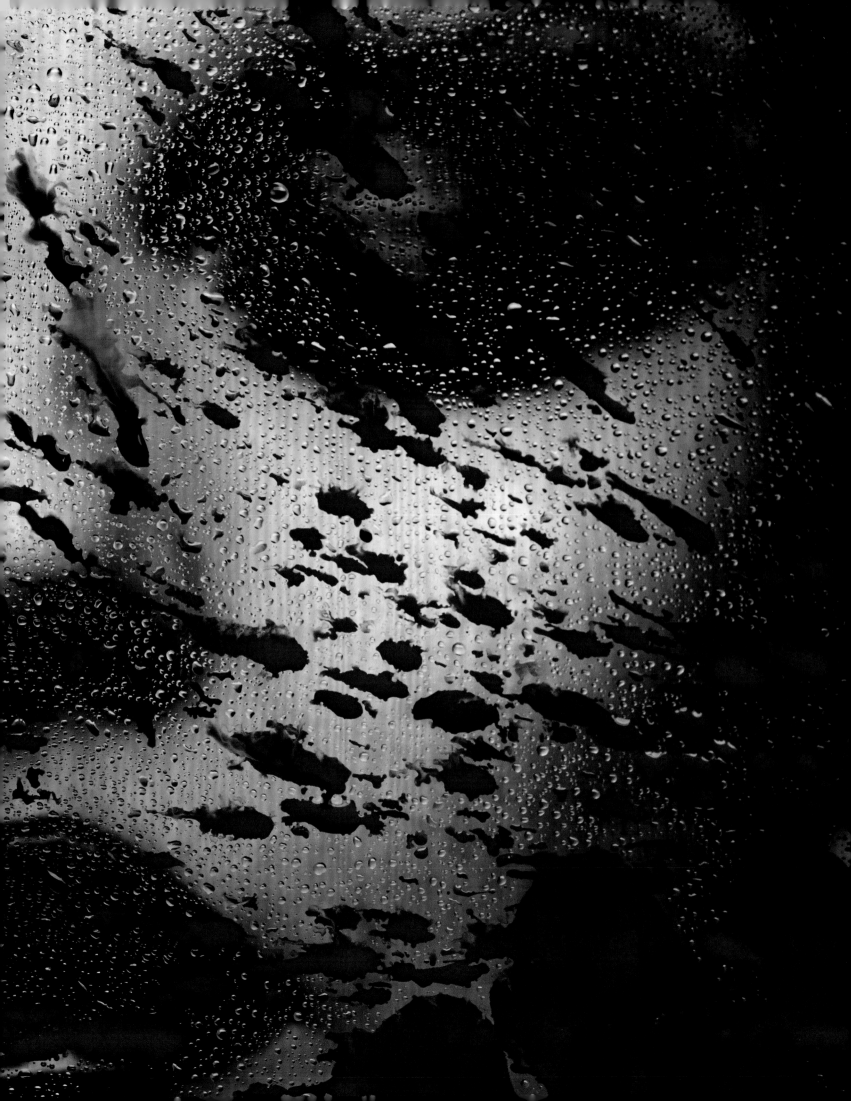

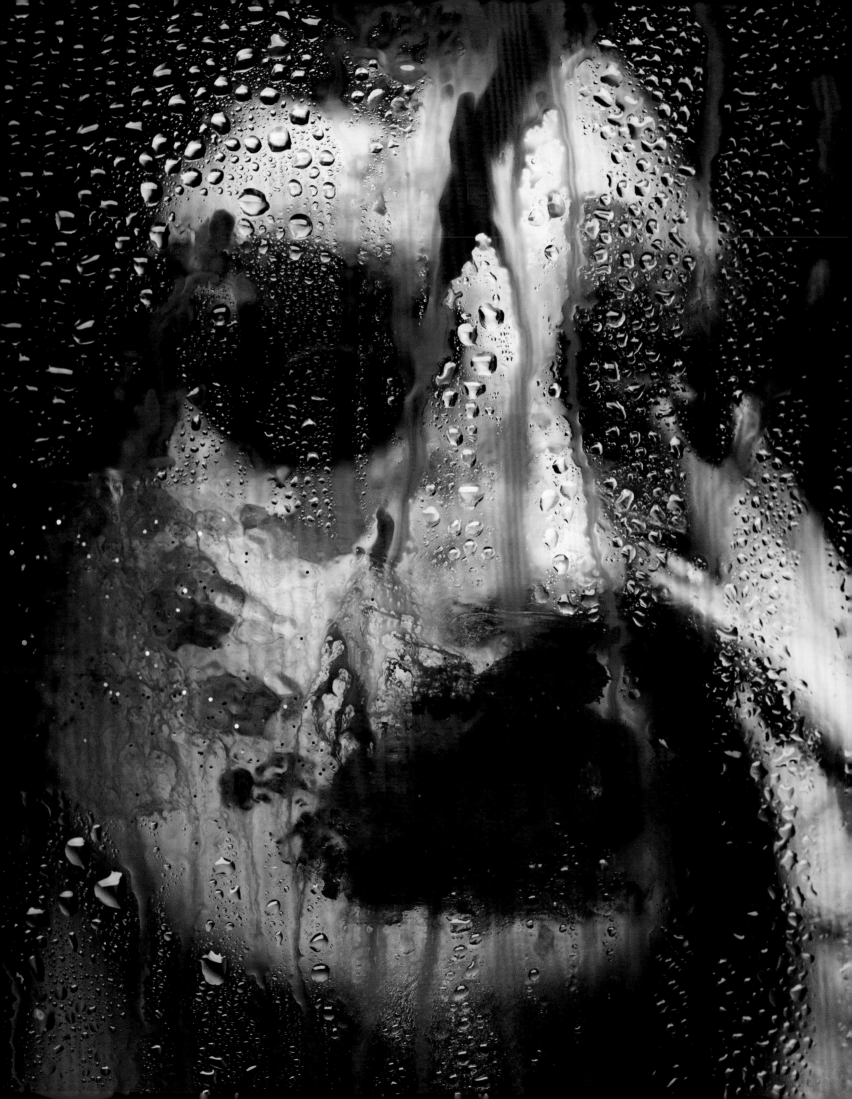

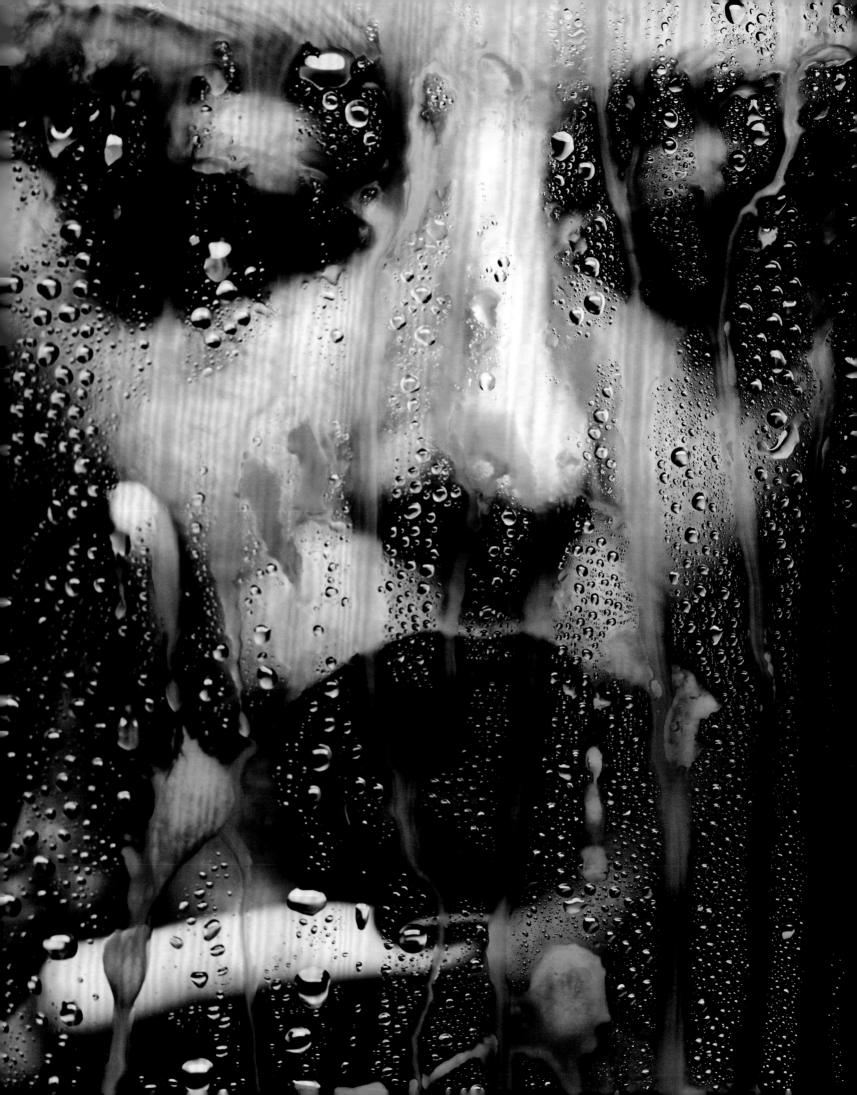

Nick is always fascinated by what goes on in the hair, makeup and styling room, and on this particular day he came in and said, 'Look, I want to shoot in here. I want to shoot among all the madness and mayhem.' So we all thought, 'Why don't we give the girls some makeup and get them to draw on themselves?' Which is what they did. This one moment of madness just really worked.

BRITISH VOGUE APRIL 2003; PHOTOGRAPHY NICK KNIGHT; FASHION EDITOR KATE PHELAN; HAIR SAM MCKNIGHT; MANICURIST MARIAN NEWMAN; MODELS FRANKIE RAYDER, ANGELA LINDVALL.

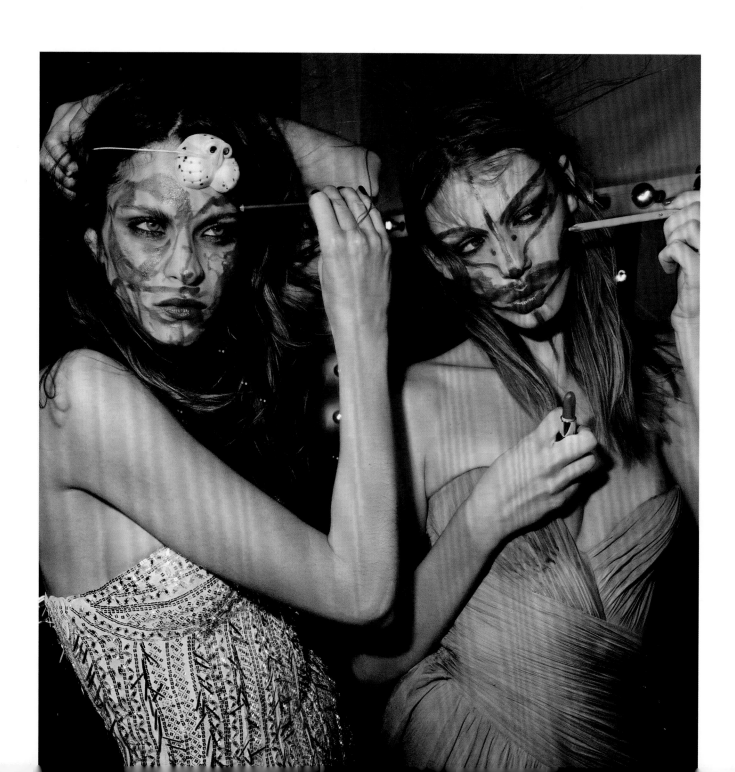

ONE
MOMENT
OF
MADNESS

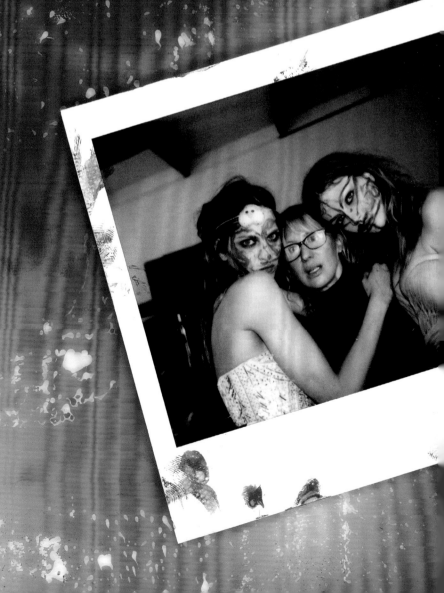

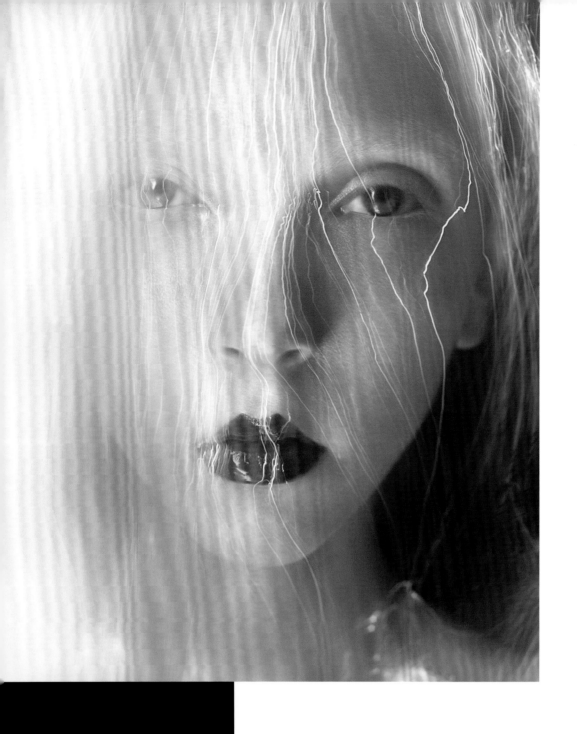

Sometimes it's just one colour,
one continuous brushstroke,
and that's it.

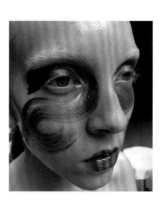

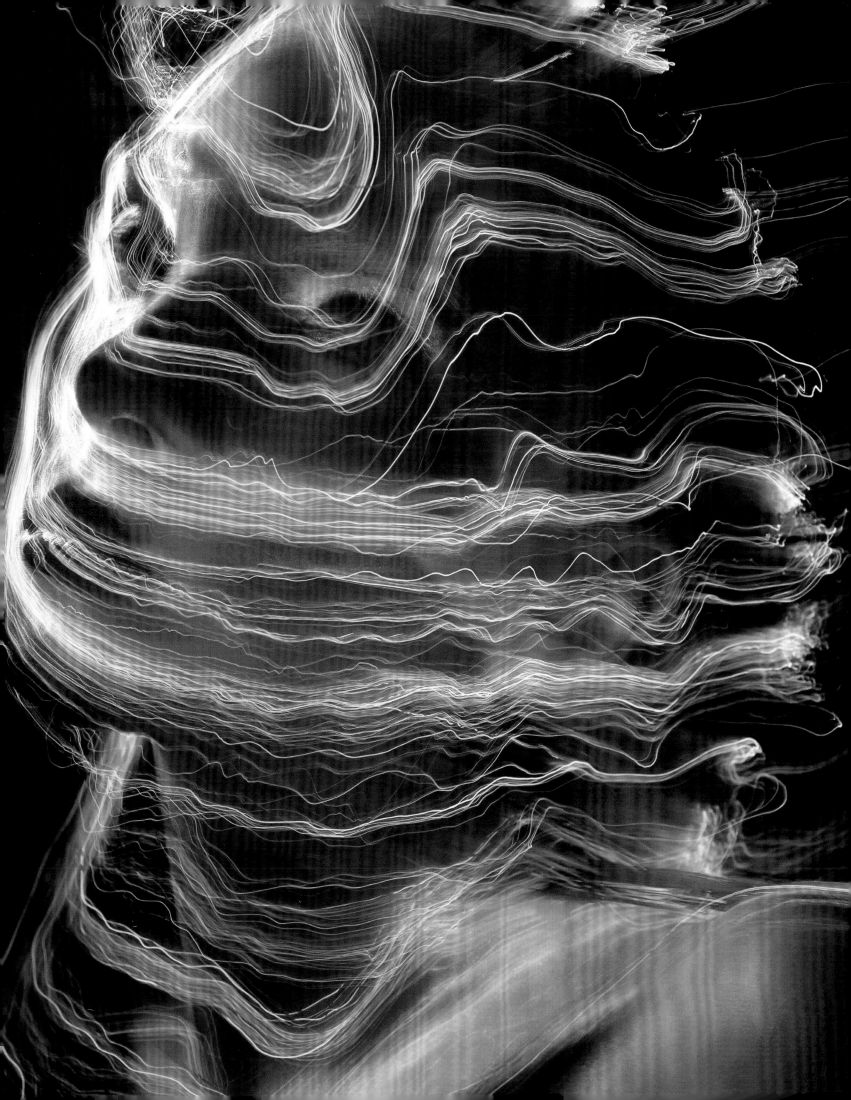

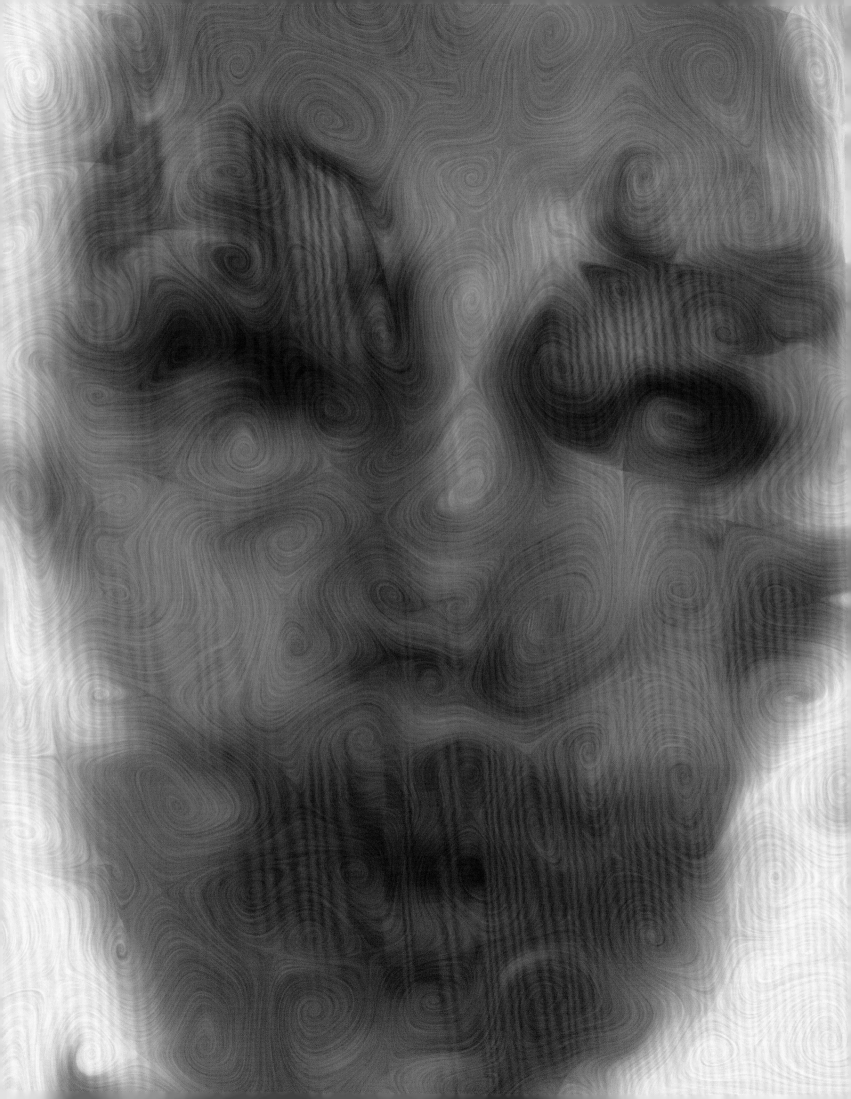

'EVERYTHING IS BECOMING MORE AND MORE THE SAME,
MORE CONFORMITY, AND THEN YOU HAVE SOMEONE AS
UNIQUE AS VAL. MAYBE UNIQUE IS A BETTER WORD THAN
DIFFERENT, BUT I ACTUALLY LIKE THE WORD DIFFERENT
MORE. I THINK "DIFFERENT" IS HEALTHY. LIKE THE WAY THAT
LEE MCQUEEN WAS DIFFERENT, JOHN GALLIANO IS DIFFERENT,
NICK KNIGHT IS DIFFERENT, SO

VAL IS DIFFERENT

I THINK YOU CAN TAP INTO THAT SOURCE, AND HAVE
A FAR MORE SPECIAL EXPERIENCE THAN IF YOU JUST SAY
"OH, I'D LOVE A SEXY GIRL".'

SØLVE SUNDSBØ

NUMÉRO 78, NOVEMBER 2006, 'L'ORIGINE DU MONDE'; PHOTOGRAPHY SØLVE SUNDSBØ; FASHION EDITOR JONATHAN KAYE; HAIR MALCOLM EDWARDS.

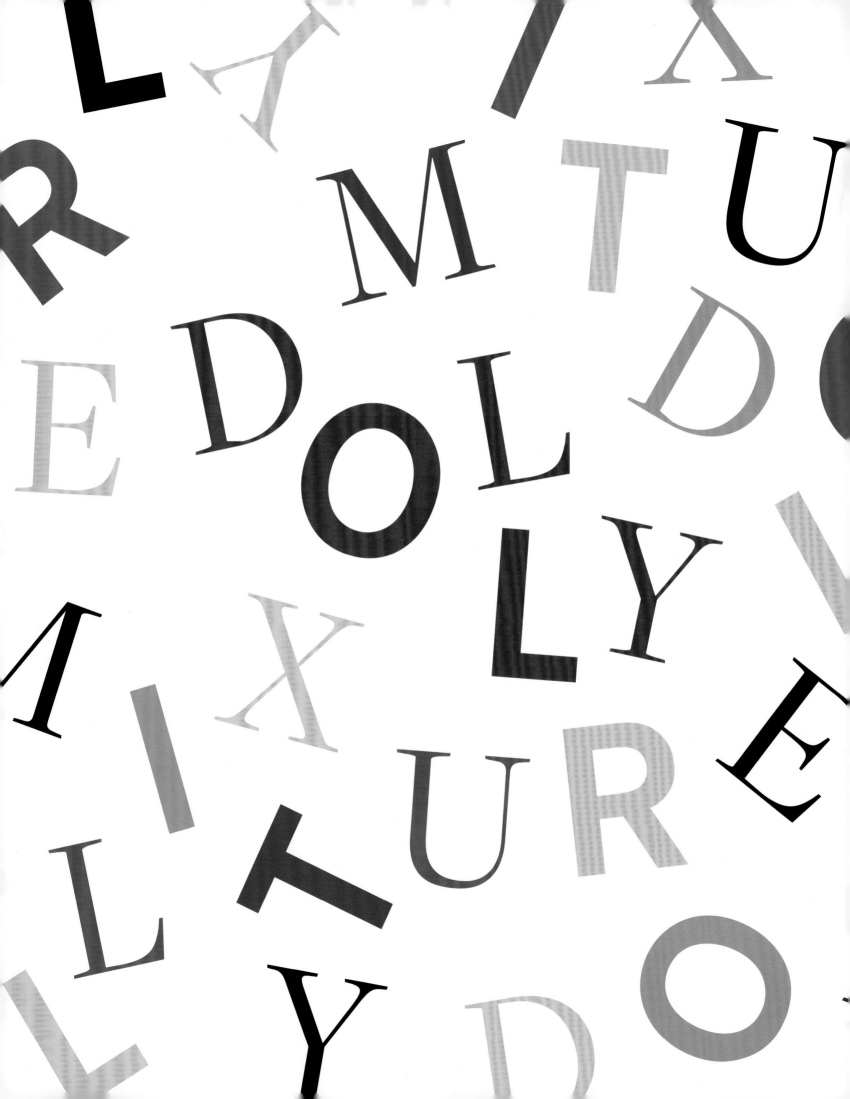

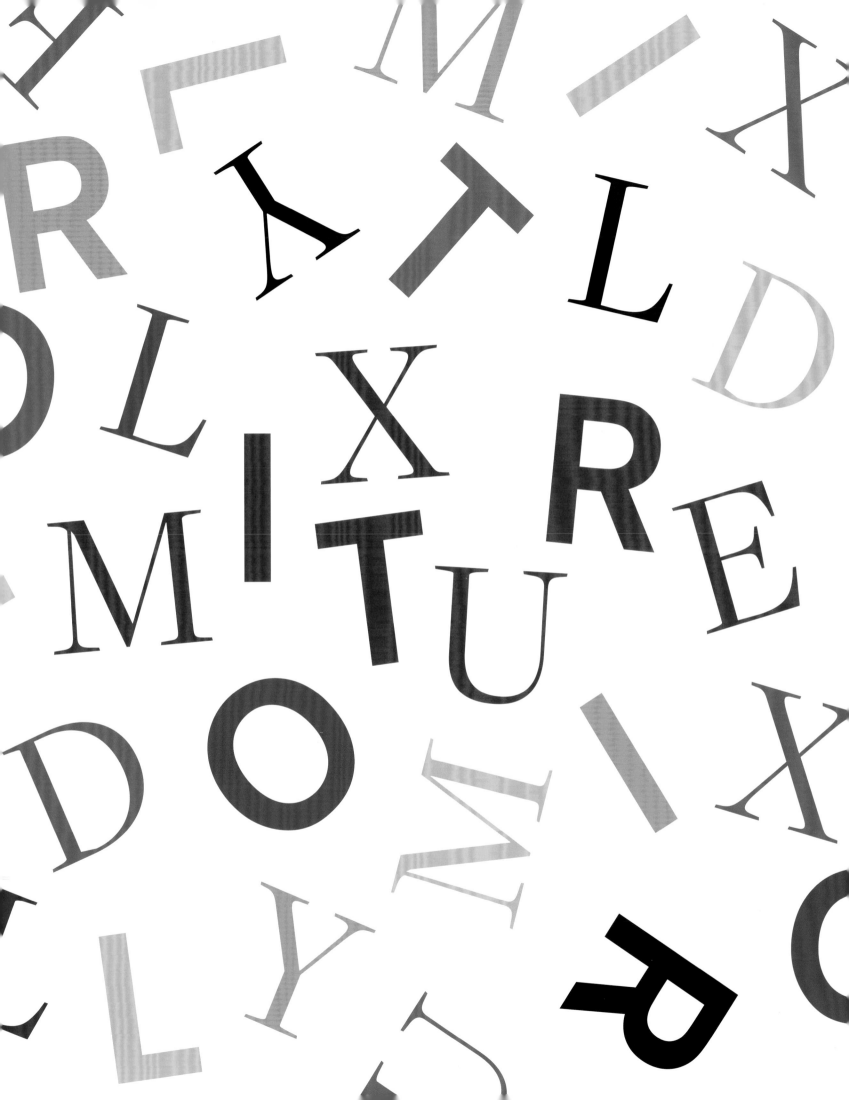

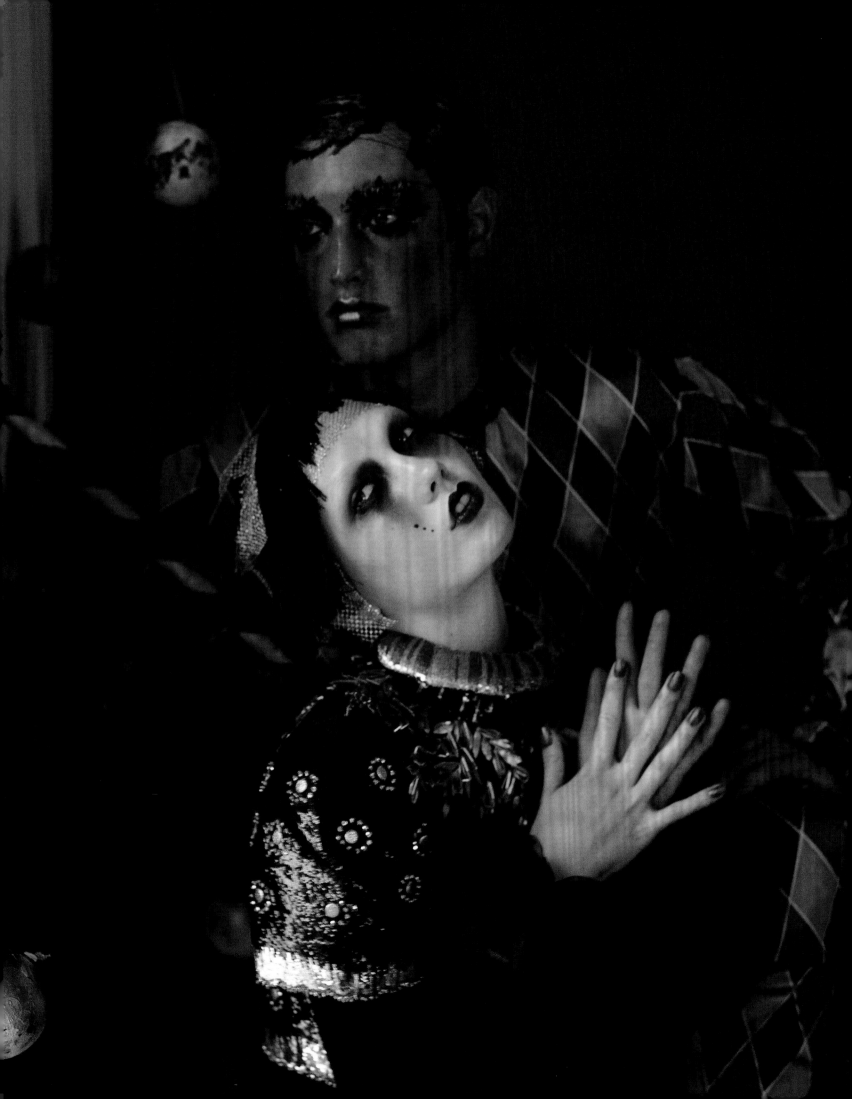

WELCOME
TO THE
DOLLHOUSE

BRITISH VOGUE OCTOBER 2010; PHOTOGRAPHY TIM WALKER; FASHION EDITOR KATE PHELAN; HAIR MALCOLM EDWARDS; MANICURIST ANATOLE RAINEY; SET DESIGN SHONA HEATH; MODEL KARLIE KLOSS.

Are you sitting comfortably? Then I'll begin. This is the story of Val's dolls. Not the immaculately arranged collection of vintage dollies that live in her London home, but the many dolls she has created with makeup. In fact, with typical creative vigour, Val has transformed some of the world's most famous models and celebrities into all manner of living dolls, from exquisitely hand-painted mannequins to strangely daubed puppets more reminiscent of Egon Schiele's expressionistic style.

As if accompanied by the twinkly tune of a Victorian music box, Val's doll-like experiments in makeup often evoke a playful spirit that feels conjured from the fragmented memories of childhood. These are indeed jolly makeup tales of cute, wide-eyed dollies – all pencil-thin brows, apples of colour for cheeks, and cutely erotic mouths. But darker dollies lurk at the back of Val's toy box, and it is in these shadowy recesses that we see the influence of artists like Hans Bellmer and his grotesquely disarticulated doll sculptures; Greer Lankton and her emaciated, freak-like doll figures; Cindy Sherman and her 'Sex Pictures', and the Chapman Brothers' in flagrante sex dolls.

But Val's doll work is not always a dichotomy of light versus dark, so it's important to note her seminal work with photographer Tim Walker on 'Mechanical Dolls' (*Vogue* Italia, 2006), a story that illustrates how the sweet and the macabre can converge. Here, living models are disturbingly transformed into vacant-looking dolls with peeling china skin, oddly broken gaits, weirdly jointed limbs and strange metal appendages for arms. These images are alluring yet shiver-inducing, conveying a melancholic beauty and bizarre sexuality that somehow renders them 'not suitable for children'.

As we stride towards making ourselves look ever more artificial, the irony is certainly not lost on Val, but her dolly masks do elicit an explosive emotional charge that seems to say, 'It's fine to be weird. It's OK to be different. You can still be loved.' Yet, unlike the dolls of mythology, the human dolls on these pages are already blessed with the gift of mortality – and, like Pygmalion, Val breathes life into our imaginations with her art. The makeup dolls she has created on these pages are there for all of us to love, adore, treasure and sometimes fear.

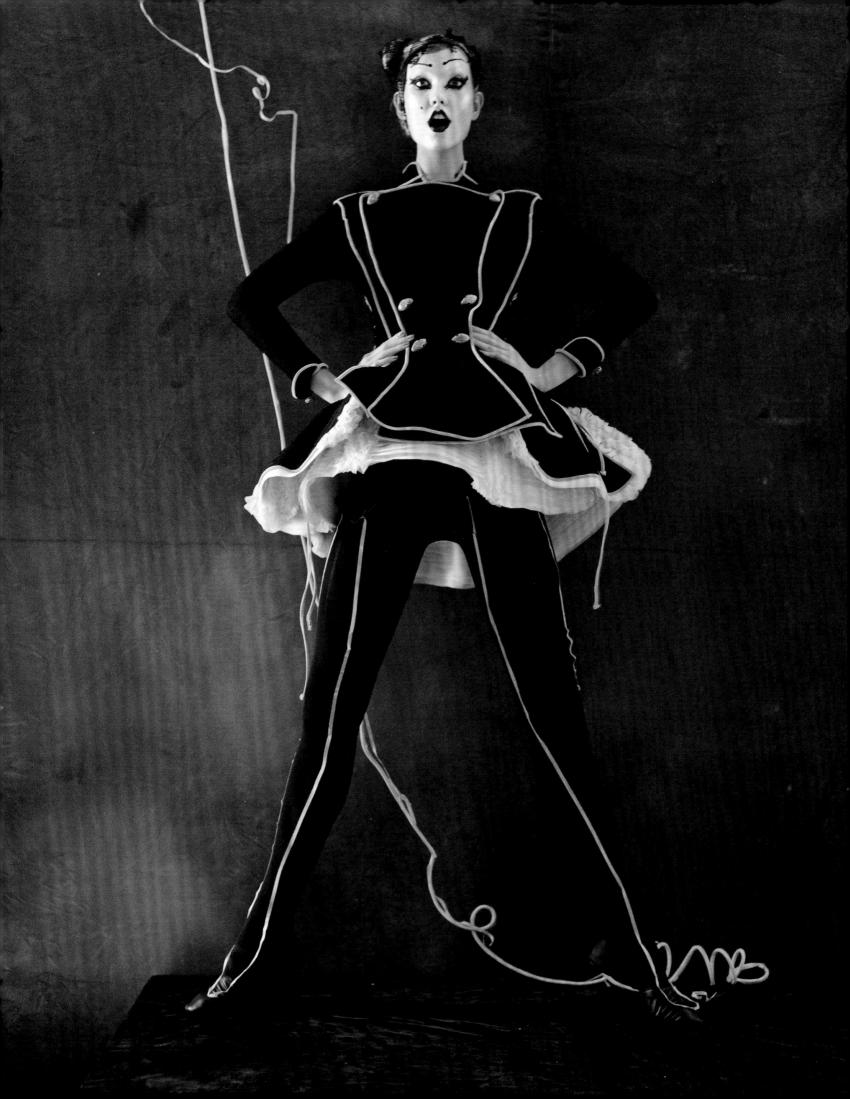

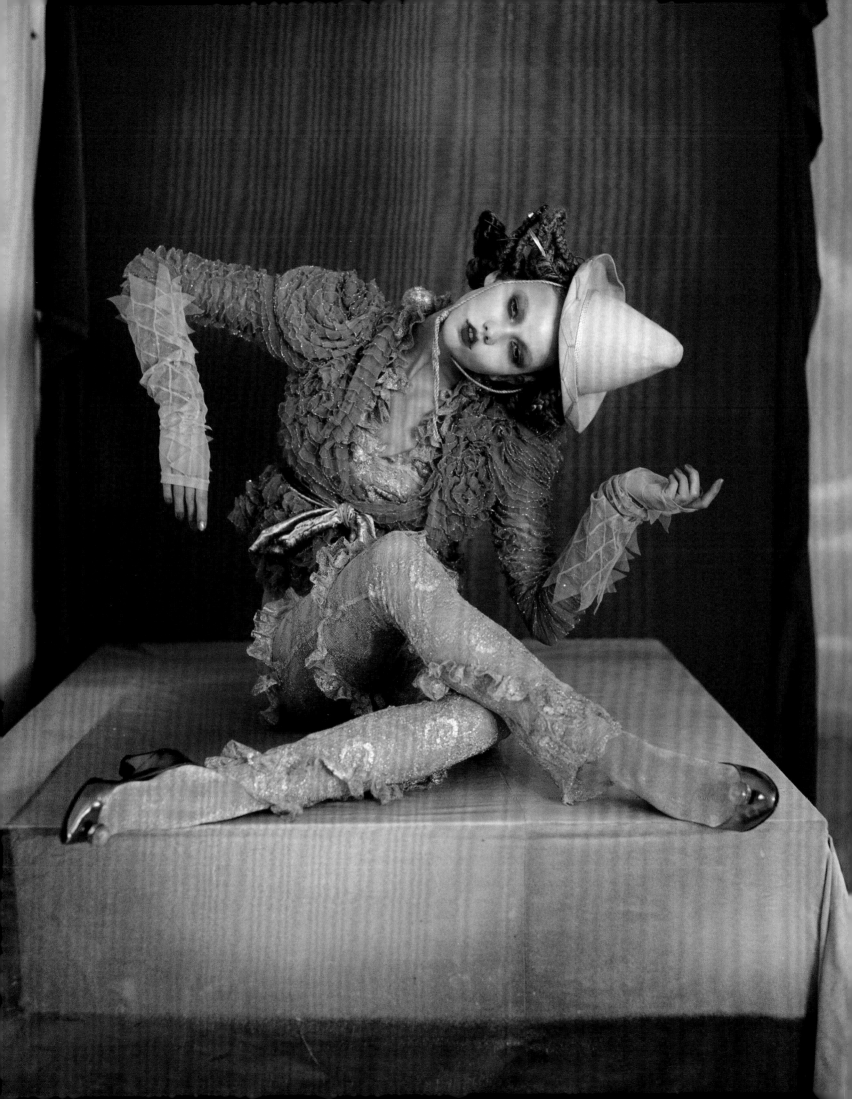

WHERE DOES YOUR FASCINATION WITH DOLLS COME FROM?

I guess from childhood. I got my first doll when I was four years old and she was called Phyllis. She became like my imaginary friend and I would tell her all my woes. I remember going to buy her with my mum. It was coming up to my birthday and we used to pass this toy shop every morning on the way to school. They had the latest 'Caroline Doll' – everybody wanted a Caroline Doll because I think she wet herself – but I didn't want her and in the dusty back of the shop was this little doll who looked really lonely in her box. I said to my mum, 'I want that doll. I want the one that's got no friends.'

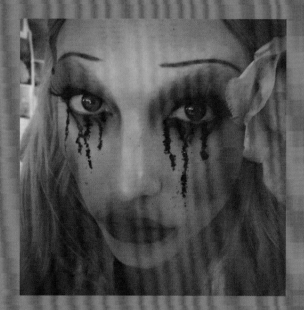

SO DID YOU LOVE PLAYING WITH DOLLS AS A CHILD?

I did. My sister had a big doll collection; she was incredibly artistic, and would always do her dolls' hair and makeup and make them look really good. But I wasn't, and Phyllis had very short, curly hair which you couldn't really do anything with, so whenever I got another doll I'd cut its hair till it was really short, so in the end they became sort of bald, really. Then I did the same thing with my sister's dolls – all of them! My mum and sister were crying and saying, 'What have you done?' and I just said, 'don't worry, it'll grow back again. It's only hair.' I must have really believed dolls were just like real people.

I think doll makeup is essentially quite colourful and could be considered 'cute', but it can also be a little dark. I like the idea of the painted face, a mask, sort of 'putting on a front'. But, you know, it's also so many other things; it's glam rock, it's disco, it's glitter, it's colour, it's paint, it's clowns ... It could even be all of the above, with a sort of really nice Margaret Thatcher hairdo!

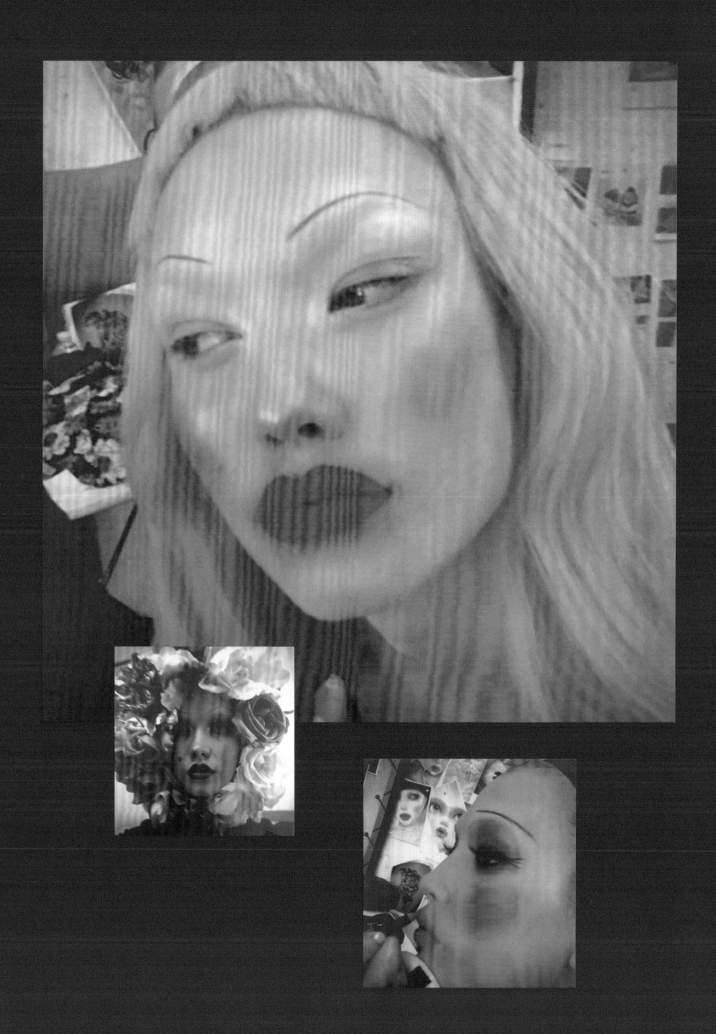

HAIR SAM MCKNIGHT. MODEL KARLIE KLOSS.

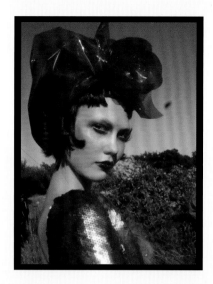

I LOVE THE ROMANCE OF 'WHERE TROUBLES MELT LIKE LEMON DROPS'.

Tim had a set built where everything was yellow, so it felt like a good space mentally, with yellow being my favourite colour. I bleached Karlie's eyebrows and turned her into a sort of vintage, thirties-inspired showgirl dolly.

Sometimes the makeup was yellow, sometimes it was orange, sometimes red – it was all in the warm spectrum. I can follow a brief, but I'd much rather be spontaneous because if it doesn't work you just take it off and do something else. I'm not precious about what I do – it's only paint. When I work with Tim we go on a journey together.

'You can take pictures on your own but if you're trying to create characters or tell stories you can't do it on your own. You have to collaborate with people that have the ability to find the essence of what you're trying to describe.'

TIM WALKER

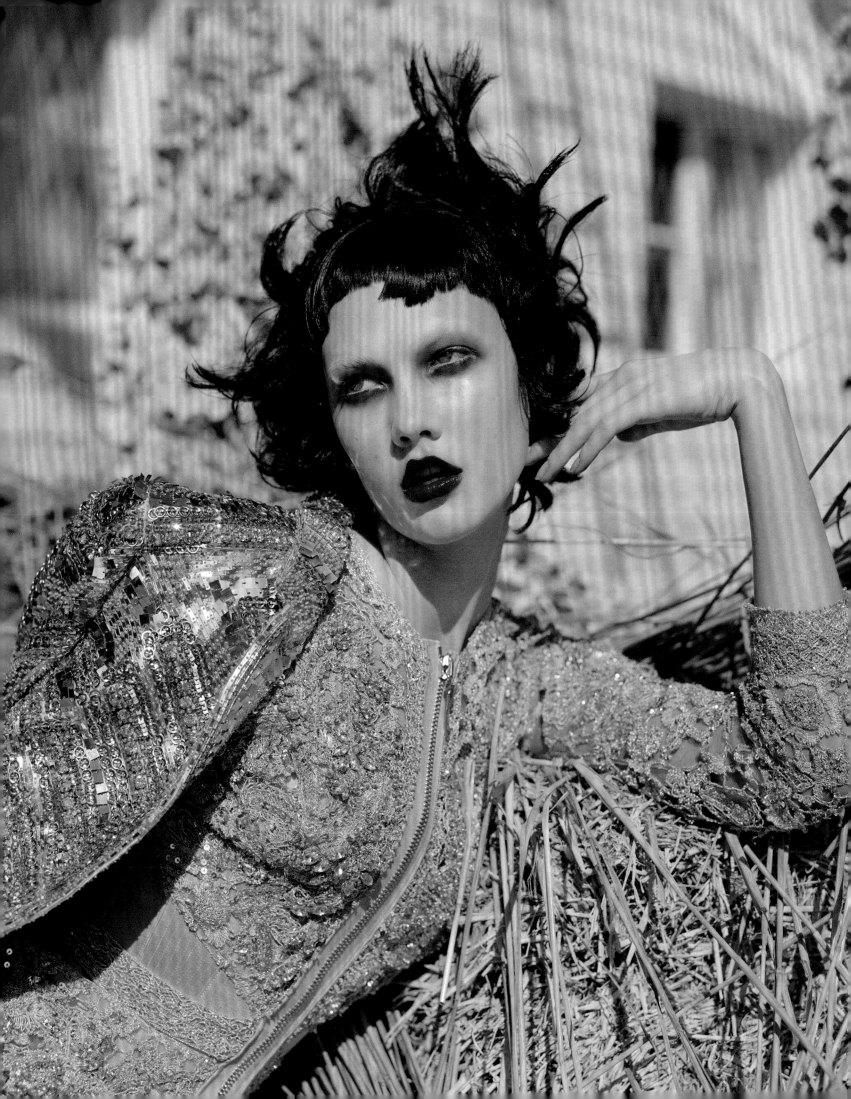

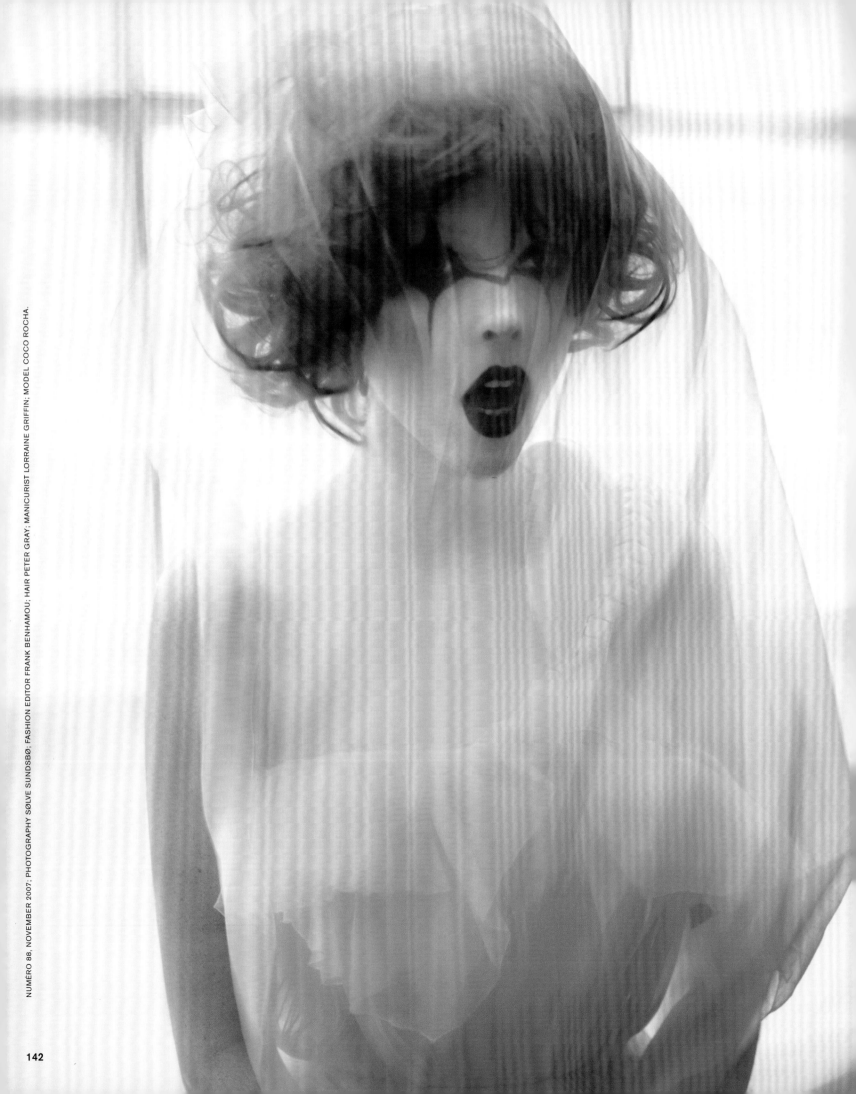

NUMÉRO 88, NOVEMBER 2007; PHOTOGRAPHY SØLVE SUNDSBØ; FASHION EDITOR FRANK BENHAMOU; HAIR PETER GRAY; MANICURIST LORRAINE GRIFFIN; MODEL COCO ROCHA.

I LOVED THE SHOCK
FACTOR OF THE
MAKEUP AGAINST
THE ROMANCE
OF EVERYTHING
ELSE. WE KIND OF
HAVE TO MIX IT UP
SOMETIMES.

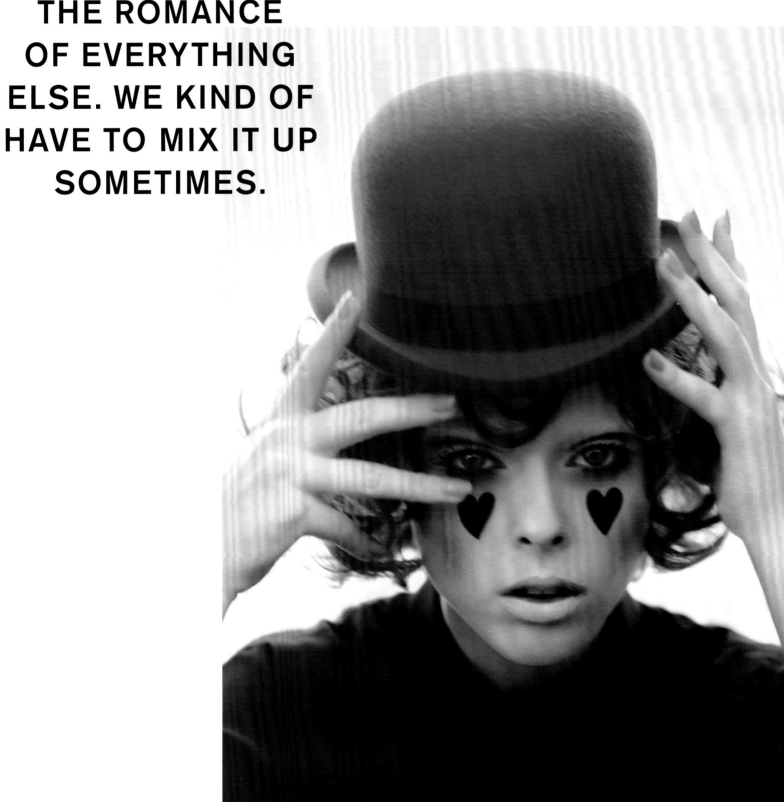

W MAGAZINE MAY 2013; PHOTOGRAPHY PATRICK DEMARCHELIER; FASHION EDITOR EDWARD ENNINFUL; HAIR MALCOLM EDWARDS; MODEL ZOE COLIVAS.

'Malcolm went in and stole this shoot. I said to him,
"You should be ashamed!", because he just stole the story.
I remember crying "It's supposed to be a beauty story!"
I called Val and she said, "Oh, let's do the hair. I'm in a hair
story." It was fun, and because she used to be a hairdresser,
there's no way she could say let's not do this. It wasn't
about her ego. No. It was about what was good for the
picture. She just went with it.'

EDWARD ENNINFUL

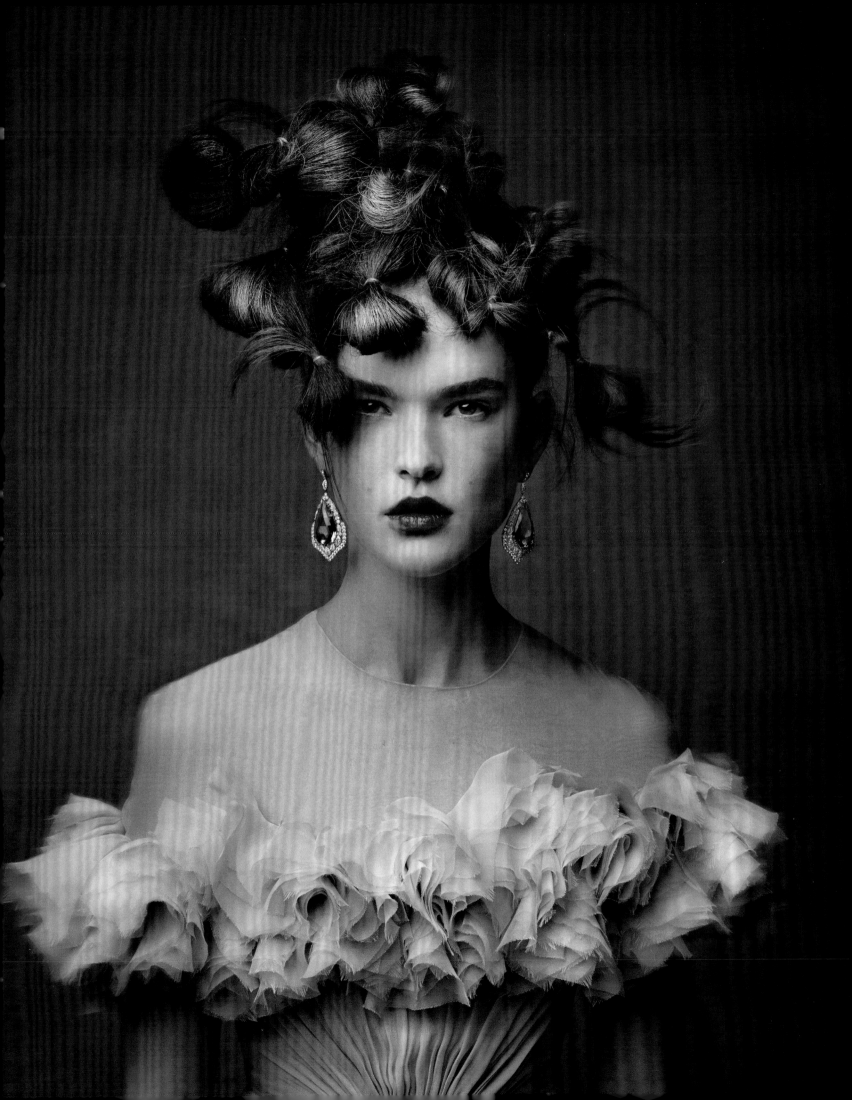

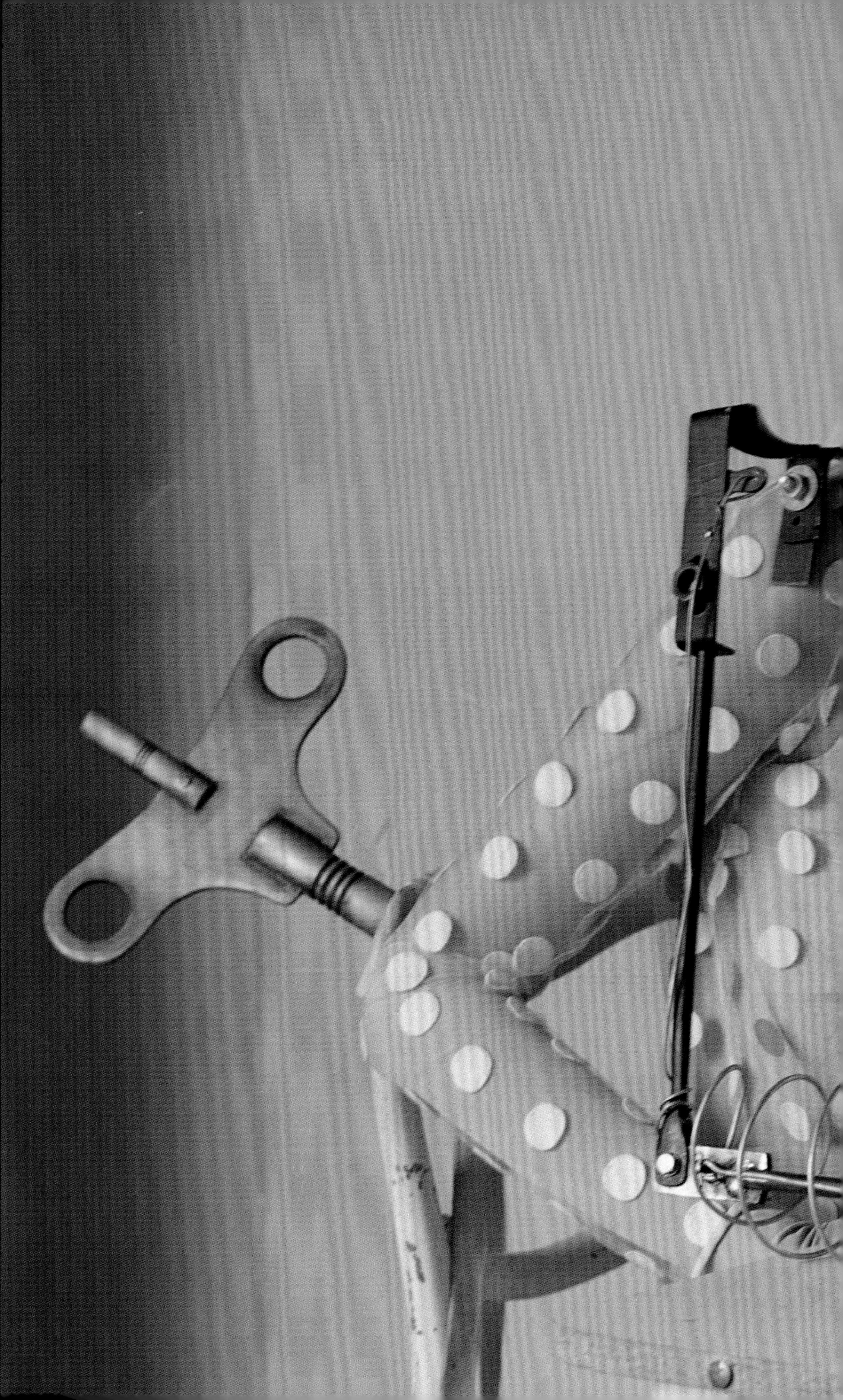

VOGUE ITALIA OCTOBER 2011; PHOTOGRAPHY TIM WALKER; FASHION EDITOR JACOB K; HAIR MALCOLM EDWARDS; MODEL KIRSI PYRHONEN; SET DESIGN RHEA THIERSTEIN.

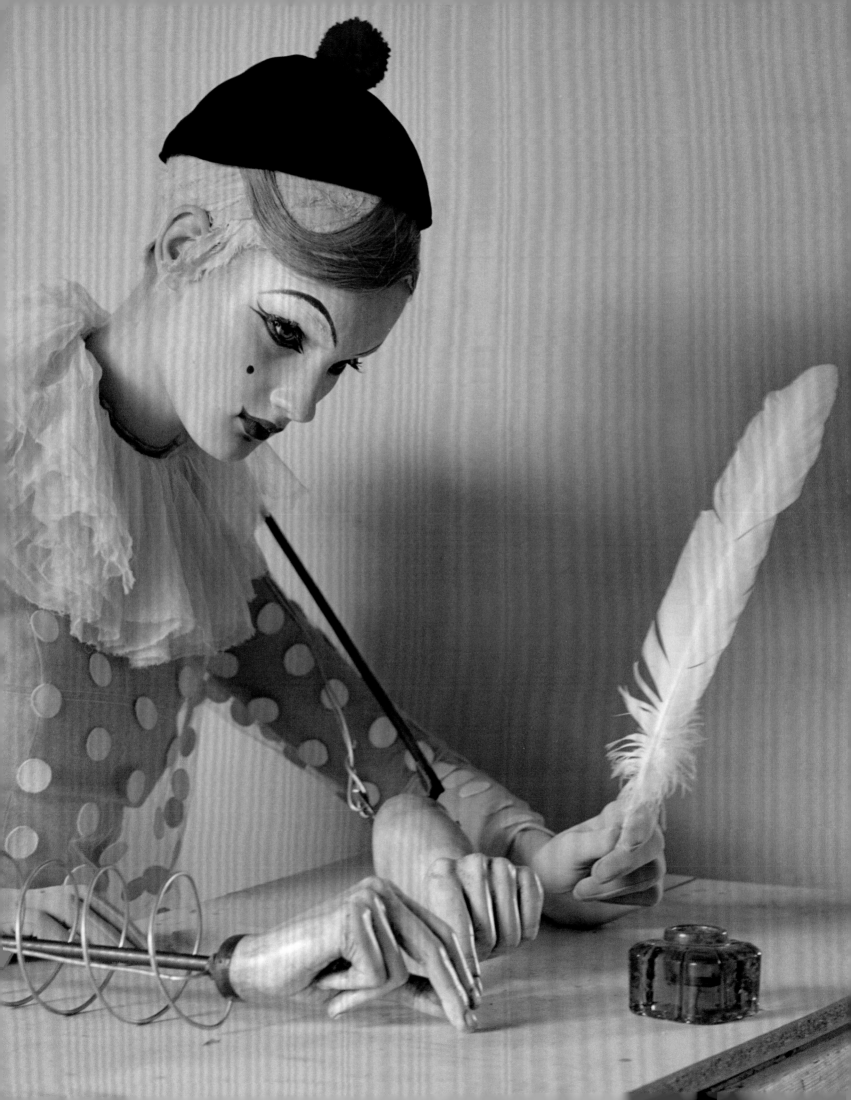

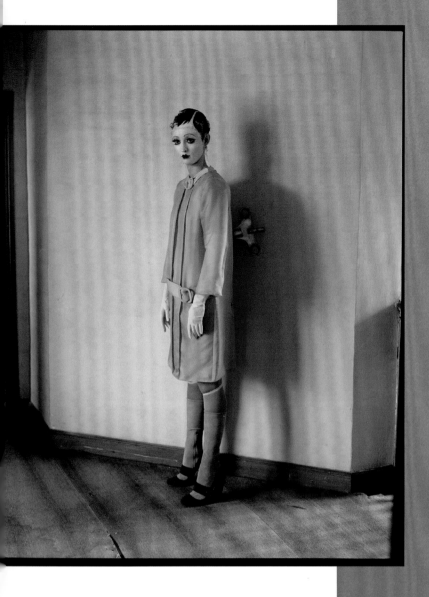

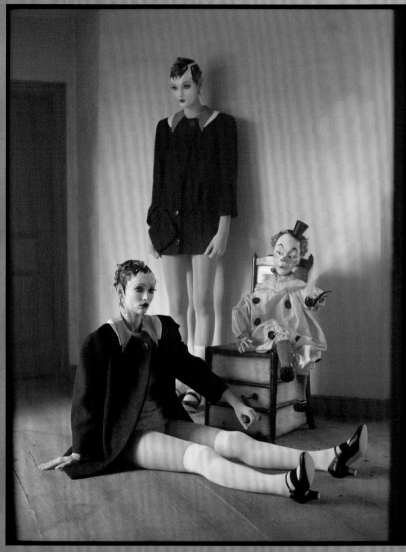

'VAL LOVES A DOLL

SO I ONLY WANTED TO WORK WITH VAL ON THIS
BECAUSE I KNEW THAT SHE'D REALLY GET IT.
I SHOWED HER MY *MECHANICAL DOLLS OF
MONTE-CARLO* BOOK AND SHE JUST SET OFF AND
DID ALL THIS RESEARCH ABOUT HOW TO GET A
CRACKLED FACE, HOW TO GET AN ANTIQUE FACE,
HOW TO MAKE A MOUSTACHE WORK ON A FACE.
VAL ALSO REALLY UNDERSTANDS THE MODEL.
SHE UNDERSTANDS SOMEONE THAT CAN
ELEVATE WHAT SHE DOES, WHICH PERFORMERS
CAN PULL OFF HER WORK, THE HAIRDRESSER'S
WORK, THE STYLIST'S WORK. AND THAT CAN
MAKE THE PICTURE.'

TIM WALKER

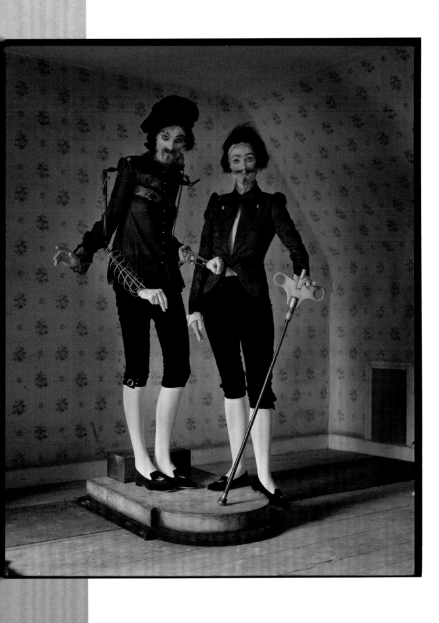

WHAT'S BEEN YOUR STRANGEST DOLL-WORK?

I did this 'Mechanical Dolls' shoot with Tim, and he wanted the models to look like little vintage Mexican figurines. He wanted it to be very painterly, very dark. There was a puppet that had been made especially by Rhea Thierstein, the set designer, and I thought at least one of the girls has to mirror that puppet, so that was my starting point. But for me the makeup ideas have to be organic and grow with the situation. Tim also wanted the girls to look like they were decayed and peeling, so that involved putting on a lot of makeup in different layers and then taking it away so it looked like it had decayed.

VOGUE ITALIA OCTOBER 2011; PHOTOGRAPHY TIM WALKER; FASHION EDITOR JACOB K; HAIR MALCOLM EDWARDS; MODELS AUDREY MARNAY, KIRSI PYRHONEN; SET DESIGN RHEA THIERSTEIN.

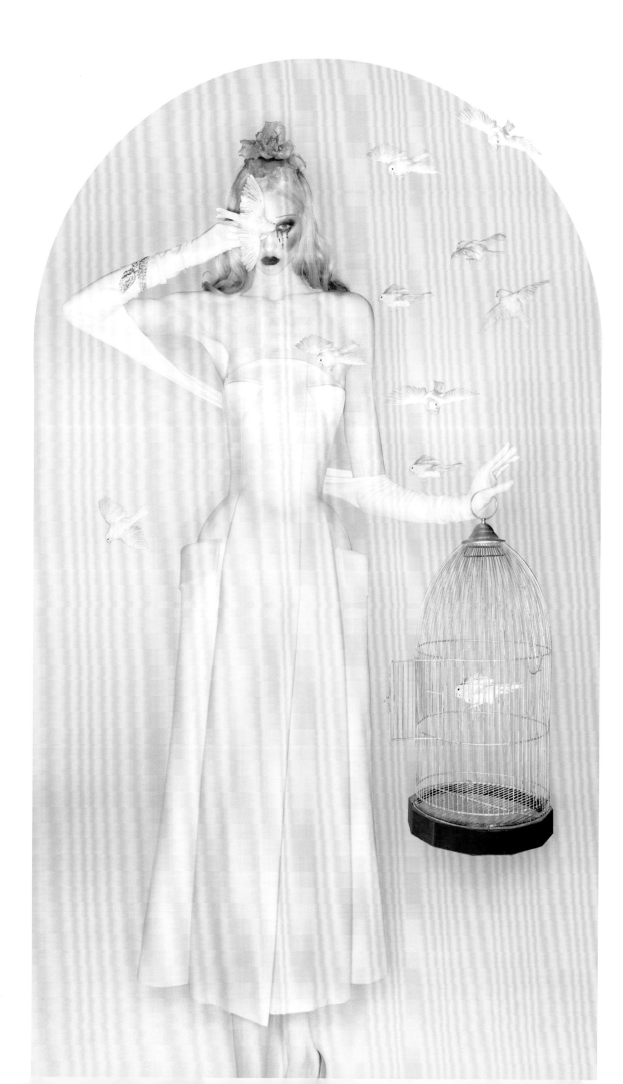

W MAGAZINE OCTOBER 2012, 'SWEET ESCAPE'; PHOTOGRAPHY NICK KNIGHT; FASHION EDITOR EDWARD ENNINFUL; HAIR SAM MCKNIGHT; MANICURIST ELSA DURRENS; MODEL KARLIE KLOSS.

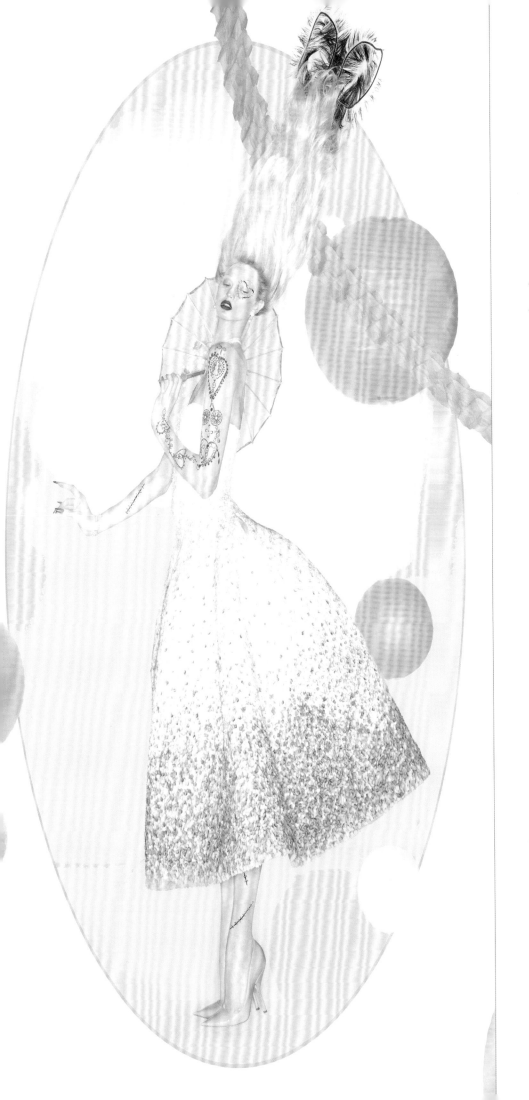

IT WAS AN AMAZING FAIRYTALE

'It was an amazing fairytale that became like illustrations, very surreal and digitally romantic. It was almost like an acid trip because Nick lengthened all the bodies and the fingers. It became about strong pastel colour and wigs. Val and I were in the dressing room just making it up as we went along.'

SAM MCKNIGHT

OPPOSITE AND FOLLOWING PAGES: W MAGAZINE JUNE 2011; PHOTOGRAPHY TIM WALKER; FASHION EDITOR JACOB K; HAIR ORLANDO PITA; MANICURIST YUNA PARK; MODEL SCARLETT JOHANSSON.

*THIS IS KIND OF THE ULTIMATE, TWISTED
DOLL MAKEUP, ISN'T IT?*

Tim wanted Scarlett Johansson to be lots of different characters,
so we photographed her as Marlene Dietrich, Buster Keaton, Tippi
Hedren in *The Birds*, and so on, but my favourite character was
Bette Davis in *What Ever Happened To Baby Jane?*

I really loved it, but this image didn't make it into the
magazine as they thought it was a bit too scary. What was great about
that particular moment was that Scarlett really got into it and literally
became Bette Davis, and if you look at the image, those are real tears.

IT'S ACTUALLY ALL A BIT WONKY

BUT I GUESS I JUST LIKE THINGS THAT ARE
A BIT WRONG
I THINK THE IDEA OF

SUPER-PERFECTION
IS BORING.

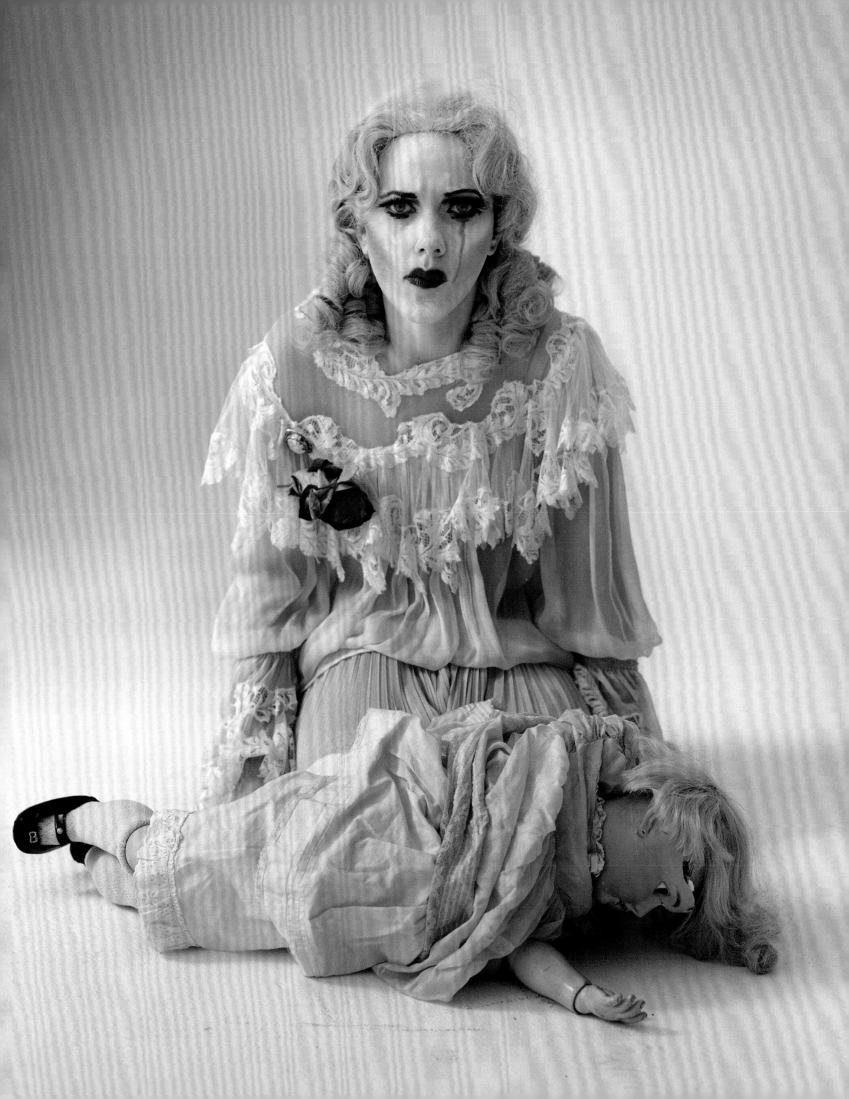

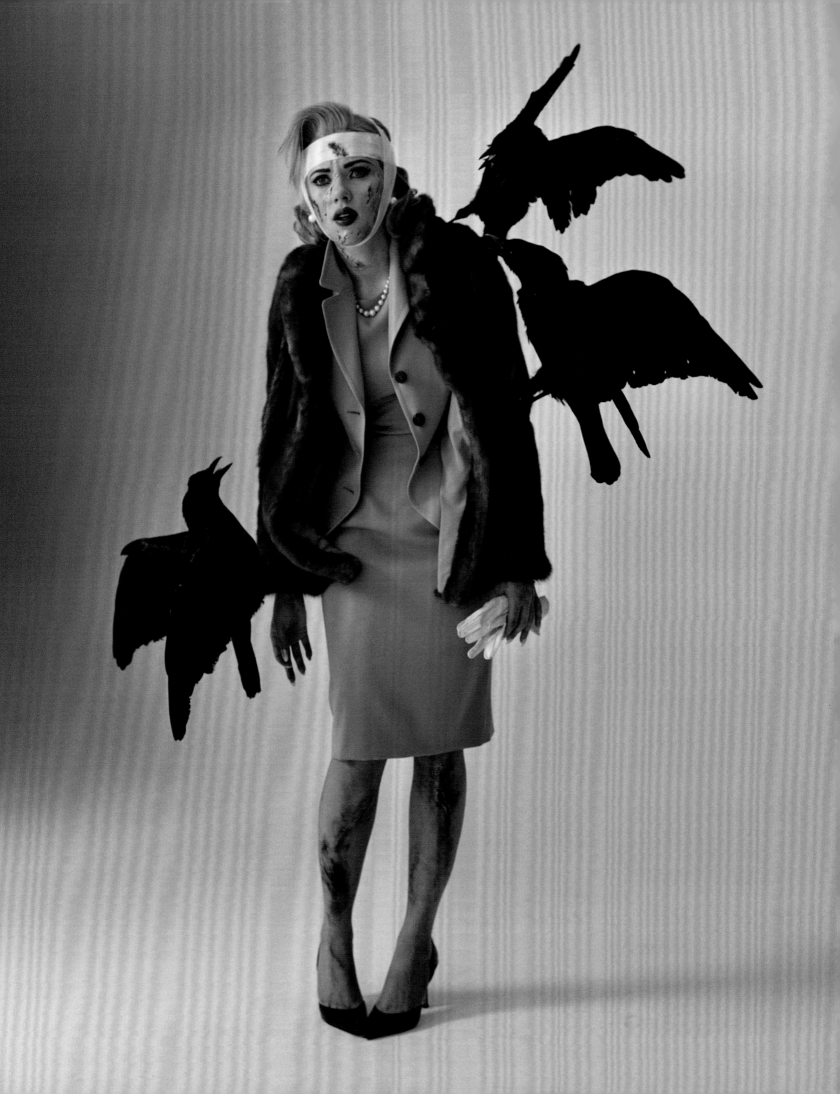

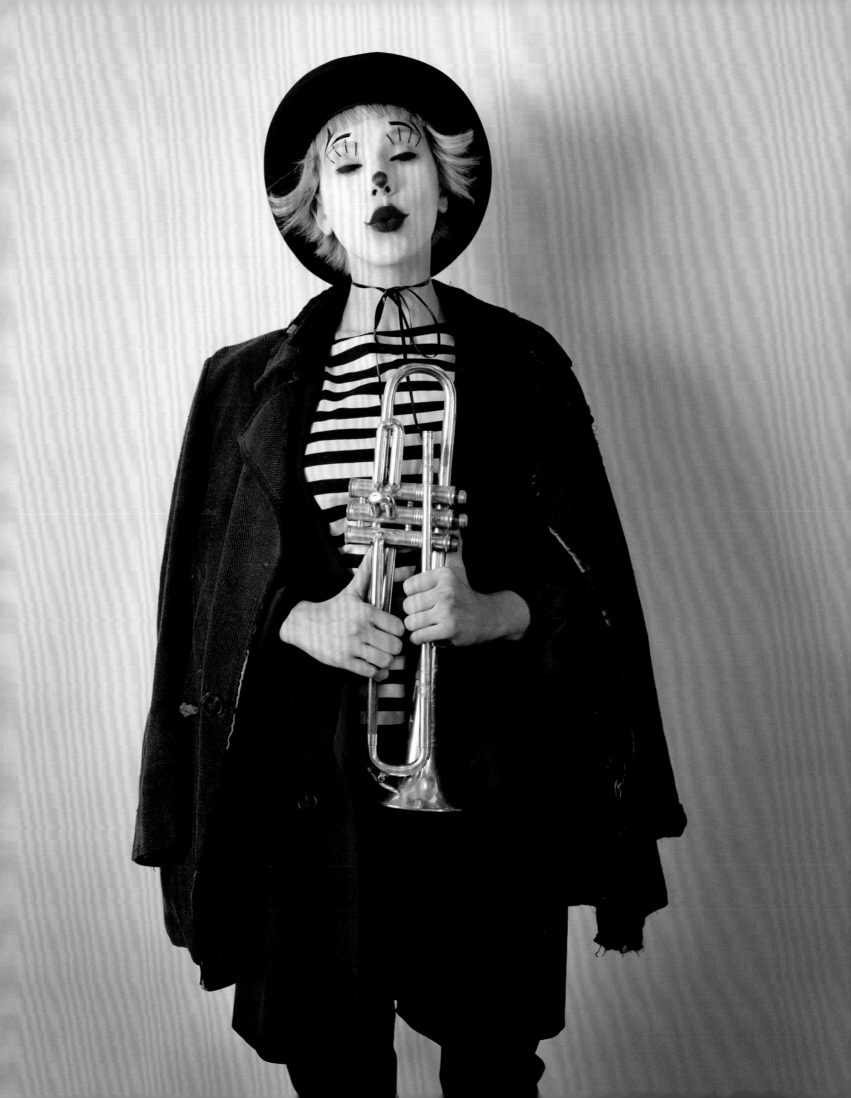

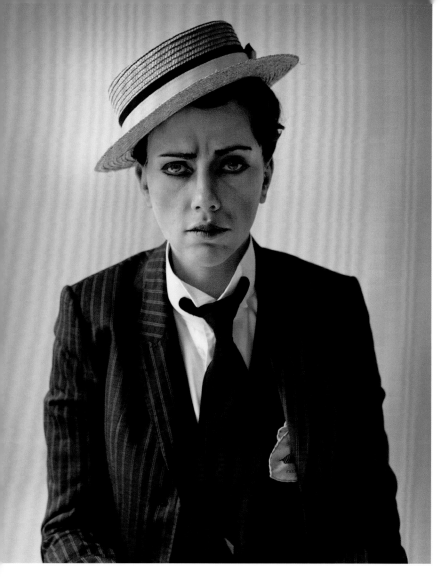

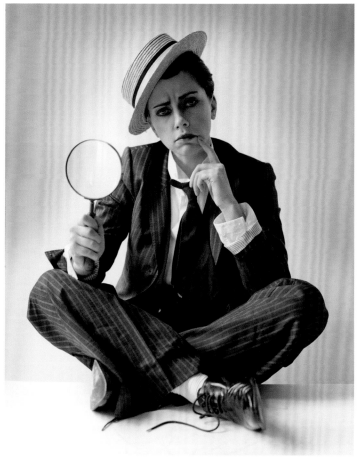

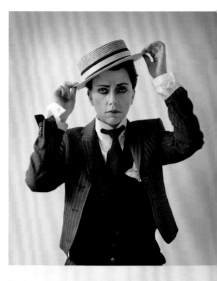

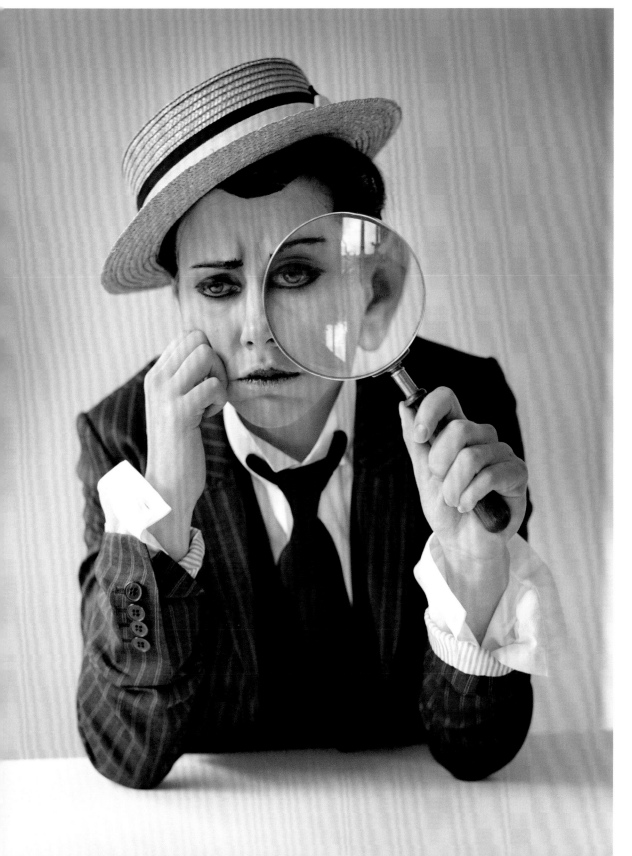

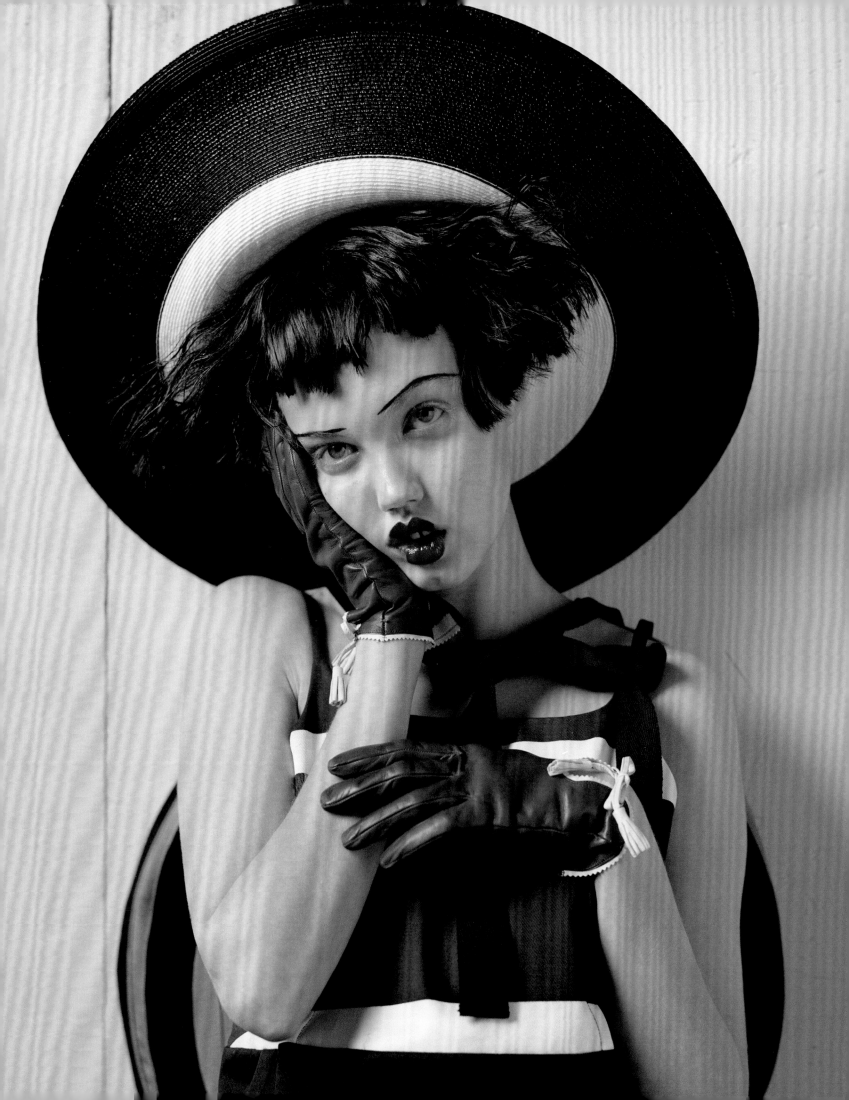

'I JUST LIKE TO DO IT, I DON'T WANT TO TALK ABOUT IT, AND IF IT DOESN'T WORK I CAN JUST CHANGE IT REALLY QUICKLY. AND I THINK VAL IS THE SAME. THAT'S WHY WE WORK WELL TOGETHER. I'M REALLY NOT OFFENDED IF SHE SAYS, "DO YOU THINK THE HAIR'S WORKING WITH THAT?" AND THEN I MAY SAY TO HER, "WELL, MAYBE NOT THE EYEBROWS."'

SAM MCKNIGHT

BRITISH VOGUE APRIL 2011; PHOTOGRAPHY TIM WALKER; FASHION EDITOR KATE PHELAN; HAIR SAM MCKNIGHT; MODEL LINDSEY WIXSON.

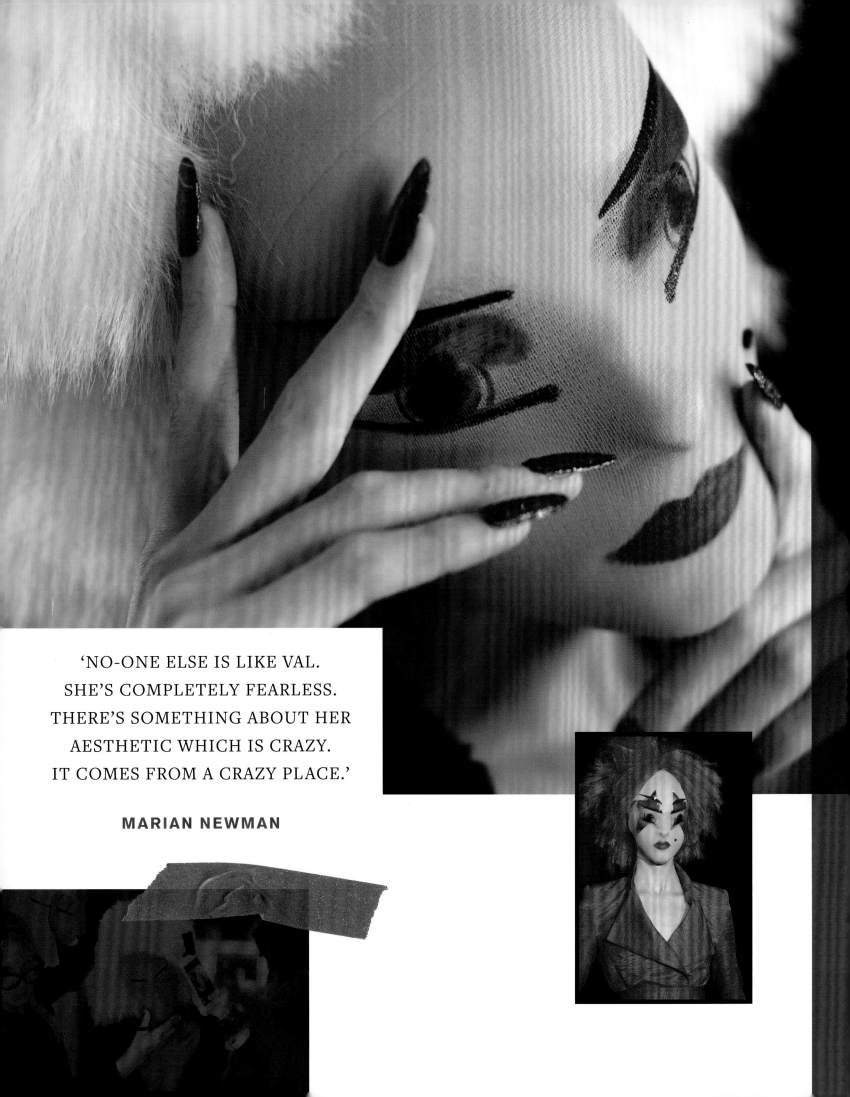

'NO-ONE ELSE IS LIKE VAL.
SHE'S COMPLETELY FEARLESS.
THERE'S SOMETHING ABOUT HER
AESTHETIC WHICH IS CRAZY.
IT COMES FROM A CRAZY PLACE.'

MARIAN NEWMAN

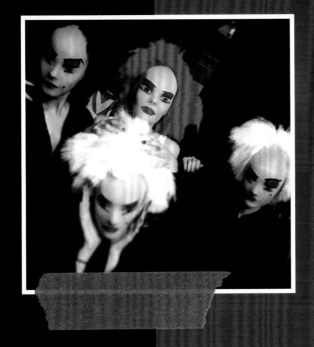

'THE HALLOWEEN AFTER THIS SHOW WAS AMAZING. SINCE WE'VE BEEN WORKING WITH VAL, EVERY HALLOWEEN THIS IS ALWAYS THE MOST COPIED LOOK.'

GARETH PUGH

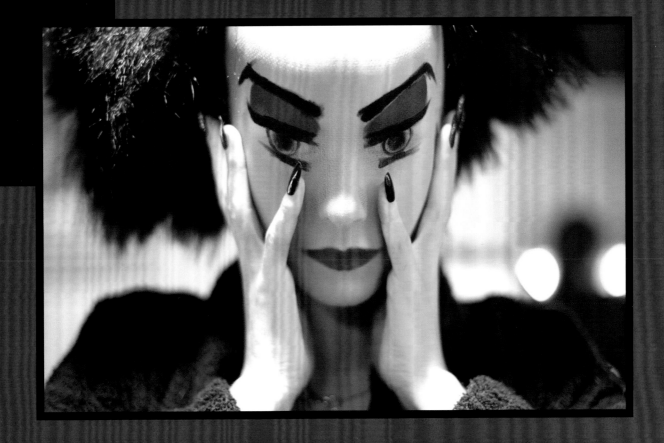

GARETH PUGH SS16: PHOTOGRAPHY LUCA CANNONIERI; FASHION EDITOR KATIE SHILLINGFORD; HAIR MALCOLM EDWARDS; MANICURIST MARIAN NEWMAN.

STIC
SE

CKY

XY

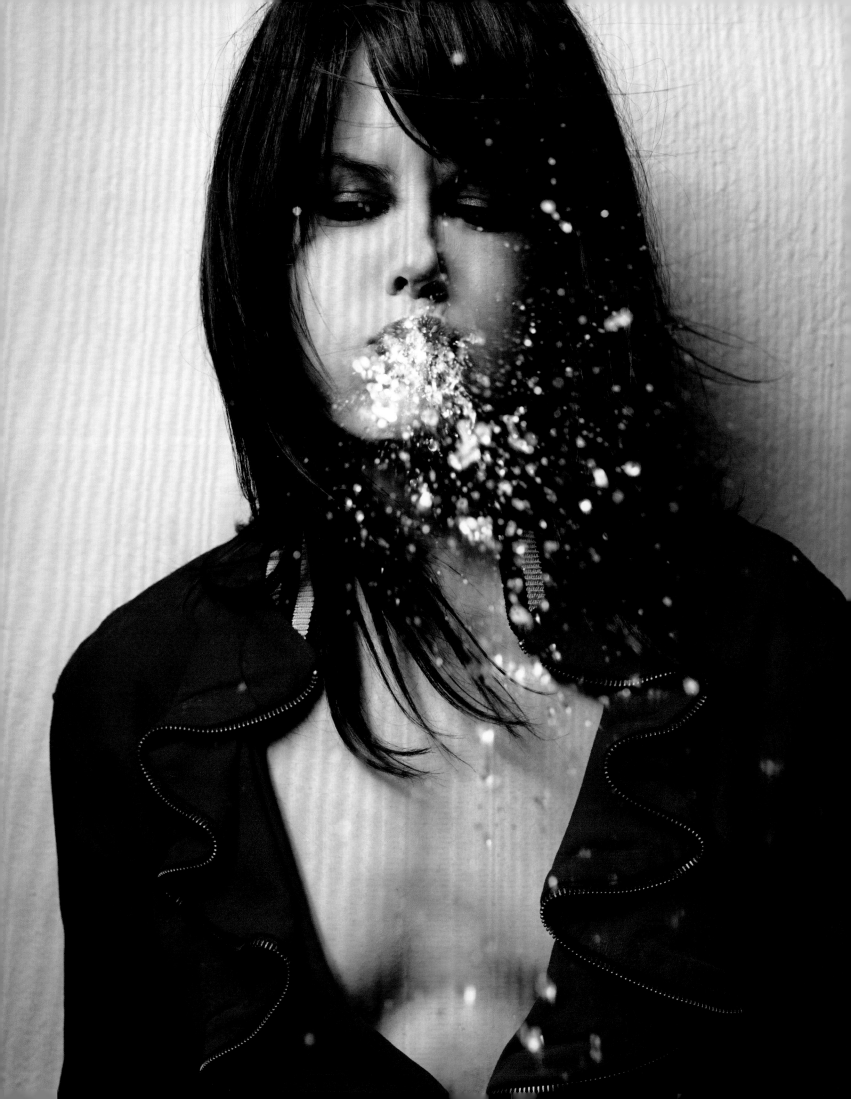

TO A
CLIMAX

Just like the stiletto heel is said to mimic the arch of a woman's foot at the height of orgasm, makeup that darkens, enhances or wets lips and eyes imitates signals of fertility and sexual allure. However, Val's erotically charged work shows us how makeup can go beyond sexy clichés and into a delicious, decadent, almost narcotic realm of the senses.

What is clear from Val's work is how, even when the model appears lost in the euphoria of climax, she is still in control. She is not submissive; she is sexually aware and powerful – a power that comes from the notion that makeup is not just a fabulous lie, it's also a weapon, a tool and even a mask that we can choose to remove. Val's more sensual journeys in makeup are broad-ranging, from the strict, uptight maitresse about to inflict dominance on her trembling charge, to the post-coital flushes of the hot-cheeked Lolita and the innocent, yearning waif.

Is Val intent on liberating us from our sexual hang-ups? Possibly, but whatever your bag, be it genteel après-midi liaisons like those enjoyed by Catherine Deneuve in *Belle de Jour*, or covert diversions into the smorgasbord of contemporary fetishes, it's interesting to note how Val's makeup addresses sexuality on so many delectable levels.

PHOTOGRAPHY CRAIG MCDEAN; ART DIRECTION ALEX WIEDERIN; FASHION EDITOR TABITHA SIMMONS; HAIR SAM MCKNIGHT; MODEL NICOLE KIDMAN.

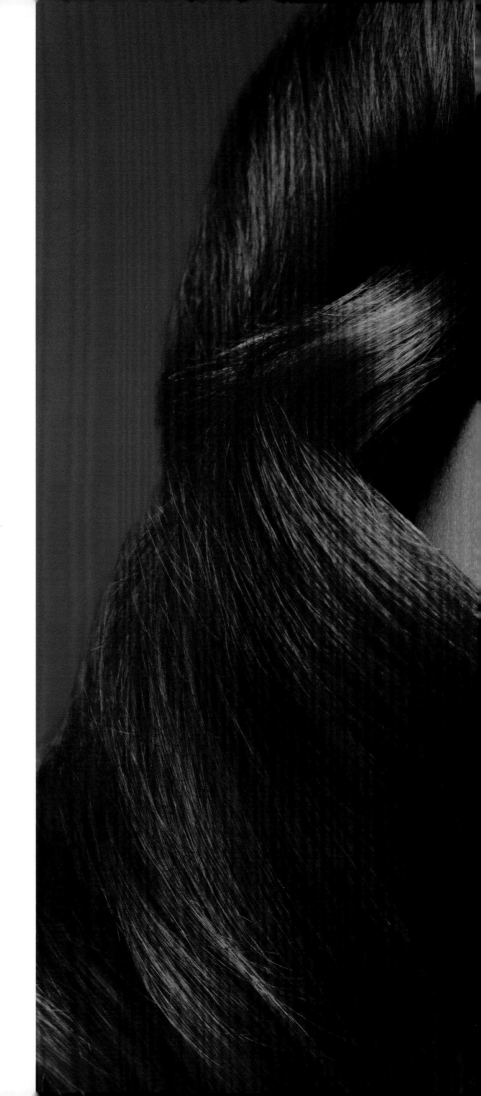

NUMÉRO 58, NOVEMBER 2004; PHOTOGRAPHY SØLVE SUNDSBØ; FASHION EDITOR JONATHAN KAYE; HAIR PETER GRAY; MODEL KAREN ELSON.

'Karen has such a canvas face.
I mean that in the nicest
possible way. "Canvas face"
sounds like a schoolyard
insult! Karen told me that
when she turns up at school in
the morning in Nashville, she
meets all these mothers who
are immaculately turned out,
and she arrives in a dressing
gown, hair all over the place,
looking like she just woke
up. She said, "I know they're
thinking, *You're the one on the
cover of American Vogue?!*"
But Karen has got it all in
her. These super, super, super
models have that capacity to
be so many different people
in one face.'

SØLVE SUNDSBØ

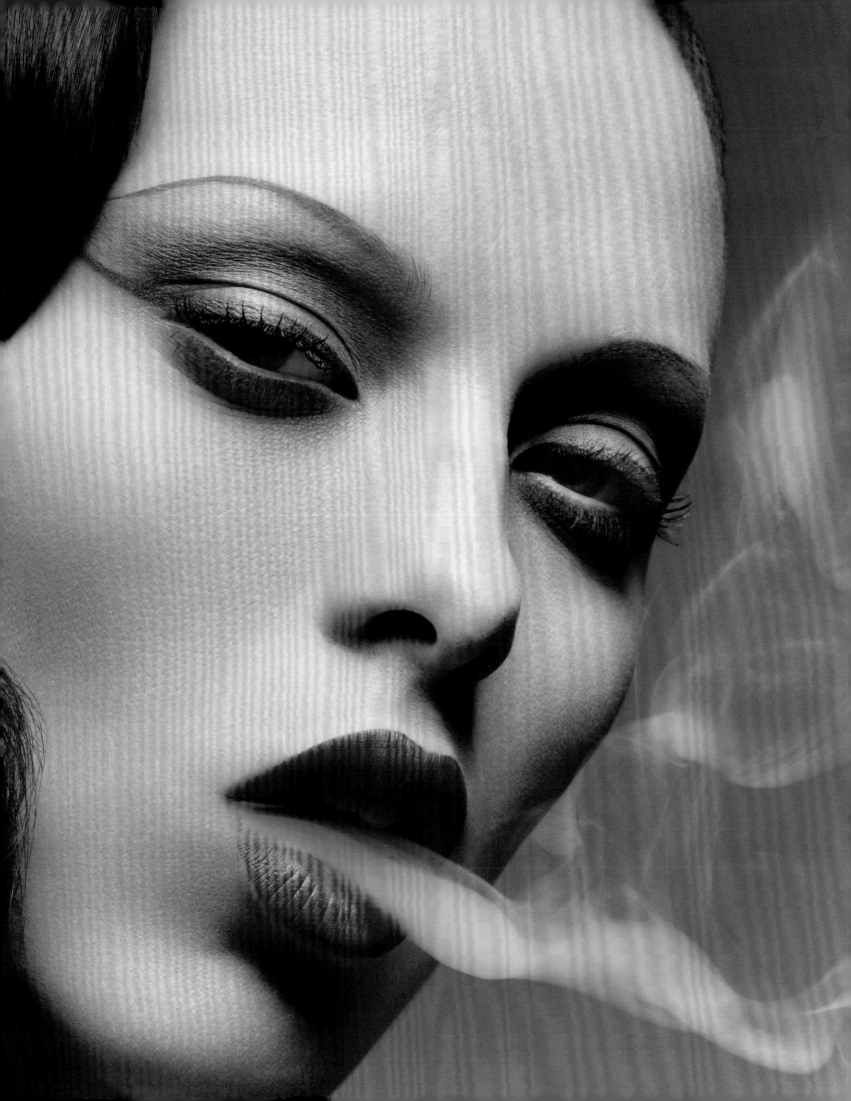

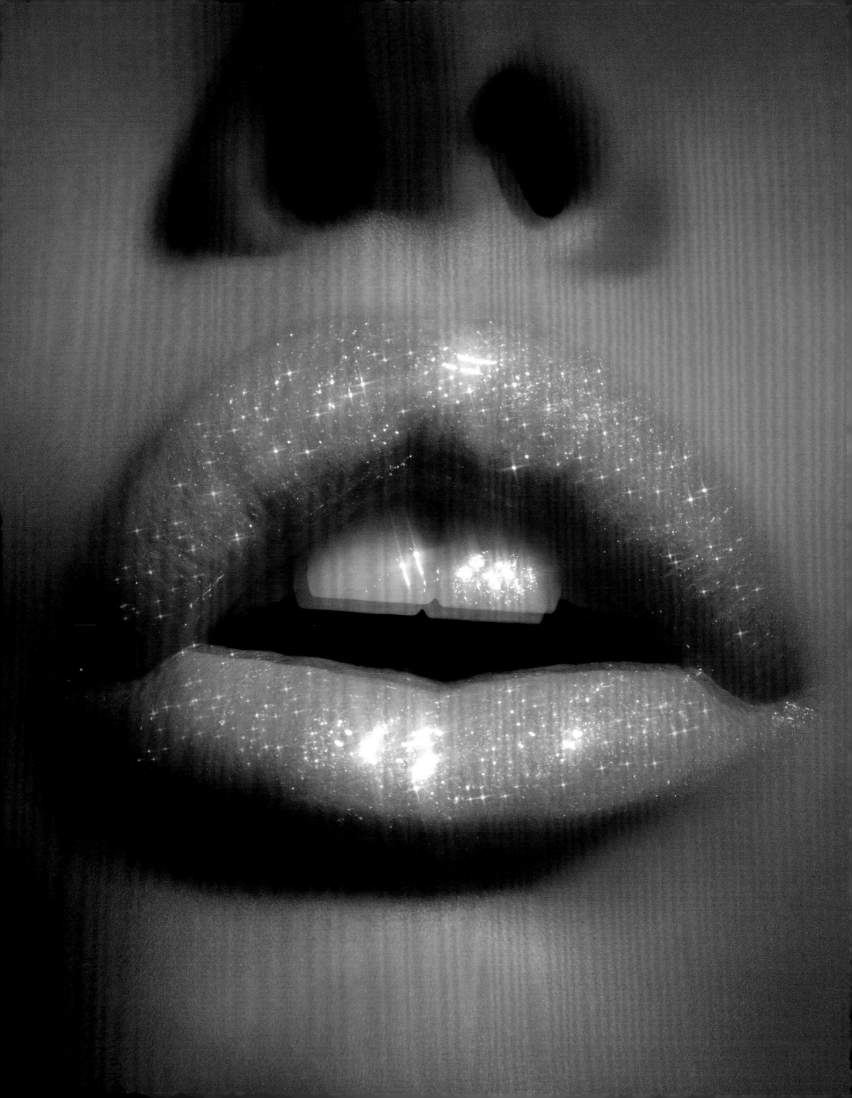

SEXY CAN BE ANYTHING.

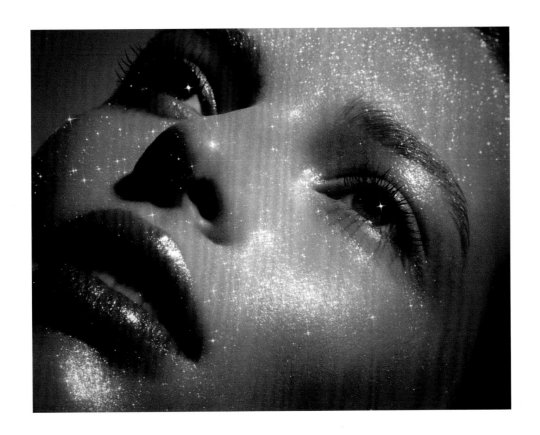

HARPER'S BAZAAR US, SEPTEMBER 2004; PHOTOGRAPHY SØLVE SUNDSBØ; HAIR PETER GRAY; MANICURIST LORRAINE GRIFFIN; MODEL POLINA KUKLINA.

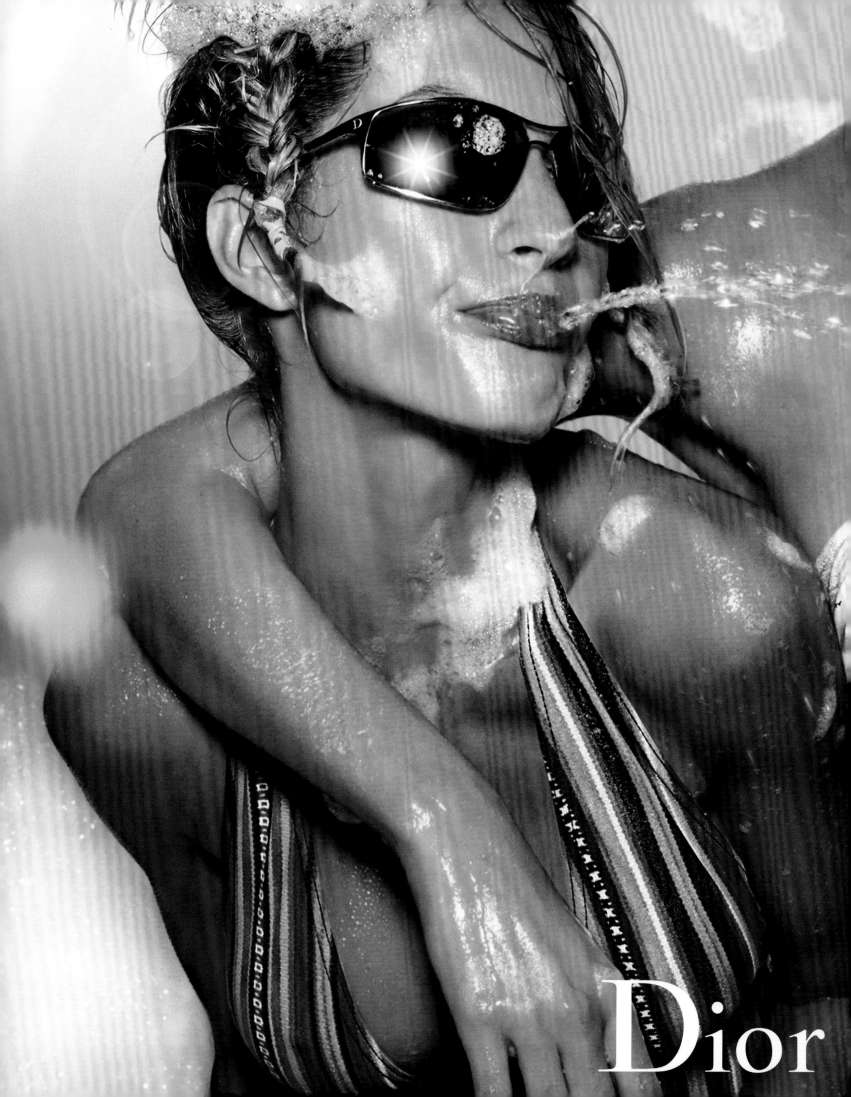

Dior

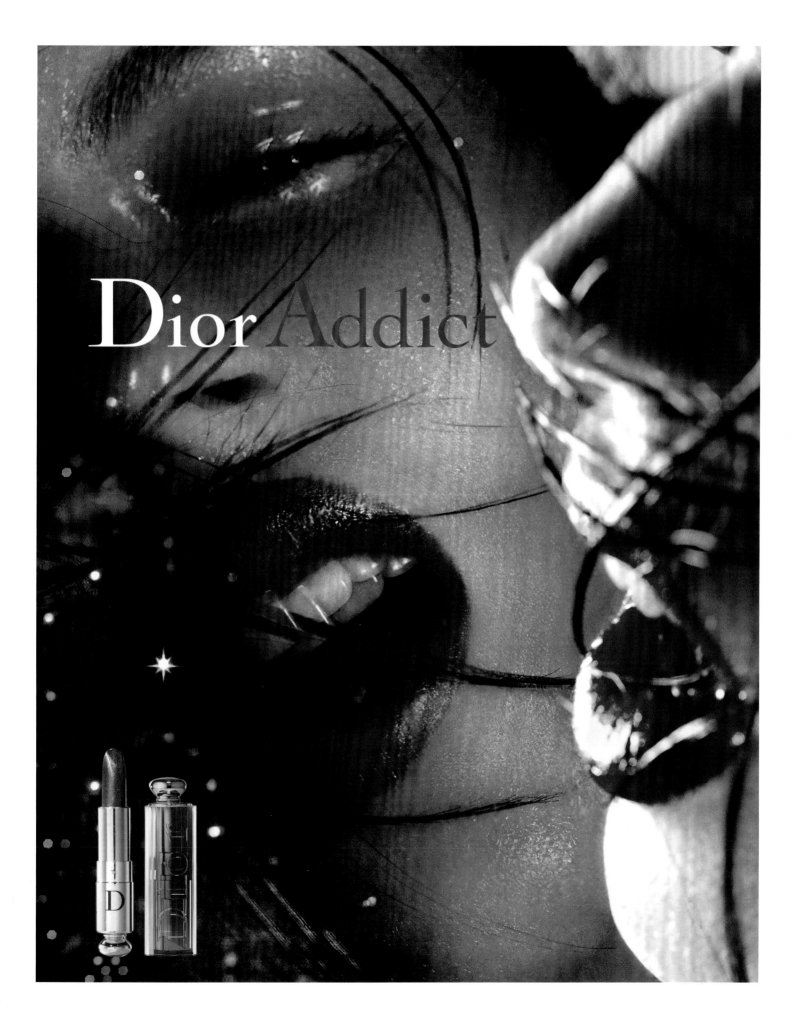

Dior Addict

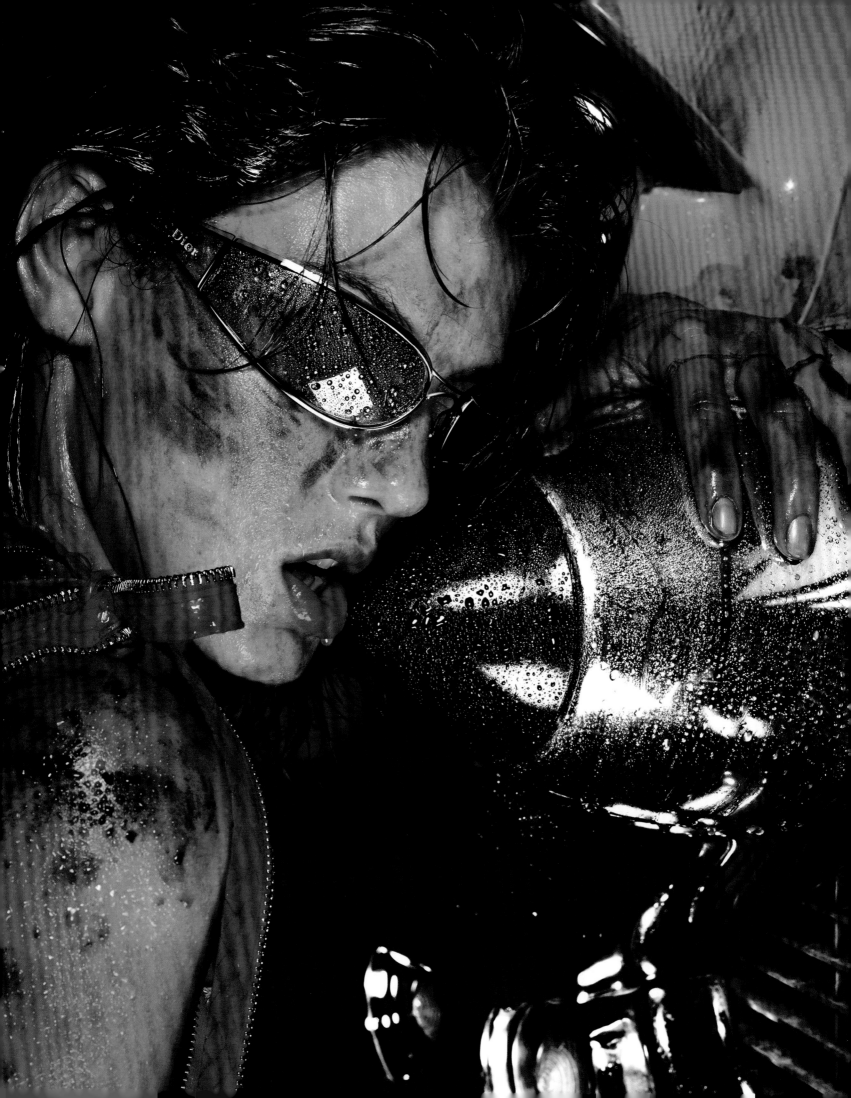

'The best time was when Nick rigged up these Cadillacs hanging upside down. The whole team had to climb over and in the cars, whether it was Sam doing the hair or Val doing touch-ups. We were just defining how the skin should look, working out the sheen, and then the glamorous dirt that Val produced was genius. It was all in a day's work for Val, she got it. And the pictures are really memorable. She's a scream, she's a laugh, she's a friend. She's a very talented person.'

JOHN GALLIANO

DIOR; DESIGNER JOHN GALLIANO; ART DIRECTION TOM HINGSTON; PHOTOGRAPHY NICK KNIGHT; FASHION EDITOR JANE HOW; HAIR SAM MCKNIGHT; MANICURIST MARIAN NEWMAN; MODEL ANGELA LINDVALL; SET DESIGN MICHAEL HOWELLS.

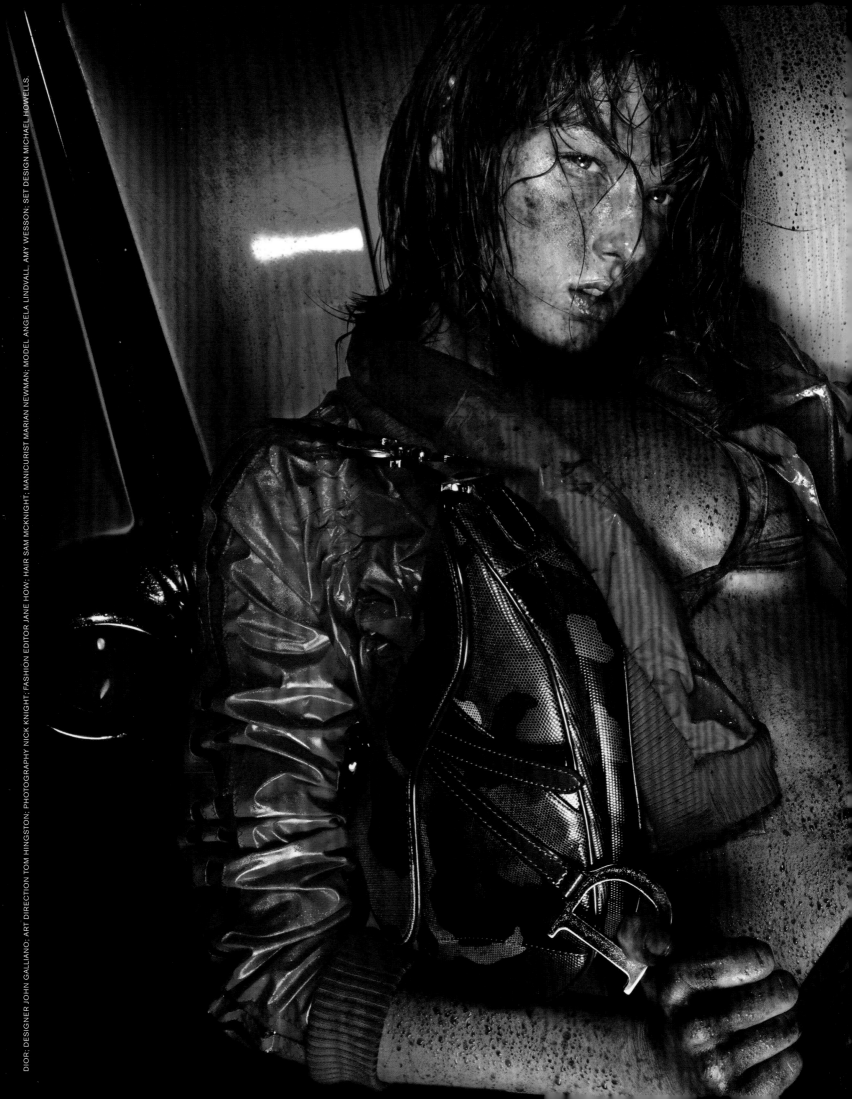

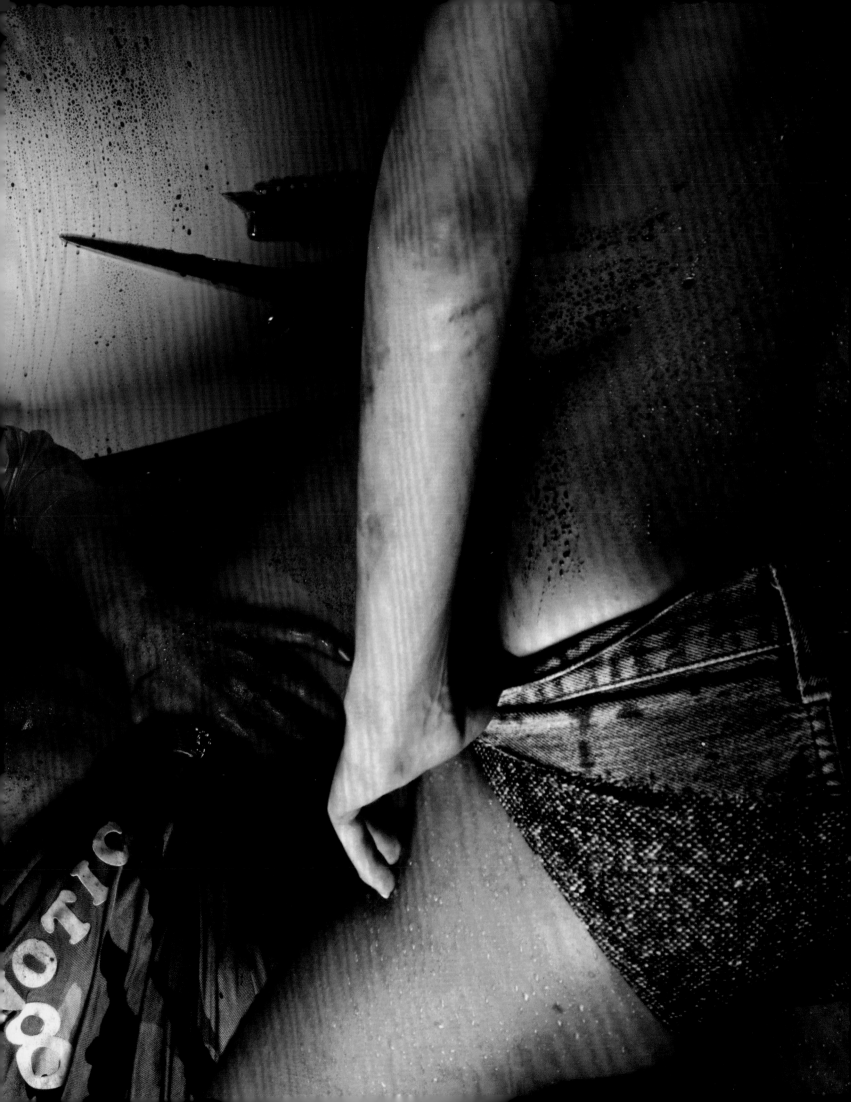

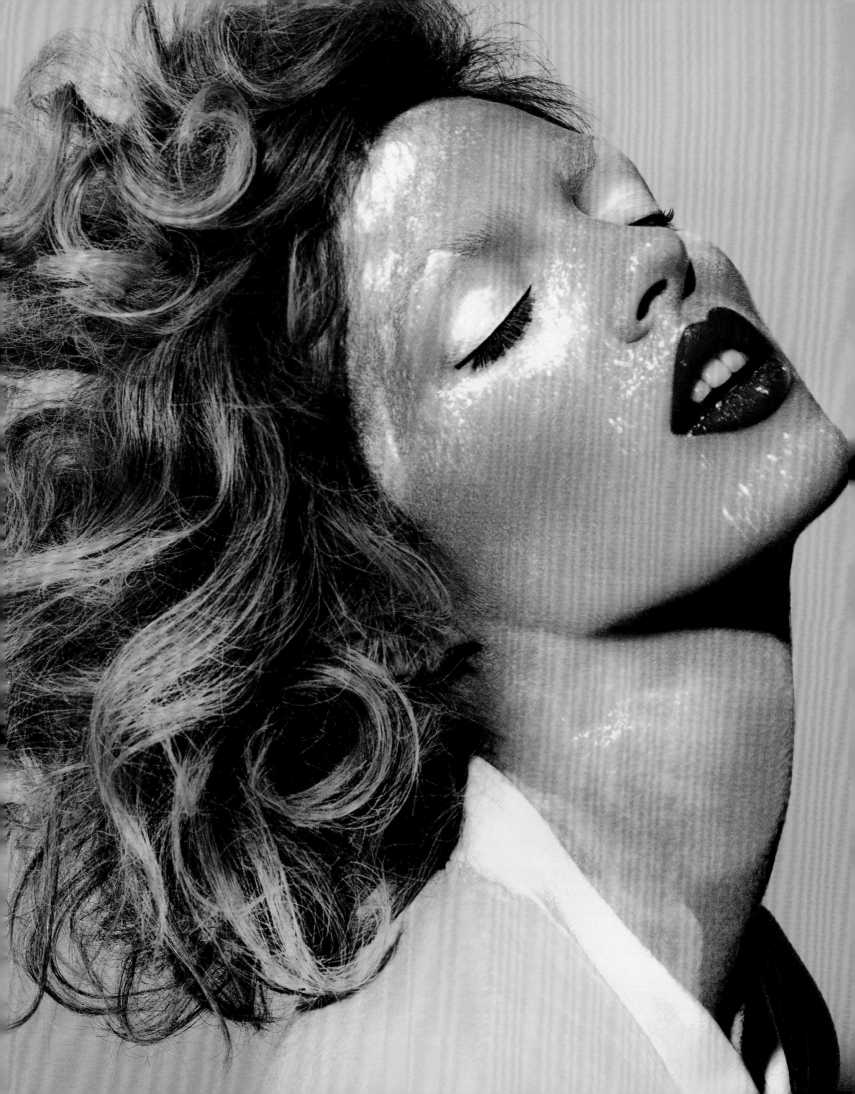

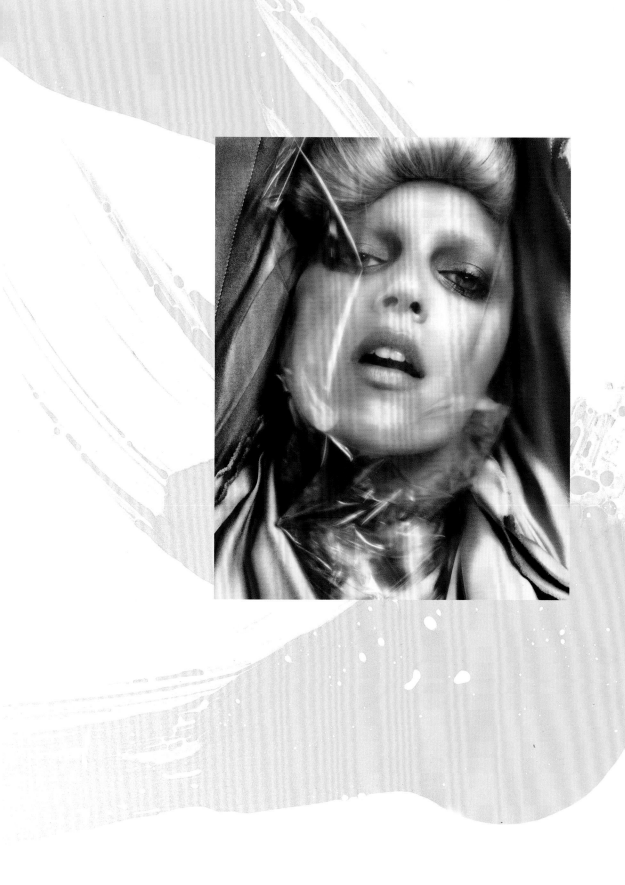

NUMÉRO 108, NOVEMBER 2009; PHOTOGRAPHY MIGUEL REVERIEGO; FASHION EDITOR CAPUCINE SAFYURTLU; HAIR KEN O'ROURKE; MODEL ANJA RUBIK.

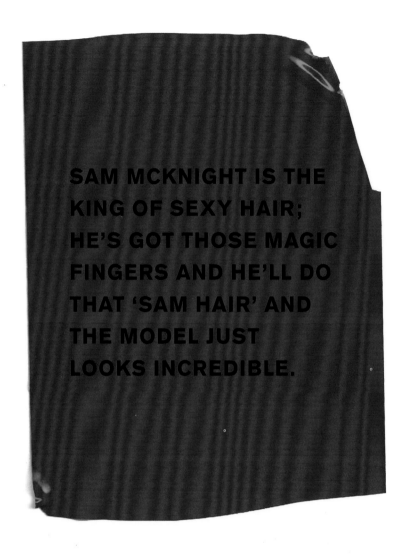

SAM MCKNIGHT IS THE KING OF SEXY HAIR; HE'S GOT THOSE MAGIC FINGERS AND HE'LL DO THAT 'SAM HAIR' AND THE MODEL JUST LOOKS INCREDIBLE.

SAM SAVES MY BACON A LOT.

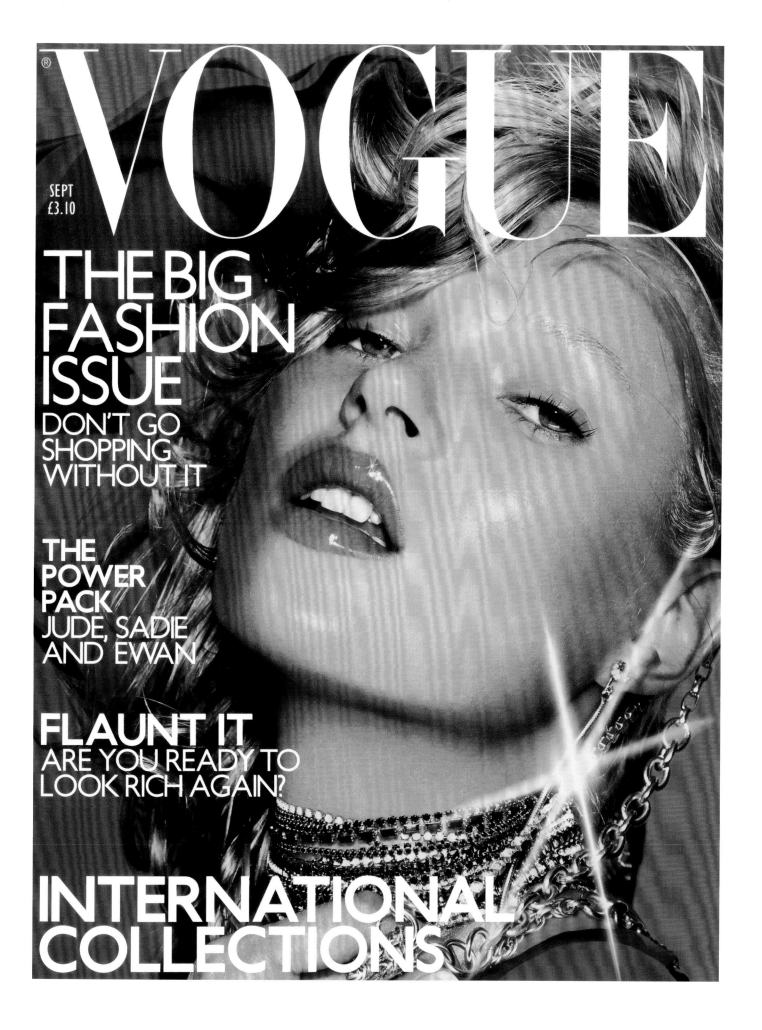

VOGUE

SEPT
£3.10

THE BIG FASHION ISSUE
DON'T GO SHOPPING WITHOUT IT

THE POWER PACK
JUDE, SADIE AND EWAN

FLAUNT IT
ARE YOU READY TO LOOK RICH AGAIN?

INTERNATIONAL COLLECTIONS

BRITISH VOGUE SEPTEMBER 2000; PHOTOGRAPHY NICK KNIGHT; FASHION EDITOR KATE PHELAN; HAIR SAM MCKNIGHT; MANICURIST MARIAN NEWMAN; MODEL KATE MOSS.

EROTIC INNOCENCE.
PURE EROTICISM.
A QUIET SENSUALITY.

LOVE MAGAZINE NO. 8; PHOTOGRAPHY TIM WALKER; FASHION EDITOR KATIE GRAND; HAIR MALCOLM EDWARDS; MODEL KATE MOSS.

THERE'S ANOTHER ANGLE ON SEX IN YOUR WORK,
LIKE THIS PURE IMAGE OF KATE MOSS.

This was for a big story that we shot over two days, so it was like 48 hours with Kate. We shot from early in the morning until late in the evening and it was about the real Kate, the purity of Kate and the innocence of Kate in many different portraits. They're about erotic innocence. Pure eroticism. A quiet sensuality. It's the vulnerable side of Kate that I think Tim has captured here. I mean, Kate's always going to be sexy.

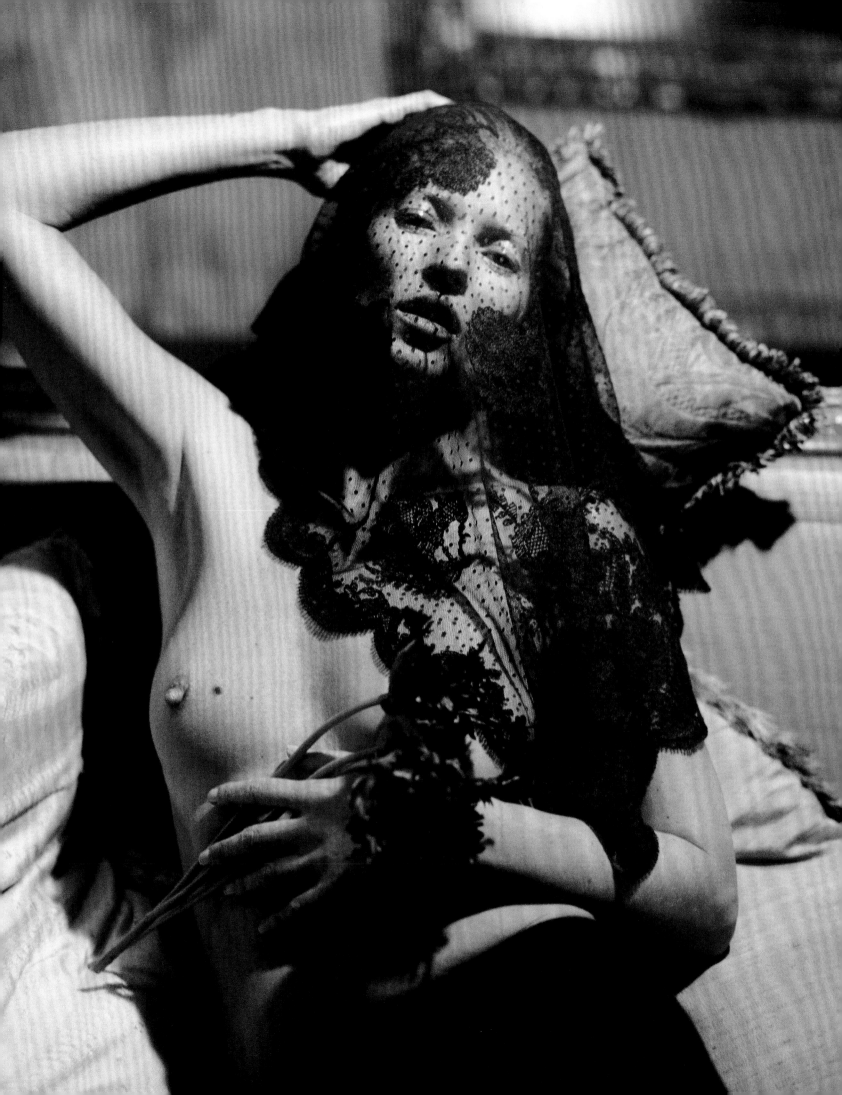

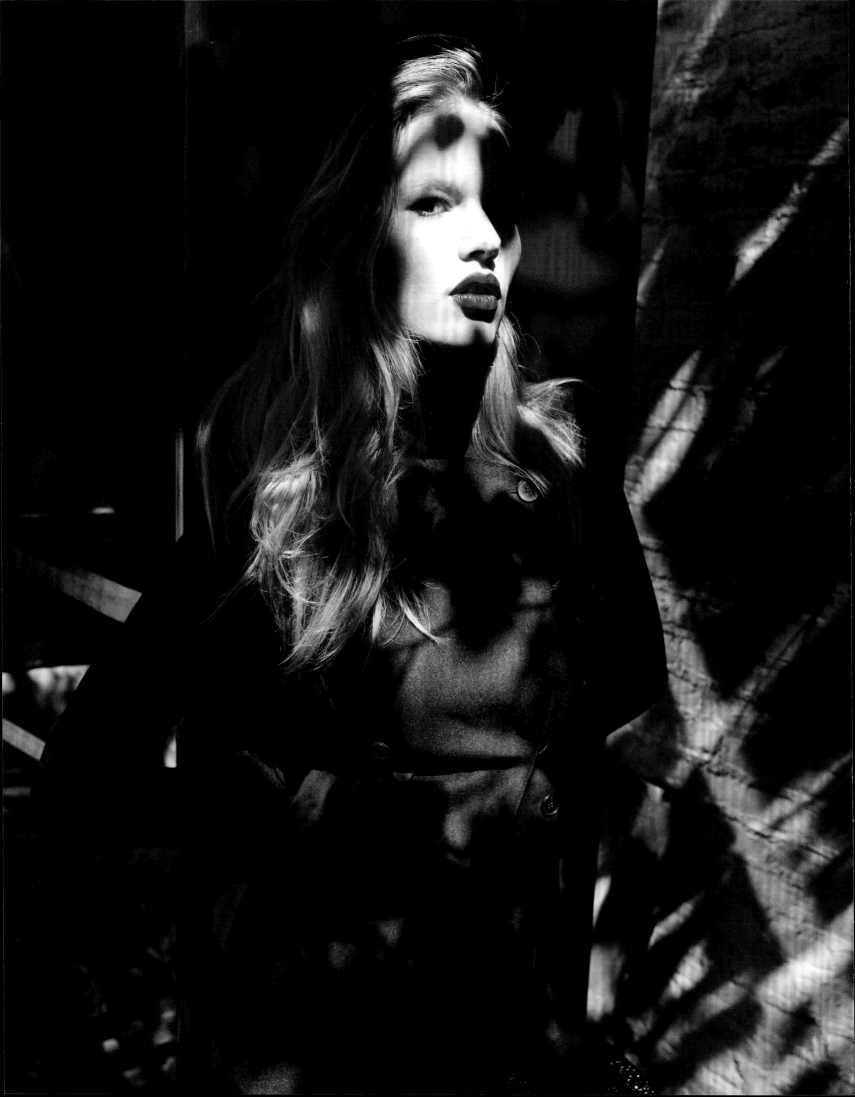

A velvet lip can look very erotic.

I love a 'femme fatale', like this image of Anna Ewers by Inez and Vinoodh. What I like about her is she looks quite disciplined, with the high neckline and the red lip. It's very matte and velvet looking, which is the polar opposite of gloss, but a velvet lip can look very erotic.

I first started doing that sort of velvet lip for a Givenchy show with Lee McQueen in 1998. We made the lip look very matte at the last minute – the models were all in the line-up, ready to go down the catwalk and they had this strong red lip. I went along the row, took some red powder and pushed that into the lipstick. Immediately it made the lips look more velvety.

VOGUE PARIS AUGUST 2015. 'SAUVAGE INNOCENCE'; PHOTOGRAPHY INEZ & VINOODH; FASHION EDITOR EMMANUELLE ALT; HAIR ODILE GILBERT; MODEL ANNA EWERS.

'VAL LIKES TO
HAVE A CERTAIN
STRICTNESS TO
HER MANNER, BUT
I THINK THAT'S HER
WAY OF DEALING
WITH A WHOLE
LOT OF PEOPLE
THAT COME IN.
AND THERE'S A
REALLY IMPORTANT
TABOO: ACTUALLY
TOUCHING
SOMEONE'S
FACE. YOU CAN'T
JUST WALK UP TO
SOMEBODY AND
TOUCH THEIR FACE.
AND OF COURSE
THAT'S EXACTLY
WHAT SHE'S DOING.
AND IT CAN BE
QUITE A STRESSFUL
PLACE BECAUSE
THESE ARE VERY,
VERY WELL-KNOWN
PEOPLE OR PEOPLE
THAT YOU REALLY
ADMIRE. AND I
THINK, FOR VAL,
THIS SLIGHTLY
SCHOOLMARMISH
PERSONA IS A BIT
OF A GAME SHE
LIKES TO PLAY.'

NICK KNIGHT

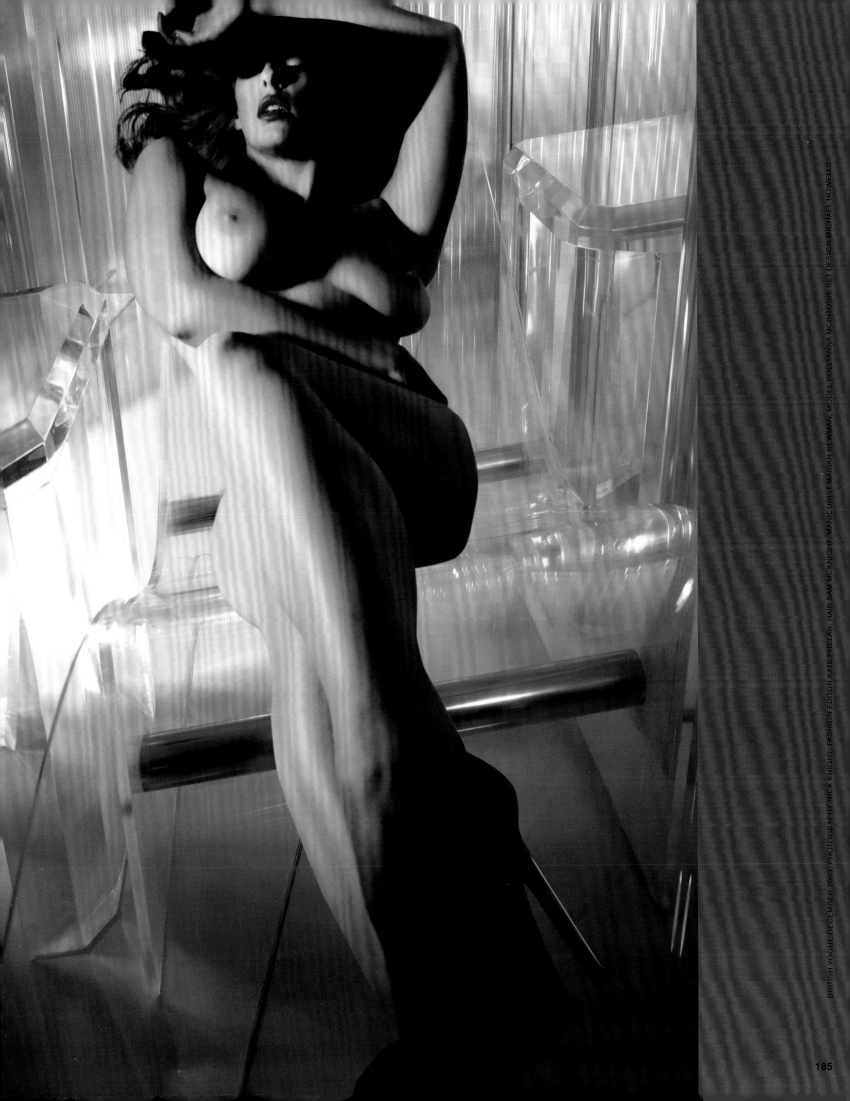

BRITISH VOGUE DECEMBER 2003. PHOTOGRAPHY NICK KNIGHT. FASHION EDITOR KATE PHELAN. HAIR SAM MCKNIGHT. MANICURIST MARIAN NEWMAN. MODEL POLLYANNA MCINTOSH. SET DESIGN MICHAEL HOWELLS

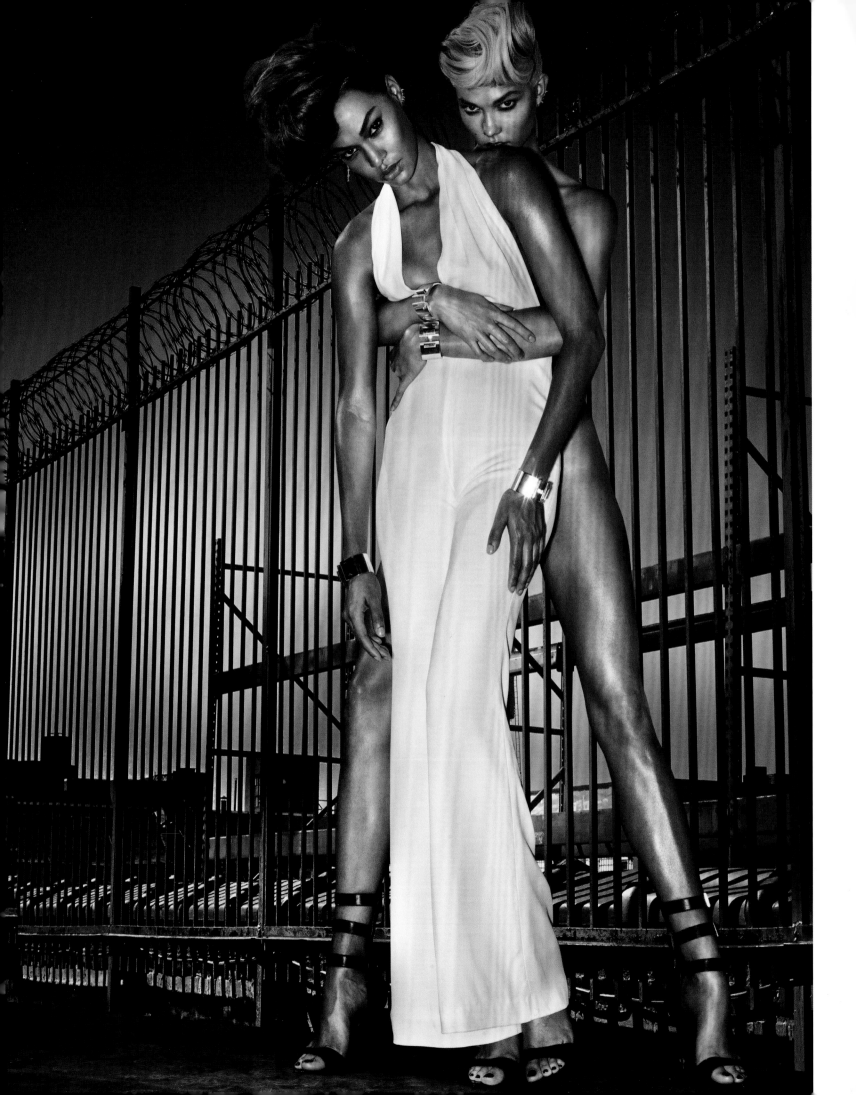

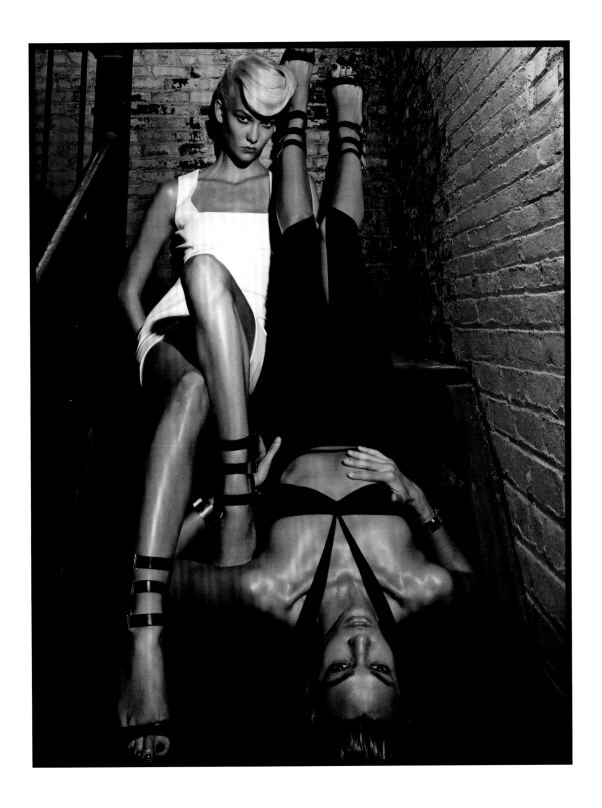

'It's like she sees with a camera lens or something. Because they looked bronzed, in real life, I remember they look golden and she just knew what effect things would have in the camera.'

EDWARD ENNINFUL

W MAGAZINE NOVEMBER 2014; PHOTOGRAPHY STEVEN KLEIN; FASHION EDITOR EDWARD ENNINFUL; HAIR SHAY ASHUAL; MANICURIST YUKO TSUCHIHASHI; MODELS JOAN SMALLS, KARLIE KLOSS.

PHOTOGRAPHY NICK KNIGHT; HAIR SAM MCKNIGHT; MANICURIST MARIAN NEWMAN; MODELS JOHN GALLIANO, ALEK WEK.

'YOU HAD THE SPACE TO PLAY AND THEY WOULD PLAY.
THEY WERE ALL QUITE EXTREME CHARACTERS. BUT THEY
WERE ALL QUITE INTERESTING CHARACTERS. YOU'VE GOT
JOHN, STEVEN, VANESSA, VAL, SAM, AND MARIAN, AND
IT'S QUITE A PLAYFUL TEAM SO THEY MUCK AROUND.
YEAH, THEY'RE DOING POLAROIDS OF EACH OTHER AND
CUTTING THEM TOGETHER AND ALL SORTS OF STUFF.
I'M THERE JUST TRYING TO LET THAT CHAOS HAPPEN.'

NICK KNIGHT

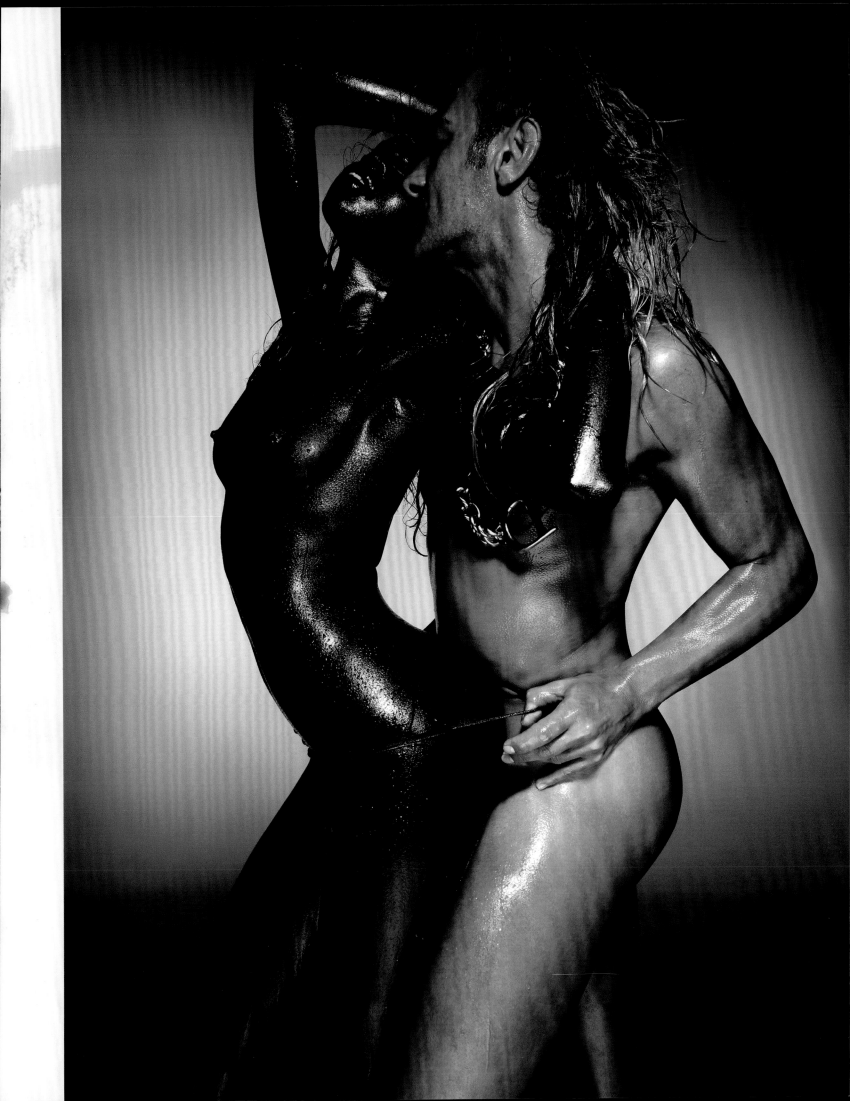

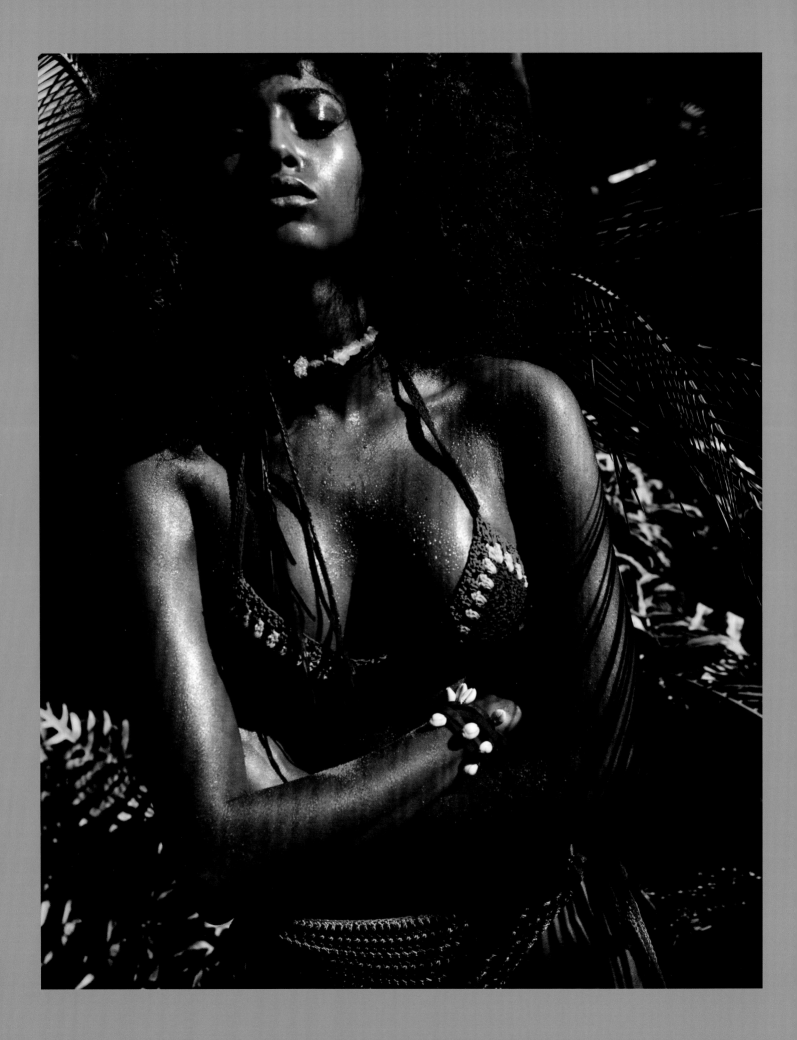

VOGUE PARIS MAY 2016: PHOTOGRAPHY MARIO TESTINO; FASHION EDITOR EMMANUELLE ALT; HAIR JAMES PECIS; MODEL IMAAN HAMMAM.

'When you are as creative as Val, you often go for the weird or strange or new or unseen before, and I'm one of those photographers who can't help being obsessed by the girl. So I often bring out the other side of Val that she can do that maybe people don't book her for as often. She's not just about the makeup. She's thinking of the image and, believe it or not, the clothes, the light, the pose, the energy, everything helps. We all have to be in tune with every aspect of the photo and it needs to take you to the exact place where you want to be.

WE BUILD A PICTURE TOGETHER.'

MARIO TESTINO

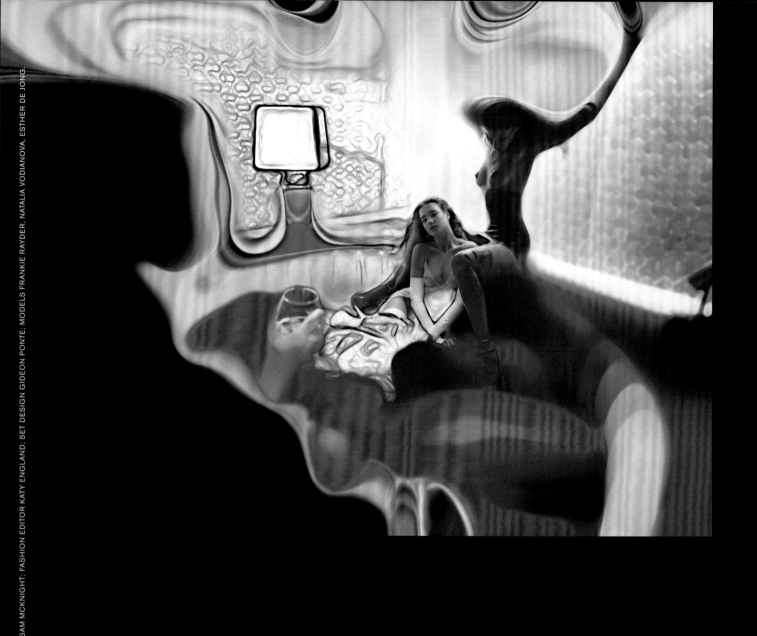

PIRELLI CALENDAR 2004; PHOTOGRAPHY NICK KNIGHT; ART DIRECTION PETER SAVILLE; HAIR SAM MCKNIGHT; FASHION EDITOR KATY ENGLAND; SET DESIGN GIDEON PONTE; MODELS FRANKIE RAYDER, NATALIA VODIANOVA, ESTHER DE JONG.

'I didn't want to do a calendar that felt like it was demeaning to women. I was talking to Peter Saville about it and he said, "Why don't you ask women for their sexual fantasies? You're empowering them to say whatever they think is sexy." So that's what we did.'

NICK KNIGHT

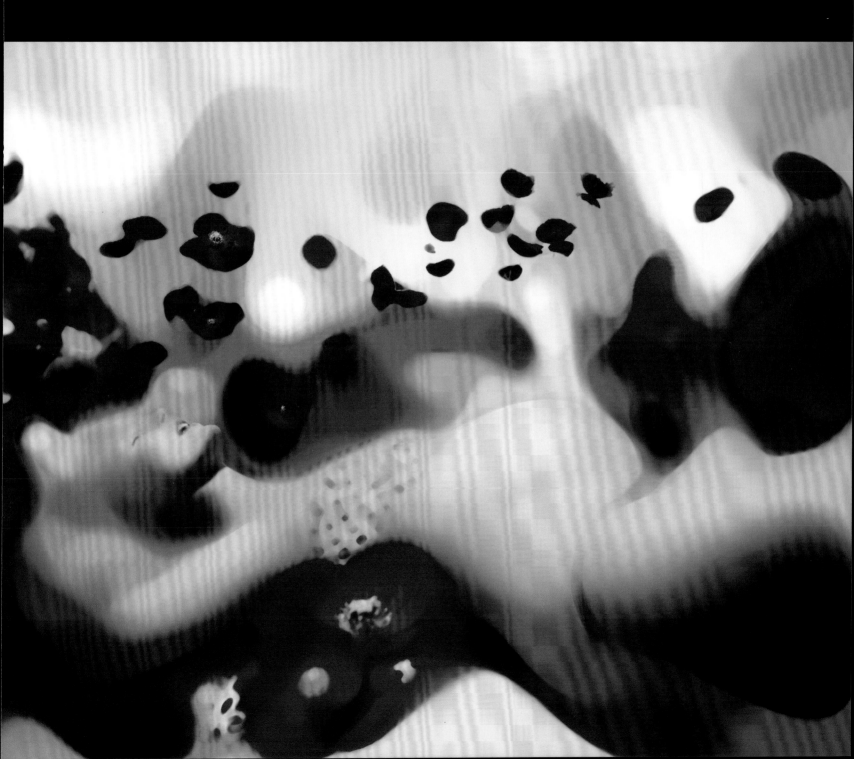

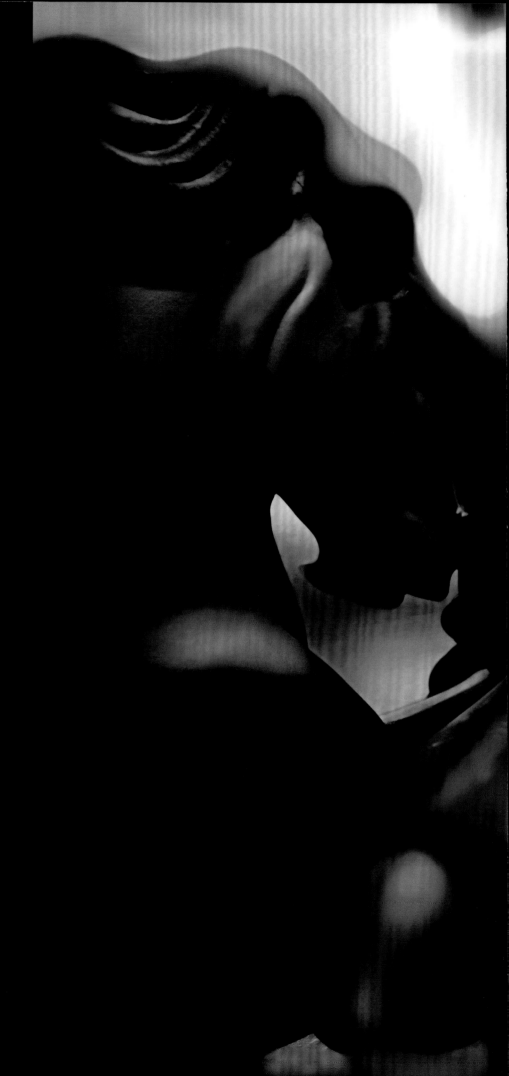

PIRELLI CALENDAR 2004; PHOTOGRAPHY NICK KNIGHT; ART DIRECTION PETER SAVILLE; HAIR SAM MCKNIGHT; FASHION EDITOR KATY ENGLAND; SET DESIGN GIDEON PONTE; MODEL KAROLINA KURKOVA.

I THINK WE HAVE TO END THIS CHAPTER WITH YOUR ULTIMATE SEXY SHOOT OF ALL TIME.

That would have to be the first and only time I did the Pirelli calendar. When the job came in we were thinking, 'Great, where are we going?' You know – what exotic location? We actually shot it in Park Royal Studios in West London.

The idea was based on conversations with 14 women, including Tracey Emin, Björk, Catherine Deneuve and Isabella Rossellini. Each was asked what they would like to see inside the calendar. Although each image illustrated one of the women's fantasies, whose idea it was was kept secret, like a masked ball.

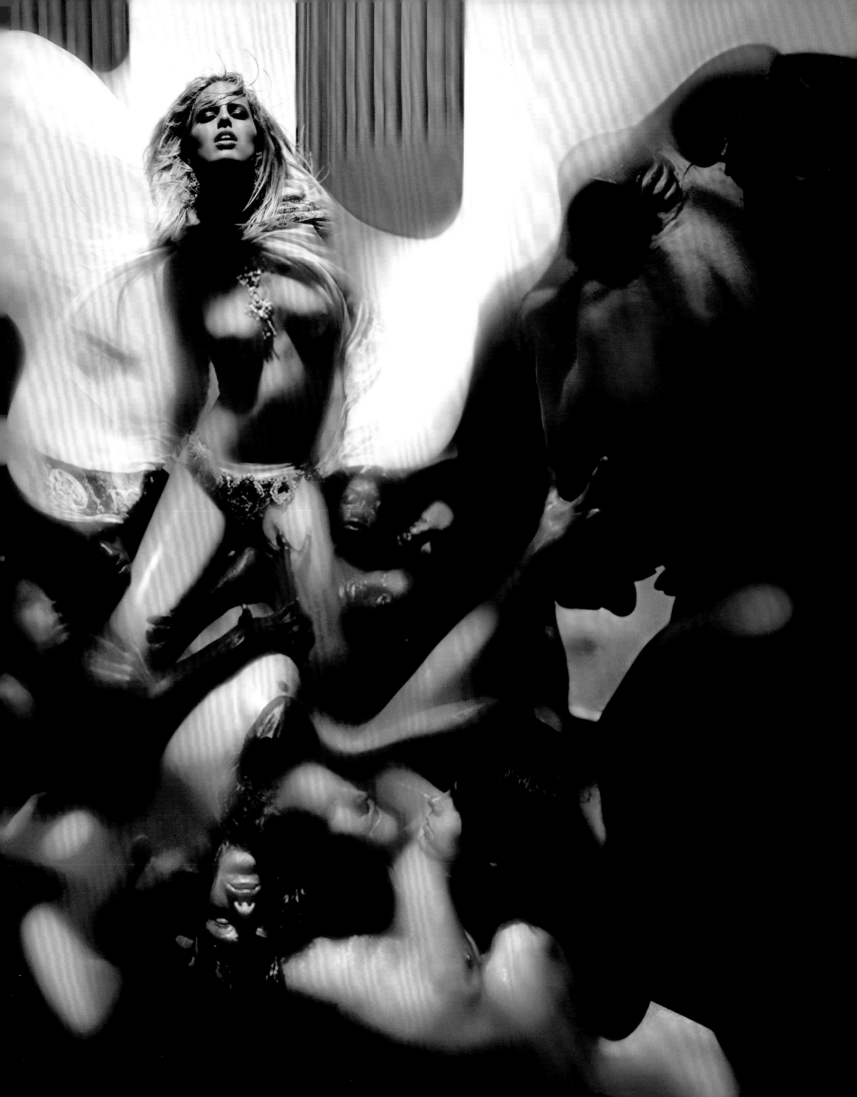

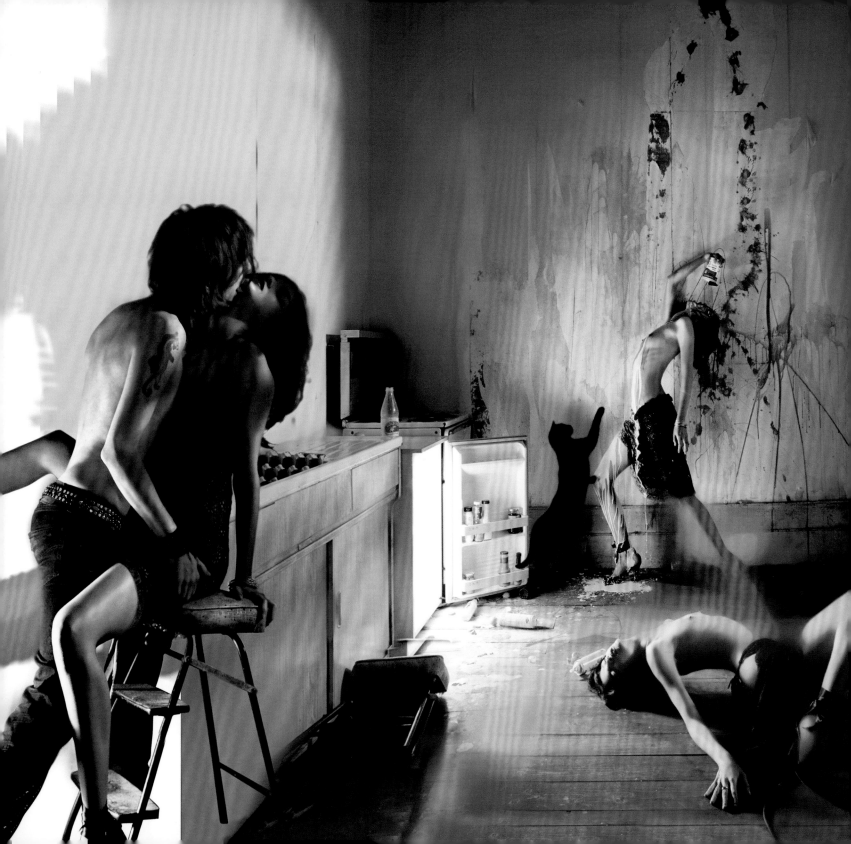

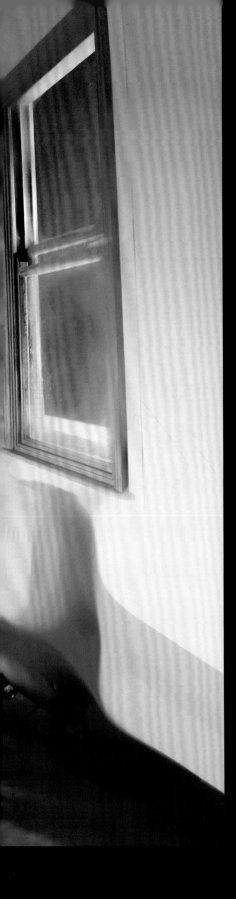

PIRELLI CALENDAR 2004; PHOTOGRAPHY NICK KNIGHT; ART DIRECTION PETER SAVILLE; HAIR SAM MCKNIGHT; FASHION EDITOR KATY ENGLAND; SET DESIGN GIDEON PONTE; MODELS MARIACARLA BOSCONO, ALISTER MACKIE.

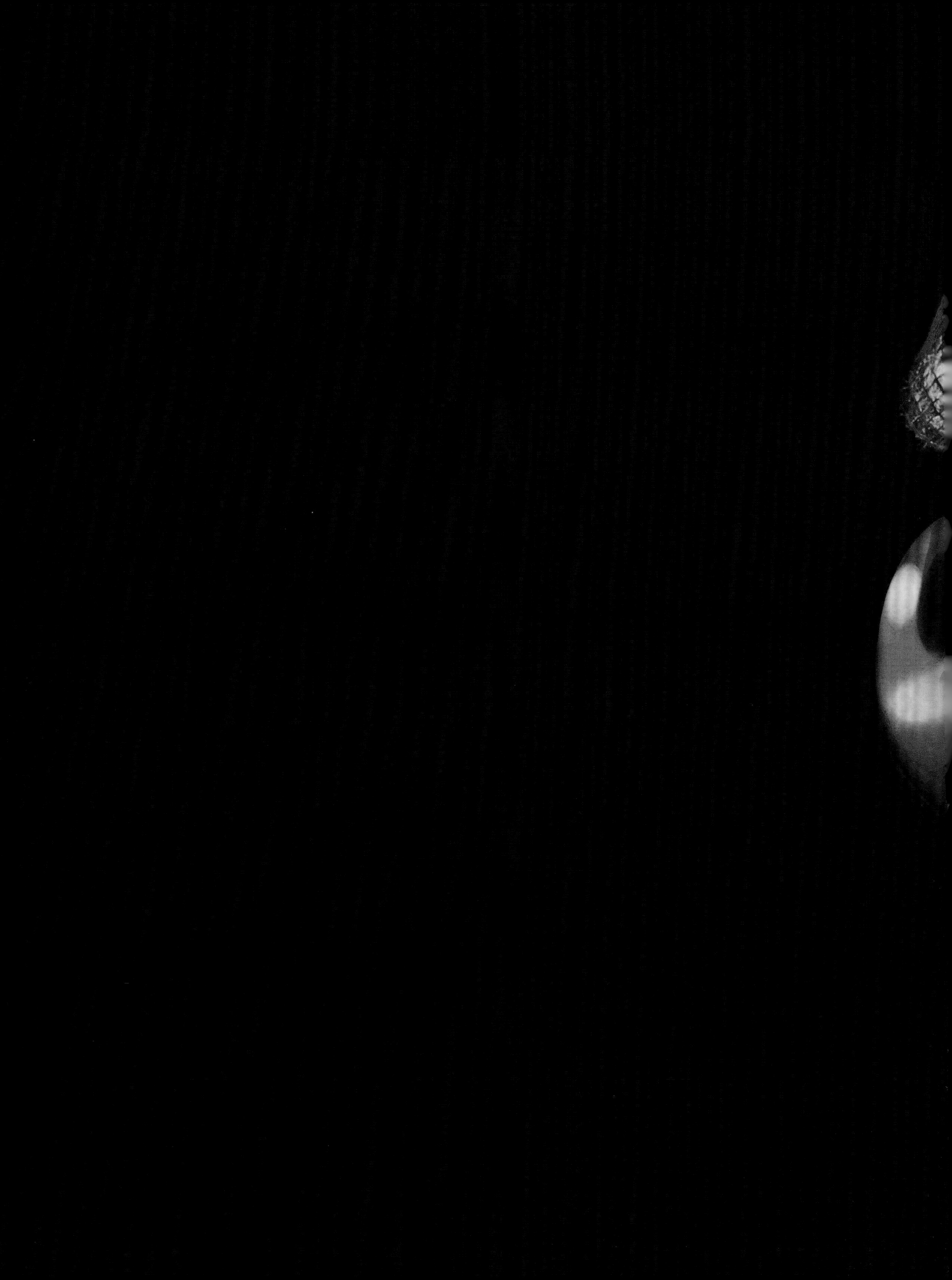

PIRELLI CALENDAR 2004; PHOTOGRAPHY NICK KNIGHT; ART DIRECTION PETER SAVILLE; HAIR SAM MCKNIGHT; FASHION EDITOR KATY ENGLAND; SET DESIGN GIDEON PONTE; MODEL ALEK WEK.

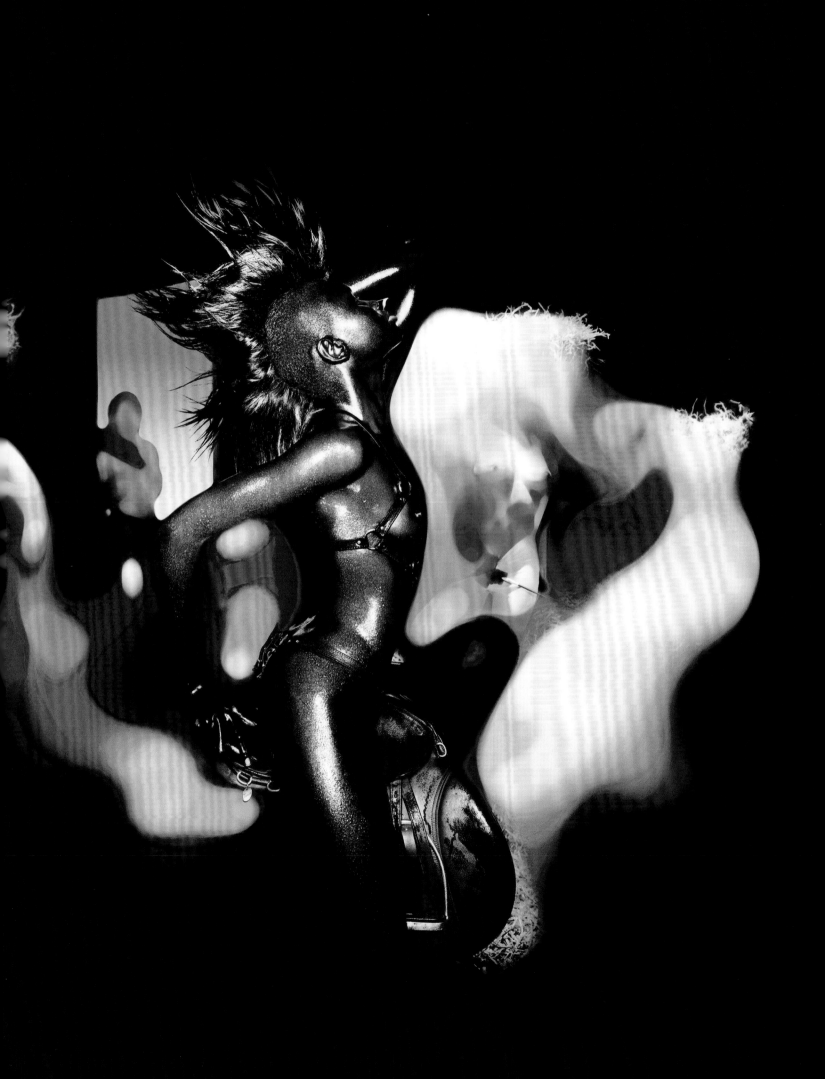

PIRELLI CALENDAR 2004; PHOTOGRAPHY NICK KNIGHT; ART DIRECTION PETER SAVILLE; HAIR SAM MCKNIGHT; FASHION EDITOR KATY ENGLAND; SET DESIGN GIDEON PONTE; MODEL LIBERTY ROSS.

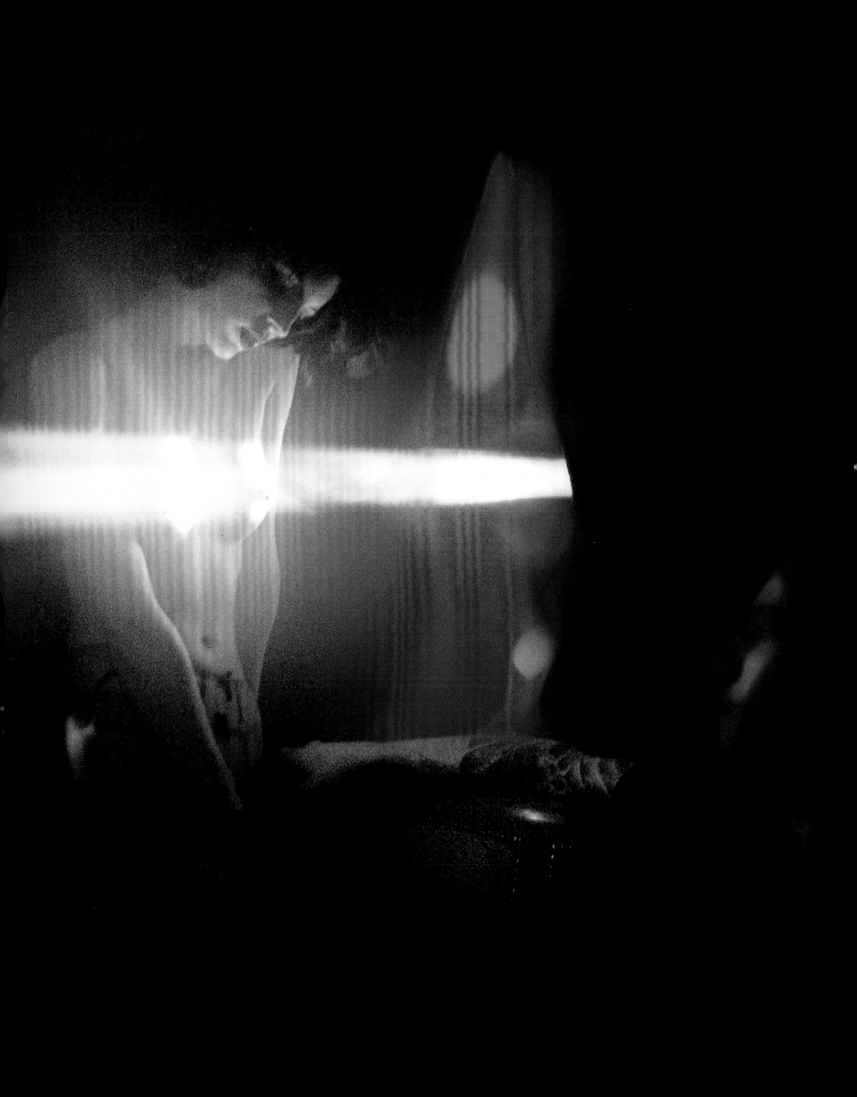

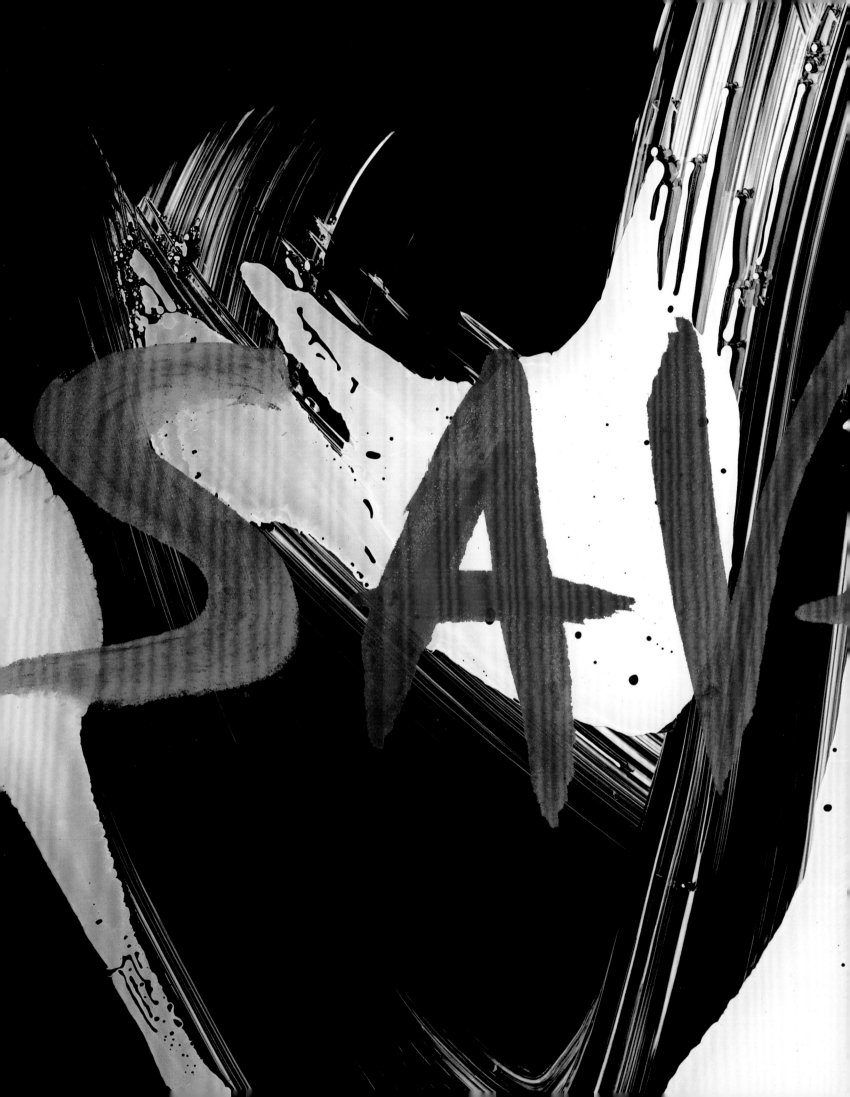

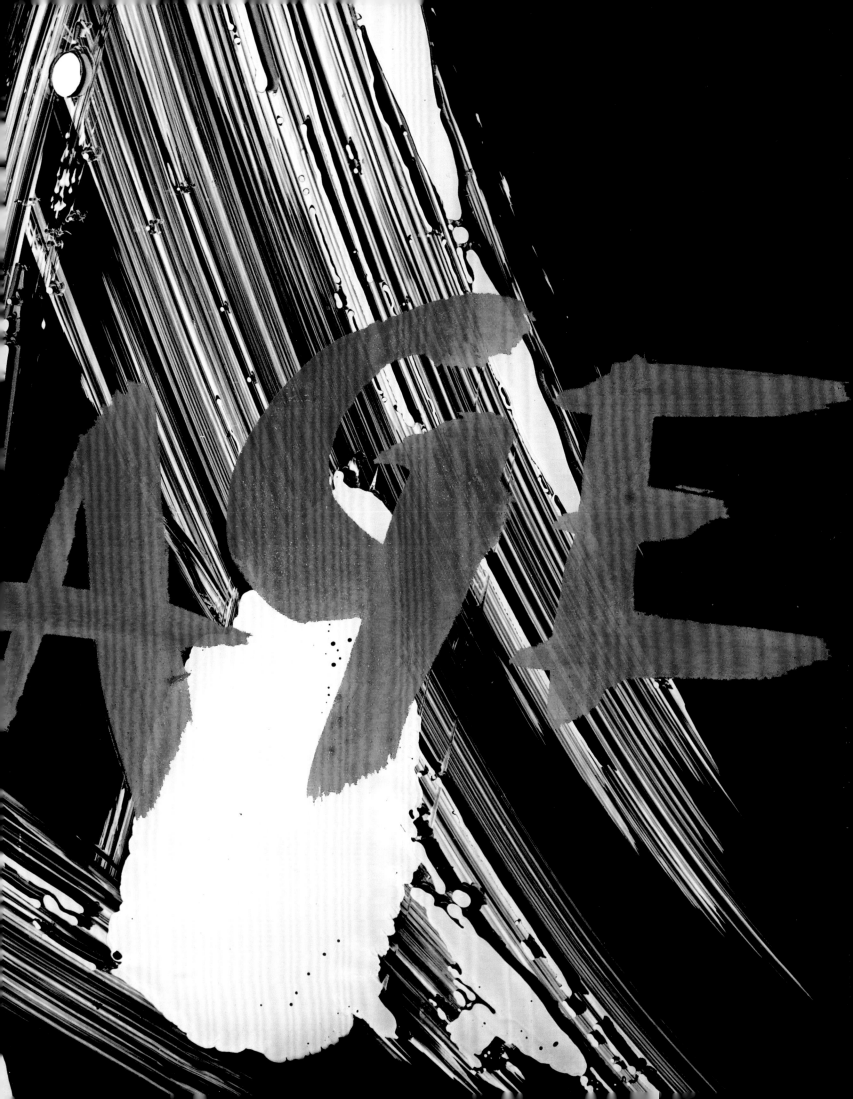

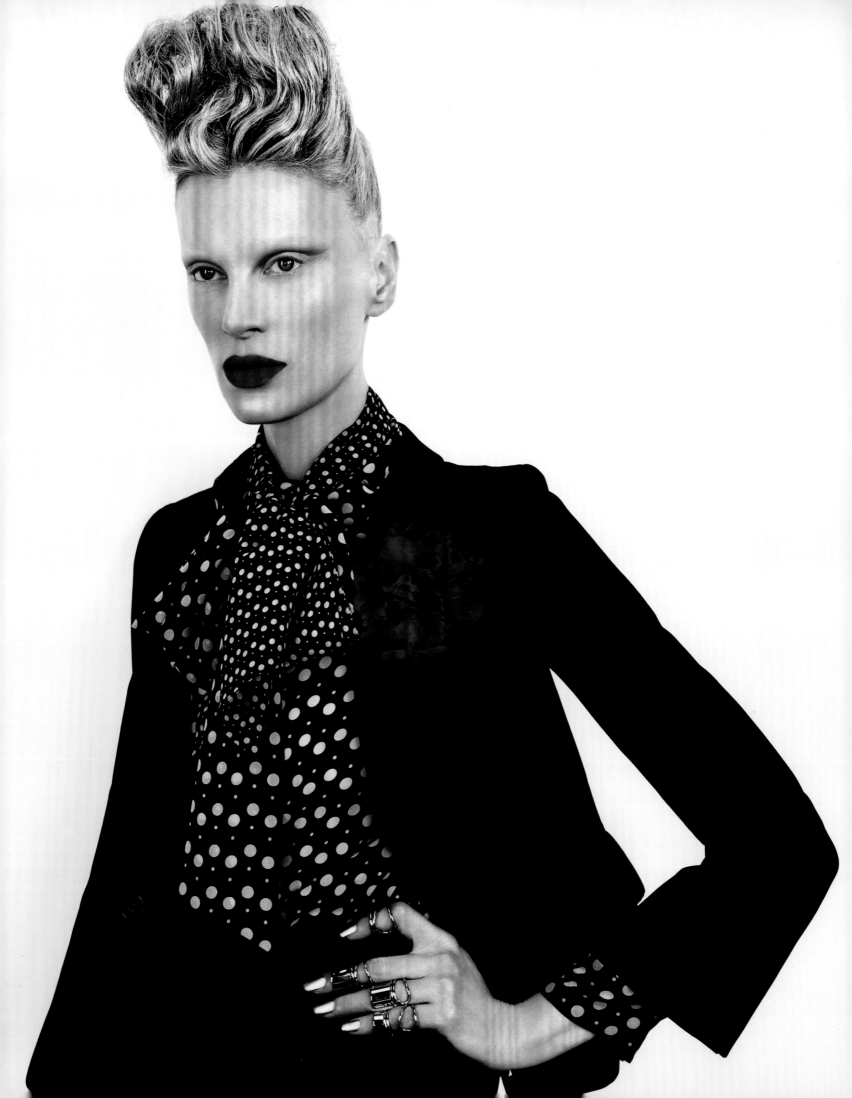

THERE BE DEVILS...

If Charles Baudelaire, the author of *Les Fleurs du Mal*, had been a modern-day punk he might have written poems about the savagely beautiful makeup in this chapter. Scratch the surface of Val's repertoire, and there be devils.

Some of Val's makeup art indicates a profligate, dark imagination, the results often raising serious questions about not only our perceptions of beauty but also our primeval fears. Throughout her career, she has shared a provocative language with many of her collaborators, including Nick Knight, Alexander McQueen and Lady Gaga. In this chapter we discover how it is possible for the words savage, beauty, romance and macabre to end up in the same sentence when discussing makeup.

Val has a truly iconoclastic approach to her art form and is an individual who is consistently prepared to smash conventions in makeup. Her work is often a vicious parody lampooning contemporary issues like the obsession with medical aesthetics and the bizarre facial landscapes that this addiction can produce.

For all the dark humour, there is a serious vein running through Val's work that often recalls religious episodes, ritualistic tribal scenes and classical paintings. These powerful images can unsettle and provoke the viewer, who is left not necessarily understanding why they like the image – or even if they should.

At her brutal best, Val seems to tap into a source of power that transforms her makeup brush into a raving avenger of punk, decadence and eroticism. If she were a poet, like Baudelaire, the makeup looks in this chapter would surely be her own flowers of evil.

W MAGAZINE MARCH 2013; PHOTOGRAPHY EMMA SUMMERTON; FASHION EDITOR EDWARD EDWARD ENNINFUL; HAIR ODILE GILBERT; MODEL KRISTEN MCMENAMY.

'Val gives me the opportunity to show people that I don't do normal nails. I do abnormal nails. She likes that I can do the weird stuff ... for *Born This Way*, Gaga was into this thing of altering the body. Because what Val was doing with the face was extreme, I did nails that had a backbone, and triple nails, so it was like three nails that had grown out of one nail.'

MARIAN NEWMAN

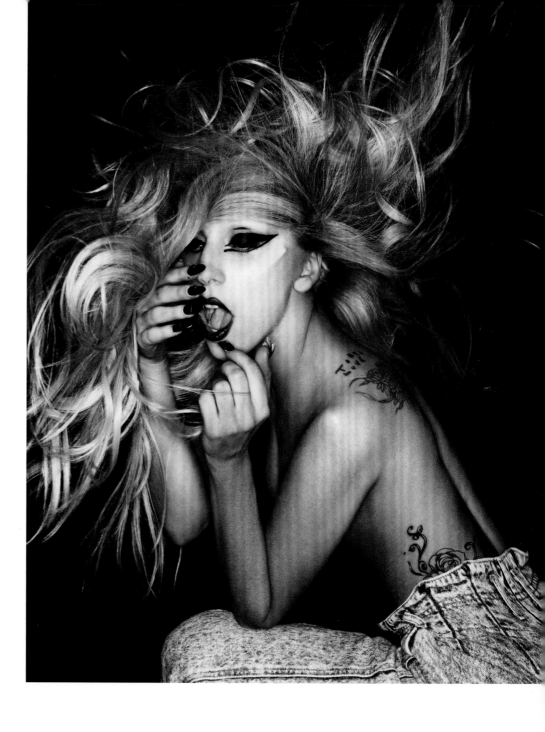

When I first met Gaga she was about 22 or 23 and she had such presence. She knew exactly what she wanted.

Gaga and her stylist, Nicola Formichetti, came to me and said, 'We're going to do an album cover with Nick Knight [*Born This Way*] and we want to do something different'. I said, 'OK, let's get rid of the eyelashes, let's get rid of your eyebrows. Let's make it more punk.' Then I thought we could try some prosthetics to pronounce her cheekbones. I took two bits

of paper and made them into little aeroplanes and just stuck them on her face. Nicola took a picture and that was the last I heard of it until three months later when we actually came to do the album cover and they said, 'Yeah, we're gonna go with that look'. They had taken my tiny bits of paper to a prosthetics expert, and, voilà, a new Gaga was born.

For the shoot for *Vogue Homme,* she turned into her alter ego, Jo Calderone. Gaga is an incredible actress; she really got into character.

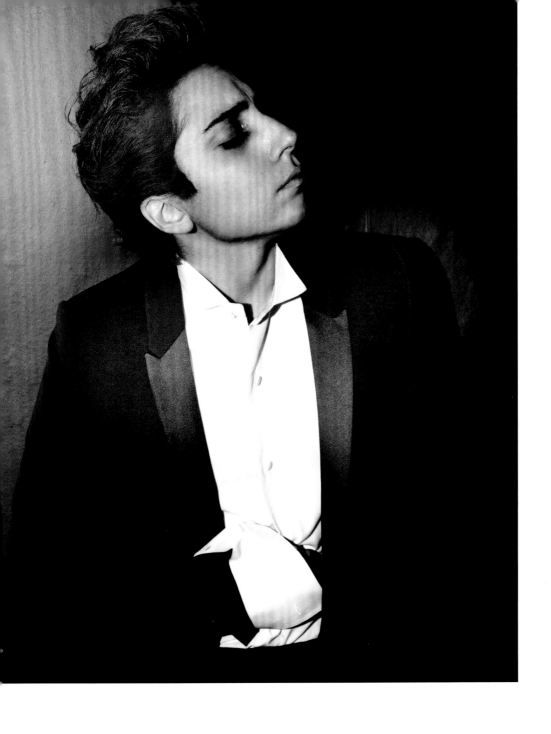

'THE SORT OF ARTISTIC STATEMENTS THAT VAL MAKES ARE QUITE PRONOUNCED, THEY'RE NOT LIGHT. I THINK THAT SHE REALLY DOES PUSH THAT SURREALISTIC PART OF HER INTERESTS.'

NICK KNIGHT

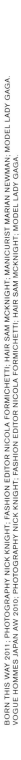

BORN THIS WAY 2011; PHOTOGRAPHY NICK KNIGHT; FASHION EDITOR NICOLA FORMICHETTI; HAIR SAM MCKNIGHT; MANICURIST MARIAN NEWMAN; MODEL LADY GAGA. VOGUE HOMMES JAPAN AW 2010; PHOTOGRAPHY NICK KNIGHT; FASHION EDITOR NICOLA FORMICHETTI; HAIR SAM MCKNIGHT; MODEL LADY GAGA.

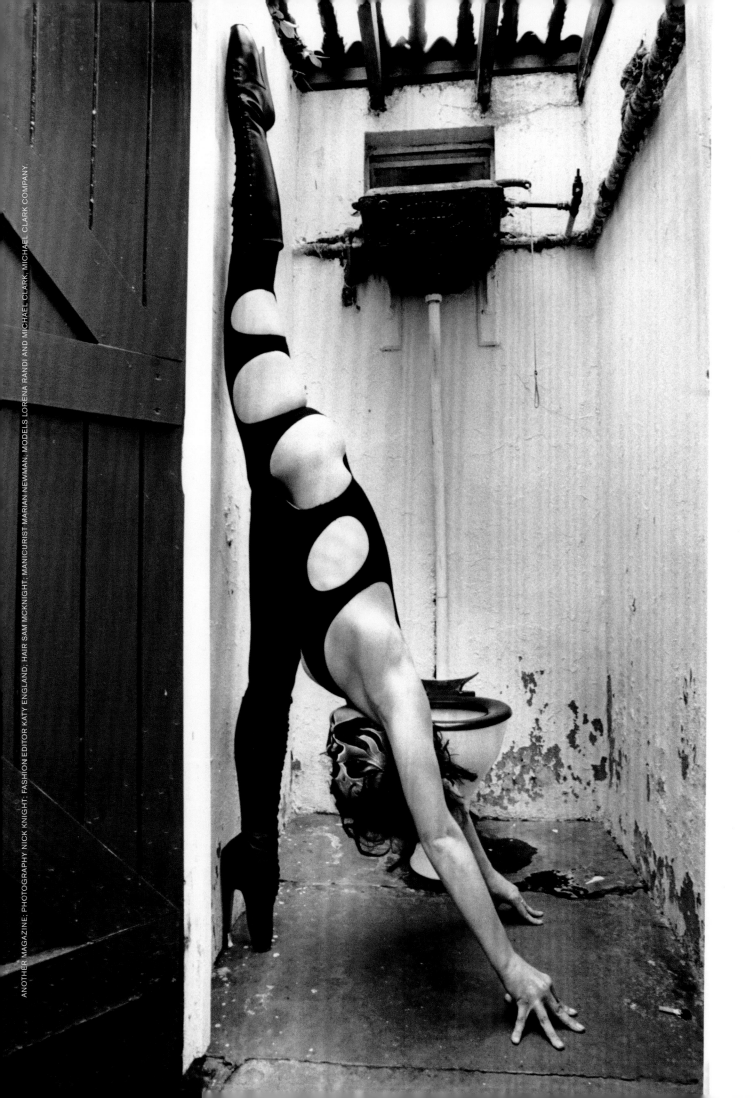

'YOU FEEL LIKE
YOU CAN THROW
ANYTHING
AT HER AND
SHE'S NOT
GOING TO SAY,
"OH, MY GOD!"
SHE'S GOING
TO GO, "AH.
OK. I'LL JUST
HAVE A LITTLE
THINK ABOUT
THAT." AND OFF
SHE GOES.
THERE'S NEVER
A NEGATIVE
WHEN YOU'RE
DOING A
CREATIVE THING
WITH VAL.'

KATY ENGLAND

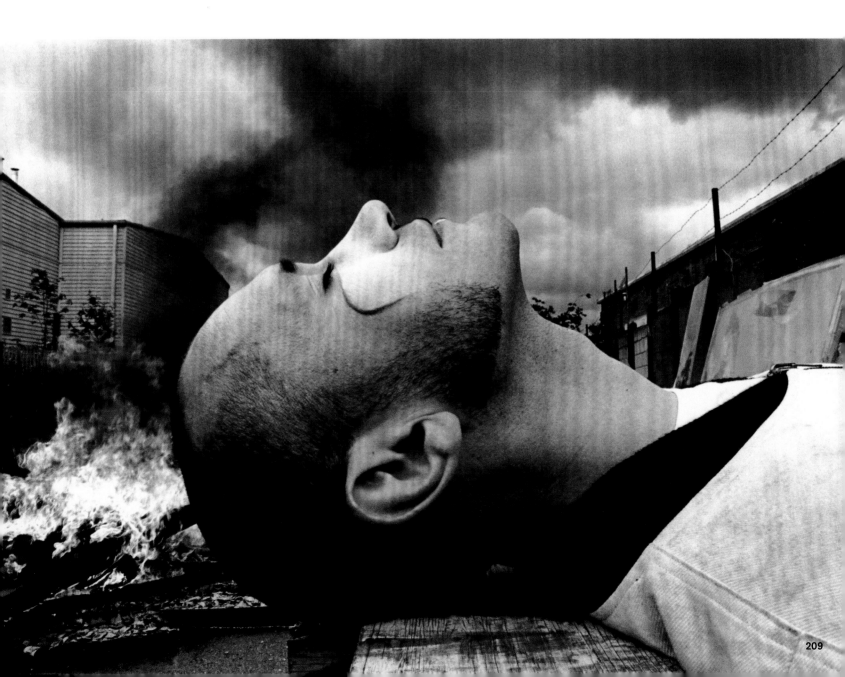

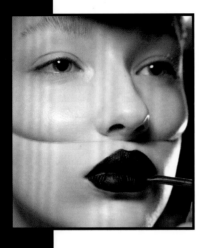

I HATE ROUTINE IN EVERYTHING.

I LIKE MOVEMENT, I LIKE CHANGING IT UP, I LIKE DOING IT WRONG.

SOMETIMES MAKING A MISTAKE CAN MAKE THE PICTURE.

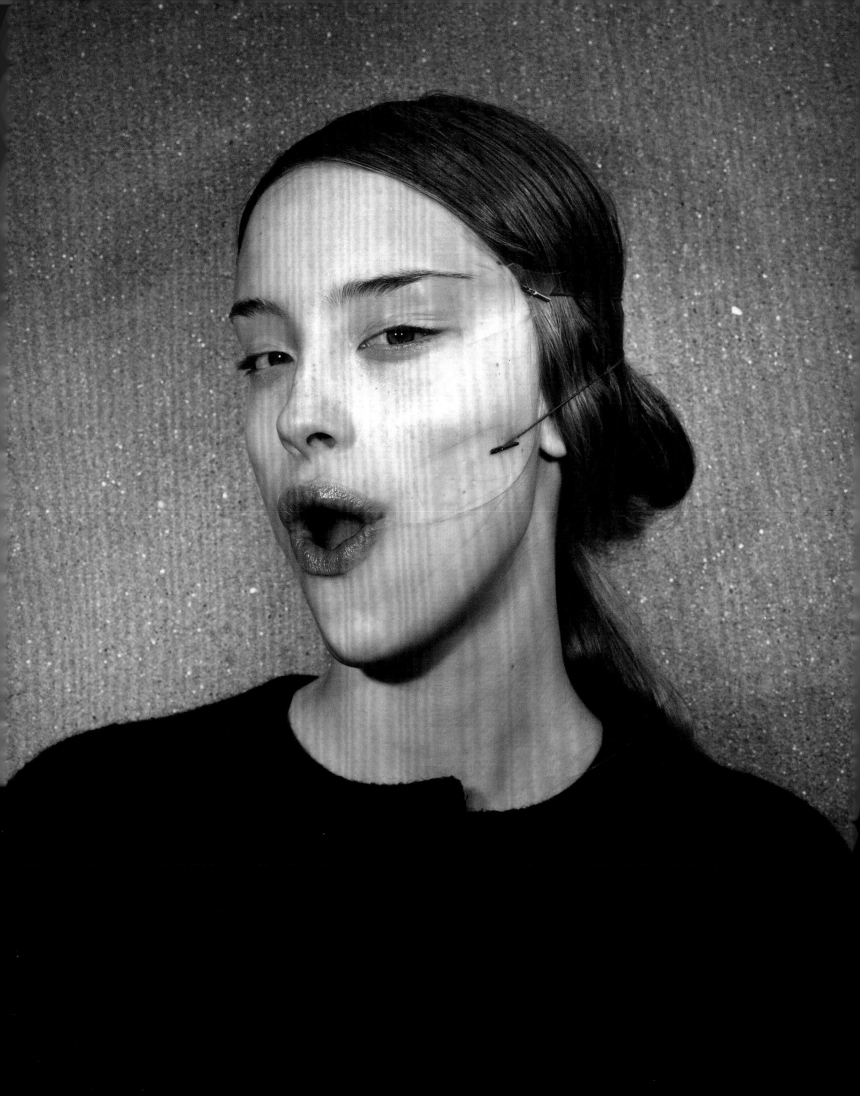

ANOTHER MAGAZINE SS 2015; PHOTOGRAPHY NICK KNIGHT; FASHION EDITOR KATY ENGLAND; HAIR SAM MCKNIGHT; MANICURIST SOPHY ROBSON; MODELS STELLA LUCIA, ARIANA LONDON, JORDON, LOUIS; SET DESIGN ANDREW TOMLINSON.

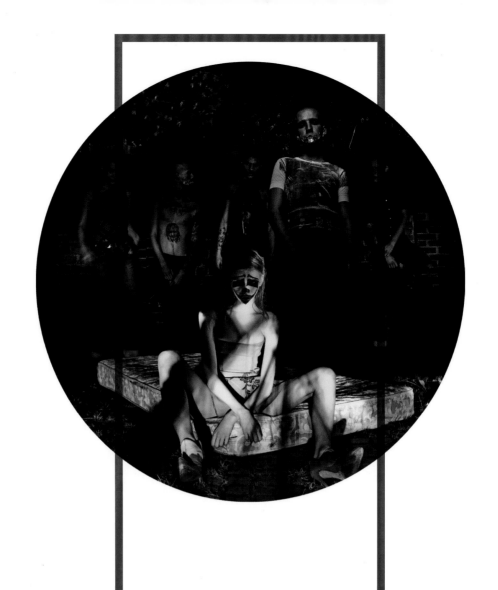

'IT WAS AN EMOTIONAL SHOOT TO DO.
THESE ARE ALL CHARACTERS YOU'RE CREATING
THROUGHOUT THE DAY WITH SAM AND VAL, WITH
ALL THESE MEMORIES, SO THEY'RE POWERFUL
CHARACTERS. YOU NEED A GREAT MAKEUP
ARTIST WHO CAN SEE THAT THROUGH AND
KNOWS WHEN TO DO ALL THE THINGS WE TALKED
ABOUT, WHEN TO PULL BACK, AND WHEN TO KIND
OF LET IT GO. AND WHO CAN UNDERSTAND WHAT
IT'S GOING TO LOOK LIKE IF WE'RE LIGHTING IT
WITH CAR HEADLIGHTS. YOU NEED SOMEBODY
TO UNDERSTAND WHAT YOU'RE DOING.'

NICK KNIGHT

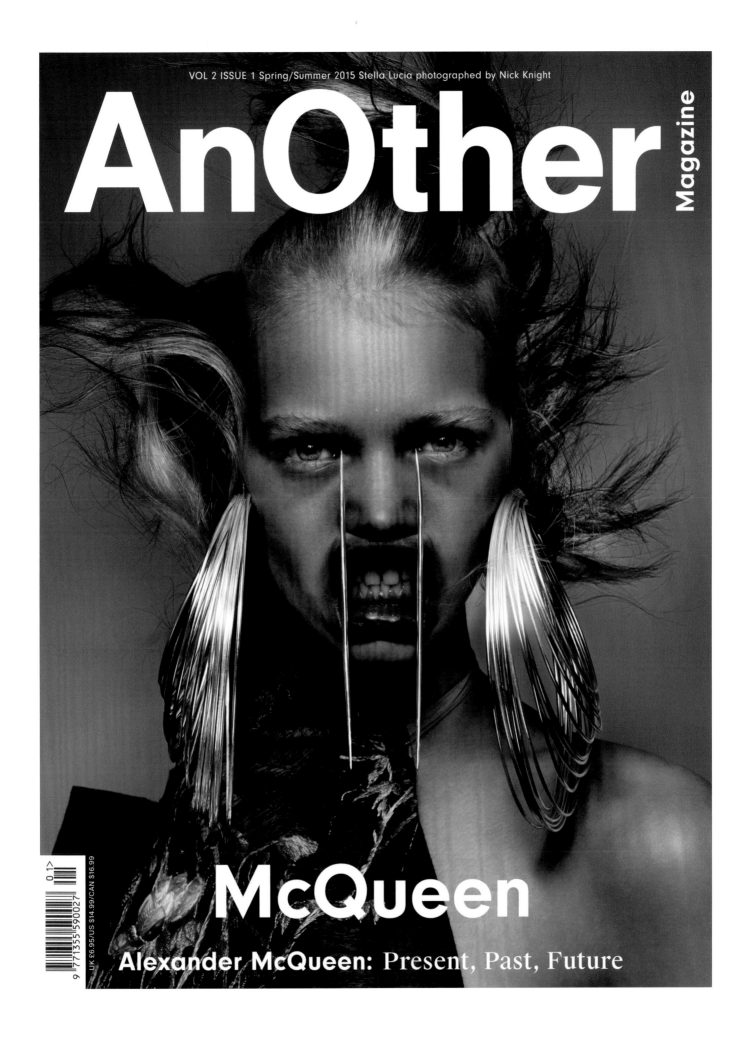

VOL 2 ISSUE 1 Spring/Summer 2015 Stella Lucia photographed by Nick Knight

AnOther

Magazine

McQueen

Alexander McQueen: Present, Past, Future

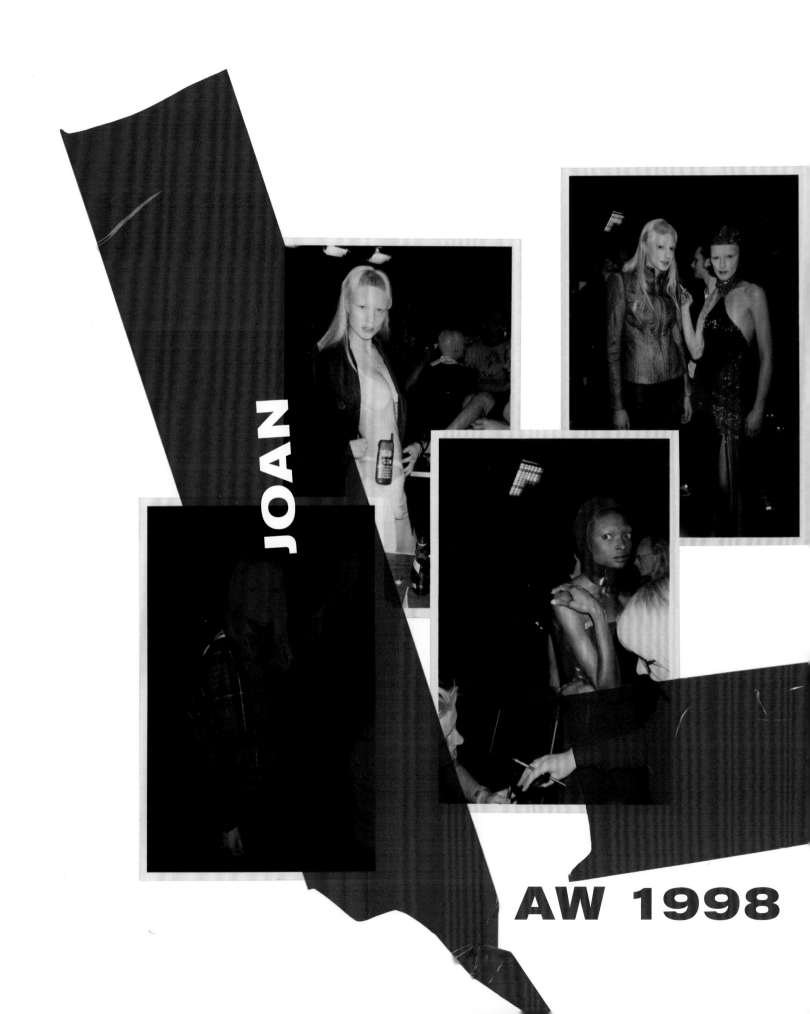

JOAN

AW 1998

LEE LOVED THE EX TREME

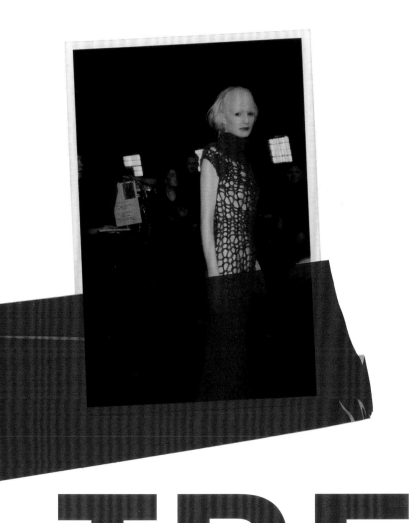

THE FACE

No 15 APRIL 1998 £2.40 US $7.50

SPEED
Suburban Motor Mayhem

SEX
Johnny Vaughan v Jamie Theakston

GORE
Resident Evil 2 and Computer Horror

AGGRO
Jerry Springer rules KO

YOU'RE NOT GOING OUT LIKE THAT!
Alexander McQueen
by Nick Knight

Jude Law
Cleopatra
Monkey Mafia

McQueen
is dead: Long live Alexander McQueen

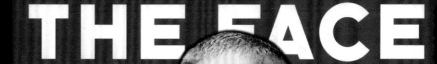

THE FACE

100
most
powerful
people in
fashion

**236 pages of
21st-century
grunge**

+

**Haircuts
Guitars
Cameras
Porno
The Matrix
Zombies
Steve-O**

Mcqueen

**Bare-knuckle genius
by Chris Heath**

NO 68 SEPTEMBER 2002 £2.90
PLATINUM ROGUE: Alexander McQueen by Vincent Peters

09

9 770263 421101

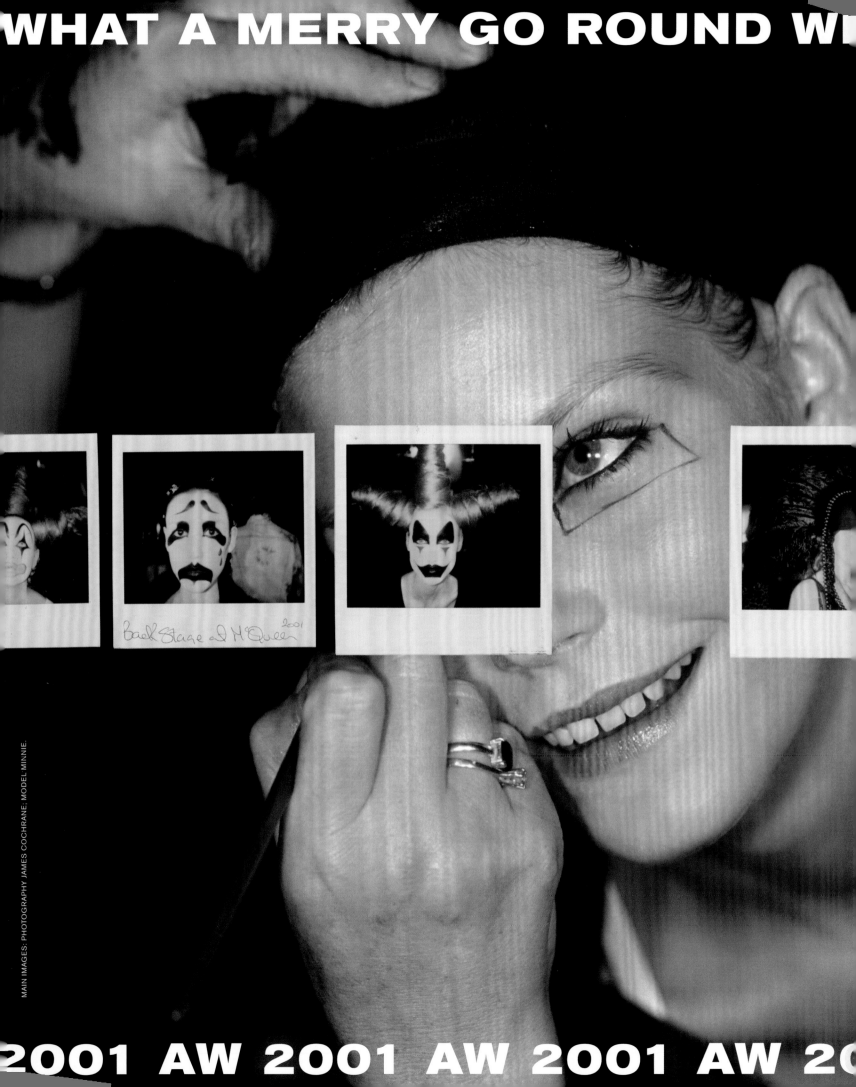

2001 AW 2001 AW 2001 AW 20

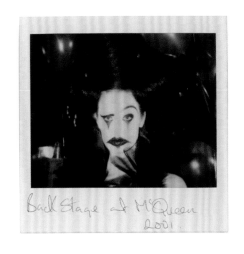

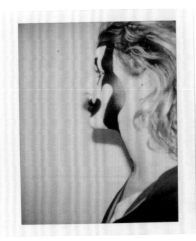

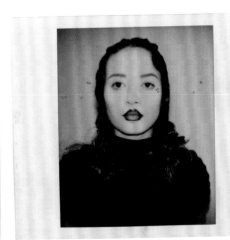

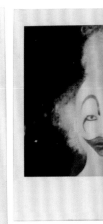

'SHE REALLY LIKES TO PLAY. AND I THINK PERHAPS THE DIFFERENCE WITH VAL IS SHE'LL REALLY GO FOR IT WITHOUT FEAR. A LOT OF PEOPLE ARE FEARFUL, LIKE, "OH, YOU KNOW THAT'S NOT VERY TRENDY RIGHT NOW. OH, NOBODY'S DOING LIPS RIGHT NOW SO WE'RE NOT GONNA DO LIPS." SHE'S LIKE, "FUCK IT!" SHE'S VERY BRAVE.'

KATY ENGLAND

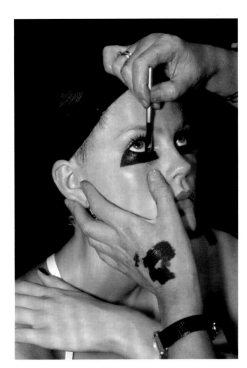

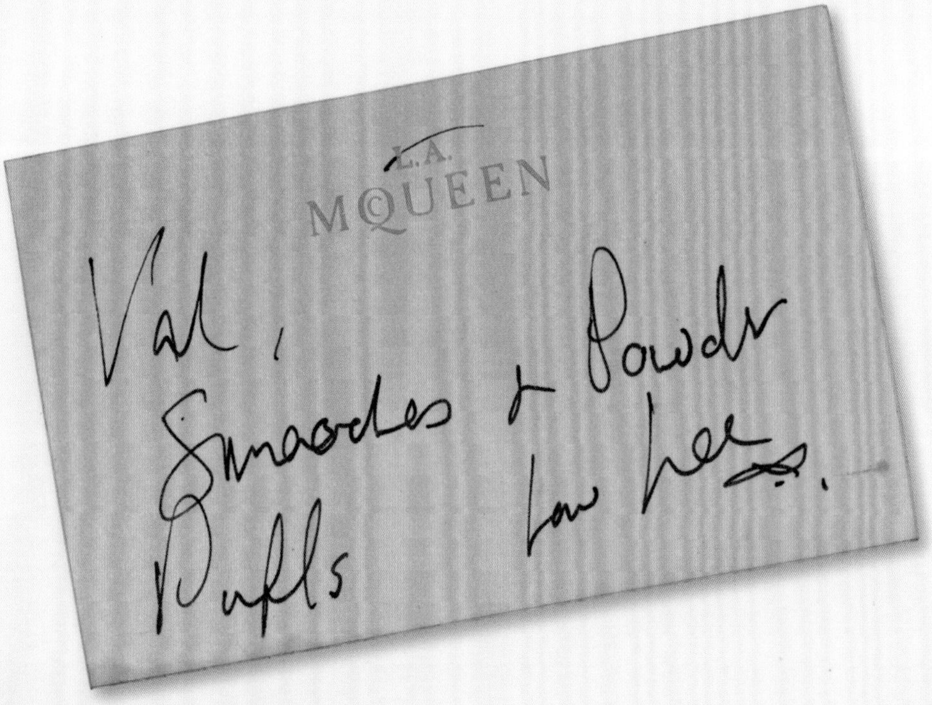
L.A.
McQUEEN

Val,
Smocks & Powder
Puffs Love Lee xx.

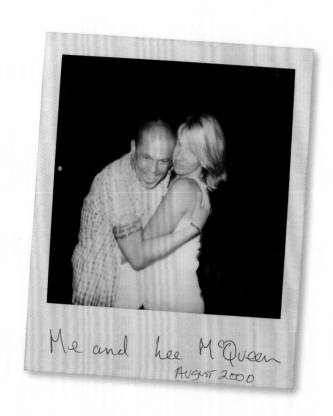

Me and Lee McQueen
AUGUST 2000

'You know, throughout history there are not a million Da Vincis,
there aren't a thousand Dalis, hundreds of Picassos, there's one.
There's one Lee McQueen. And when they're gone, they're gone.
And you think of all the things that could have been.'

NICK KNIGHT

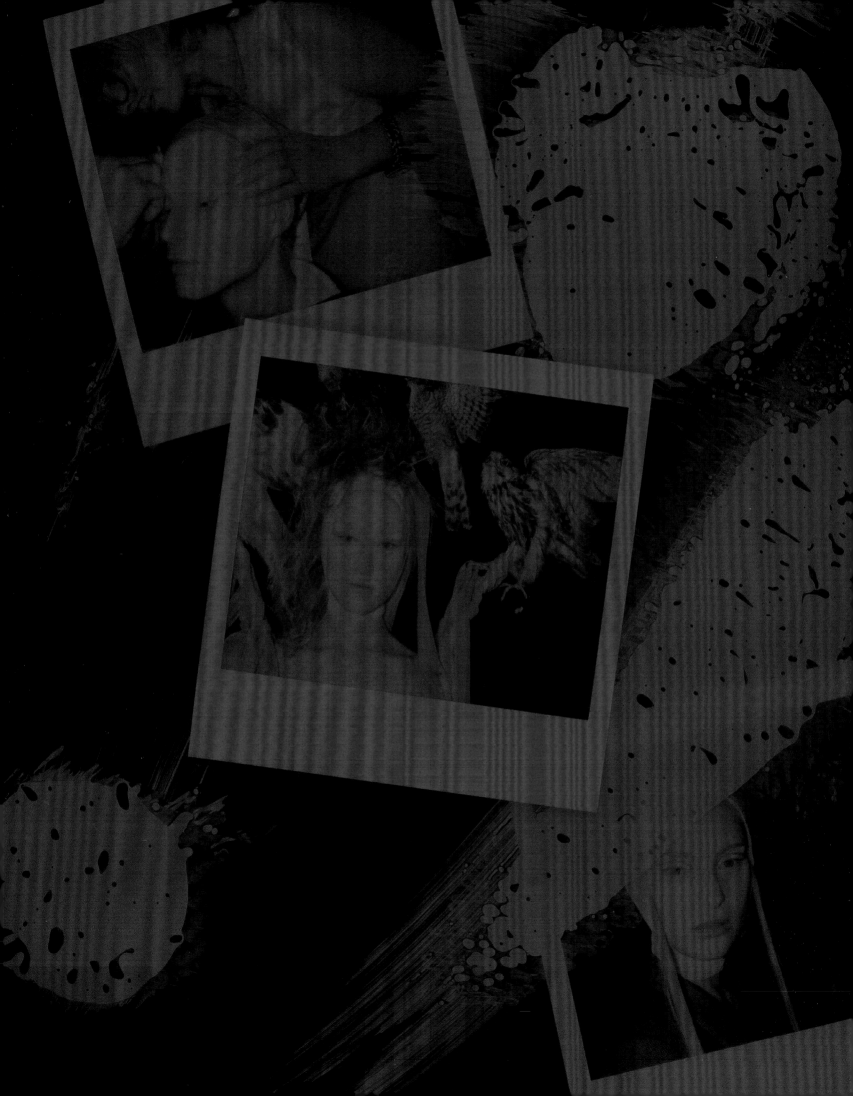

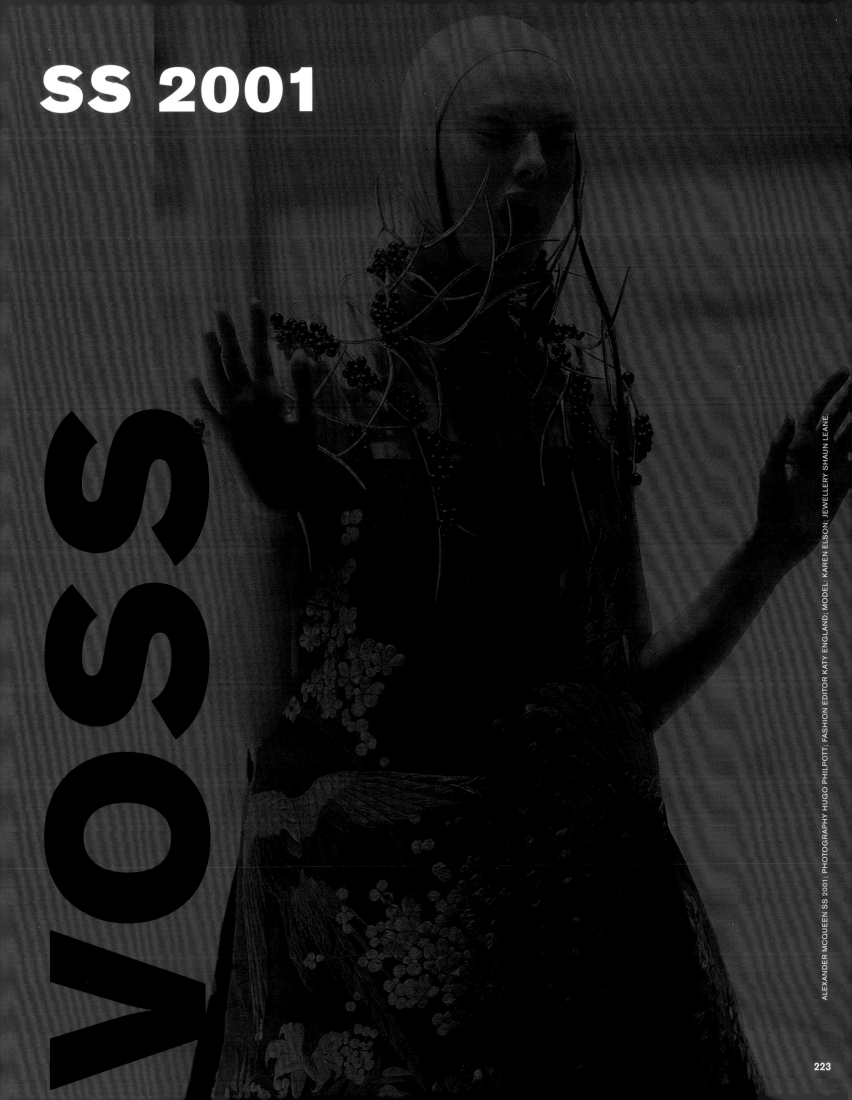

SS 2001

VOSS

ALEXANDER MCQUEEN SS 2001; PHOTOGRAPHY HUGO PHILPOTT; FASHION EDITOR KATY ENGLAND; MODEL: KAREN ELSON; JEWELLERY SHAUN LEANE.

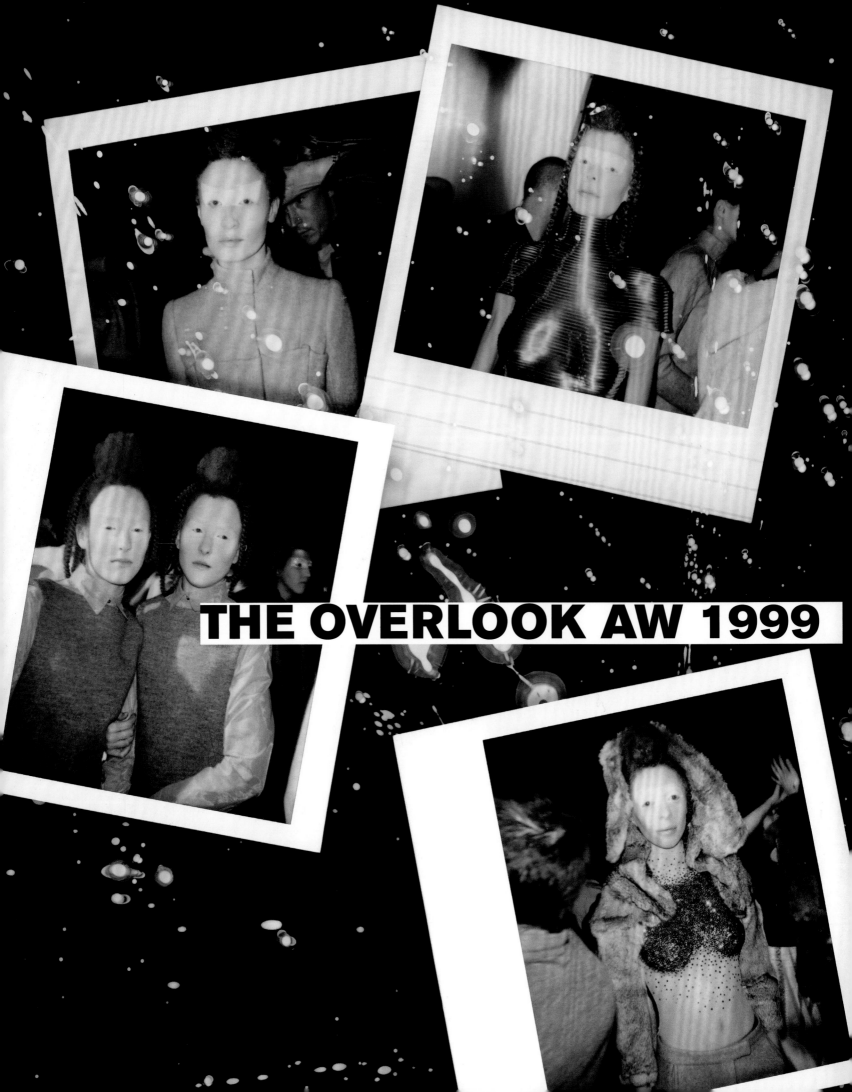

THE OVERLOOK AW 1999

I WOULD THINK I HAD GONE FAR ENOUGH, AND LEE WOULD SAY, 'THAT IS NOT INTERESTING YET'.

YOU COME FROM A PUNK BACKGROUND.
DO YOU THINK LEE SENSED THAT IN YOU?

I think he sensed that in all the people that were around him in the beginning, like Katy England. It was people who were prepared to 'go there'; you needed to be that person. And I think, with him, if you were slightly safe it wasn't going to work. I didn't always know what was inside Lee's head. The thing is, if somebody wants to go there, I will go there with them. In fact, the great thing about Lee was that I would think I had gone far enough, and Lee would say, 'That is not interesting yet'.

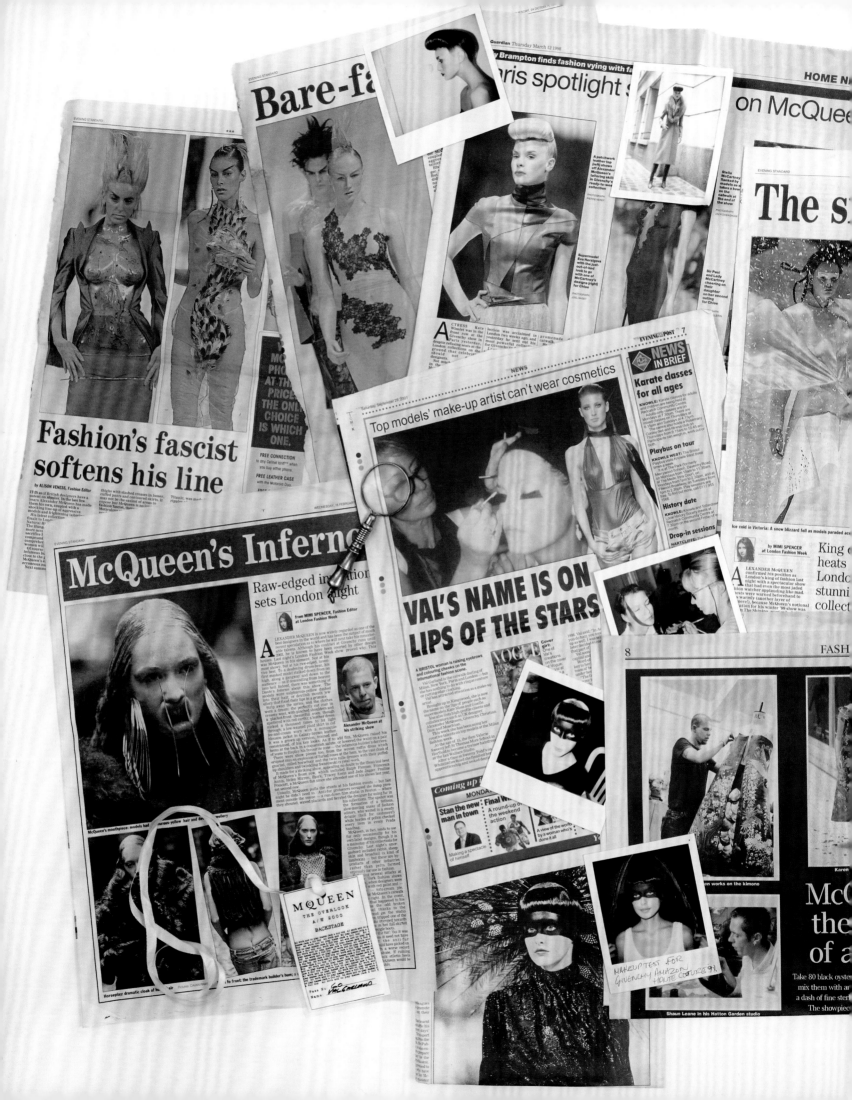

Bare-fa

The Guardian Thursday March 12 1998

by Brampton finds fashion vying with fa

Paris spotlight s

on McQueen

The s

Fashion's fascist softens his line

by ALISON VENESS, Fashion Editor

McQueen's Inferno

Raw-edged in ation sets London ght

from MIMI SPENCER, Fashion Editor at London Fashion Week

Alexander McQueen at his striking show

Horseplay: dramatic cloak of

MCQUEEN
THE OVERLOOK
AW 2000
BACKSTAGE

Saturday September 29, 2001

Top models' make-up artist can't wear cosmetics

NEWS IN BRIEF

Karate classes for all ages

Playbus on tour

History date

Drop-in sessions

VAL'S NAME IS ON LIPS OF THE STARS

A BRISTOL woman is raising eyebrows and colourful cheeks on the international fashion scene

Coming up t

MONDA

Stan the new man in town

Final W
A round-up o the weekend action

A view of the world by a woman who's done it all

Making a spectacle of himself

by MIMI SPENCER at London Fashion Week

King o heats London stunni collect

FASH

8

MAKEUP TEST FOR GIVENCHY AMAZON HAUTE COUTURE 98

Shaun Leane in his Hatton Garden studio

en works on the kimono

McC the of a

Take 80 black oyster mix them with a a dash of fine ster The showpiec

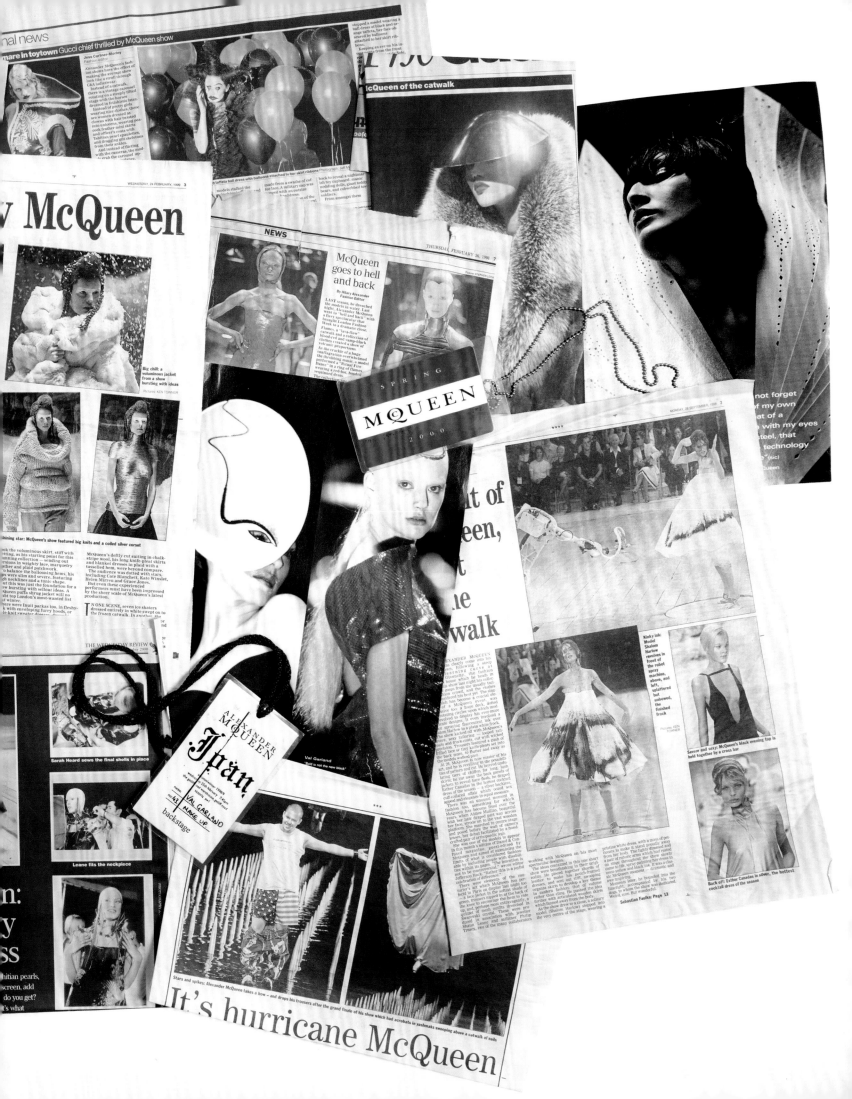

Gucci chief thrilled by McQueen show

Jess Cartner-Morley
Fashion editor

McQueen of the catwalk

McQueen

Big chill: a voluminous jacket from a show bursting with ideas

shining star; McQueen's show featured big knits and a coiled silver corset

THE WEDNESDAY REVIEW

NEWS

THURSDAY, FEBRUARY 26, 1998

McQueen goes to hell and back

By Hilary Alexander
Fashion Editor

SPRING

MCQUEEN

2000

Sarah Heard sews the final shells in place

Leane fits the neckpiece

ALEXANDER
MCQUEEN

Japan

Val Garland
MAKE UP
backstage

Val Garland
'Gold is not the new black'

of en, walk

Stars and spikes: Alexander McQueen takes a bow – and drops his trousers after the grand finale of his show which had acrobats in yashmaks swooping above a catwalk of nails

It's hurricane McQueen

Kinky ink: Model Shalom Harlow revolves in front of the robot spray machine, above, and, left, splattered but unbowed, the finished frock

Severe and sexy: McQueen's black evening top is held together by a cross bar

Back off: Esther Canadas in silver, the hottest cocktail dress of the season

Sebastian Faulks: Page 13

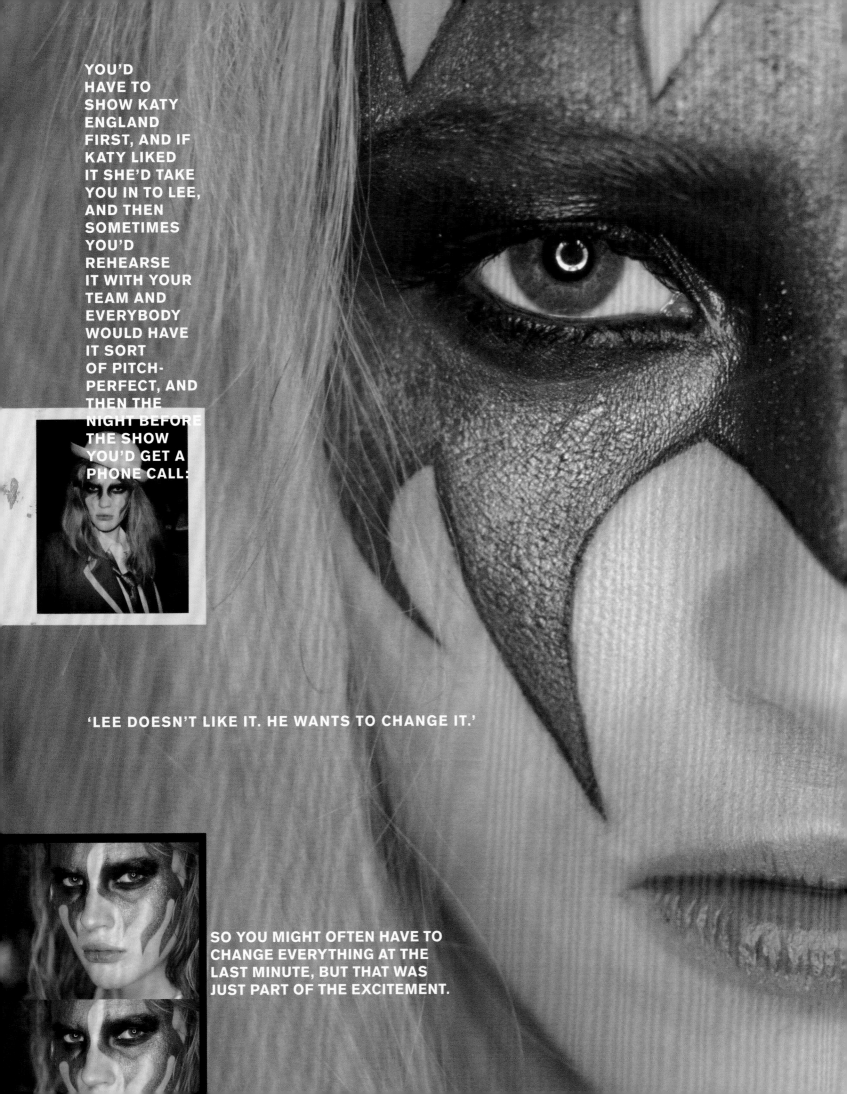

YOU'D HAVE TO SHOW KATY ENGLAND FIRST, AND IF KATY LIKED IT SHE'D TAKE YOU IN TO LEE, AND THEN SOMETIMES YOU'D REHEARSE IT WITH YOUR TEAM AND EVERYBODY WOULD HAVE IT SORT OF PITCH-PERFECT, AND THEN THE NIGHT BEFORE THE SHOW YOU'D GET A PHONE CALL:

'LEE DOESN'T LIKE IT. HE WANTS TO CHANGE IT.'

SO YOU MIGHT OFTEN HAVE TO CHANGE EVERYTHING AT THE LAST MINUTE, BUT THAT WAS JUST PART OF THE EXCITEMENT.

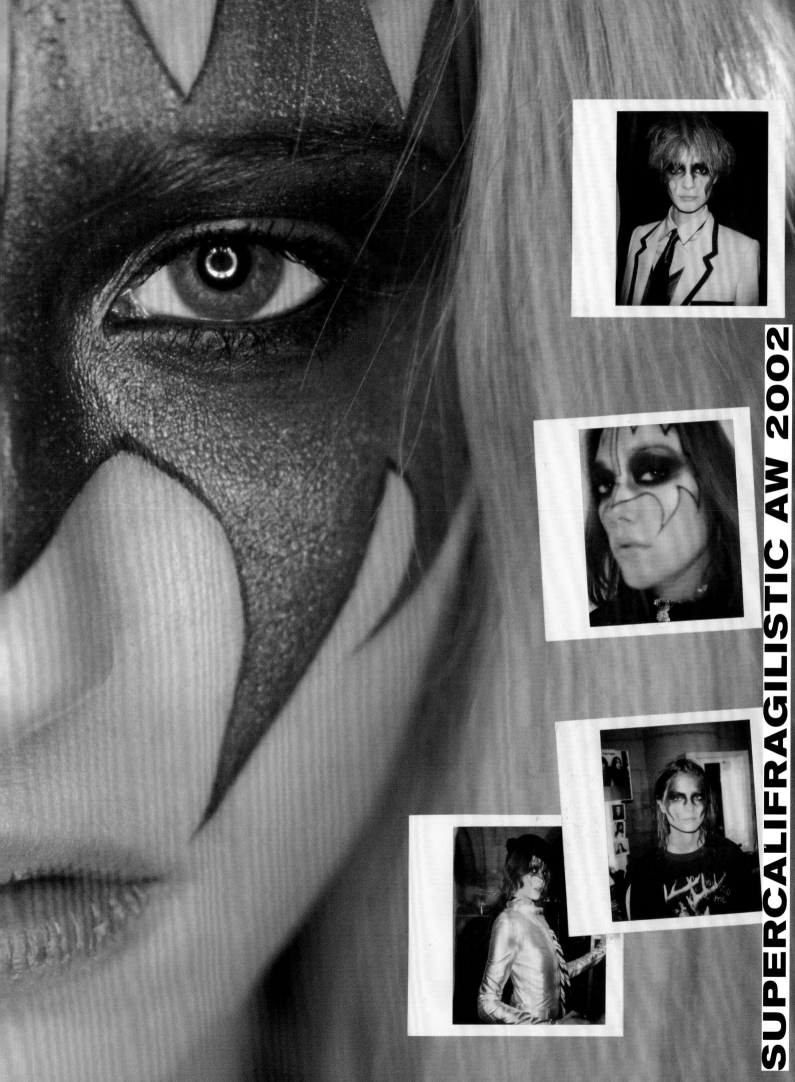

SUPERCALIFRAGILISTIC AW 2002

MAIN IMAGES: PHOTOGRAPHY JAMES COCHRANE.

ESHU AW 2002
ESHU AW 2002
ESHU AW 2002
ESHU AW 2002
ESHU AW 2002
ESHU AW 2002
ESHU AW 2002
ESHU AW 2002
ESHU AW 2002
ESHU AW 2002
ESHU AW 2002
ESHU AW 2002
ESHU AW 2002
ESHU AW 2002
ESHU AW 2002
ESHU AW 2002
ESHU AW 2002
ESHU AW 2002
ESHU AW 2002
ESHU AW 2002
ESHU AW 2002

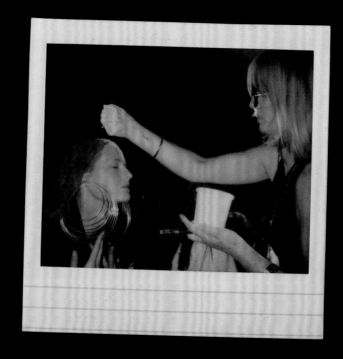

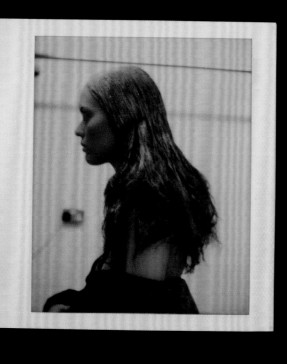

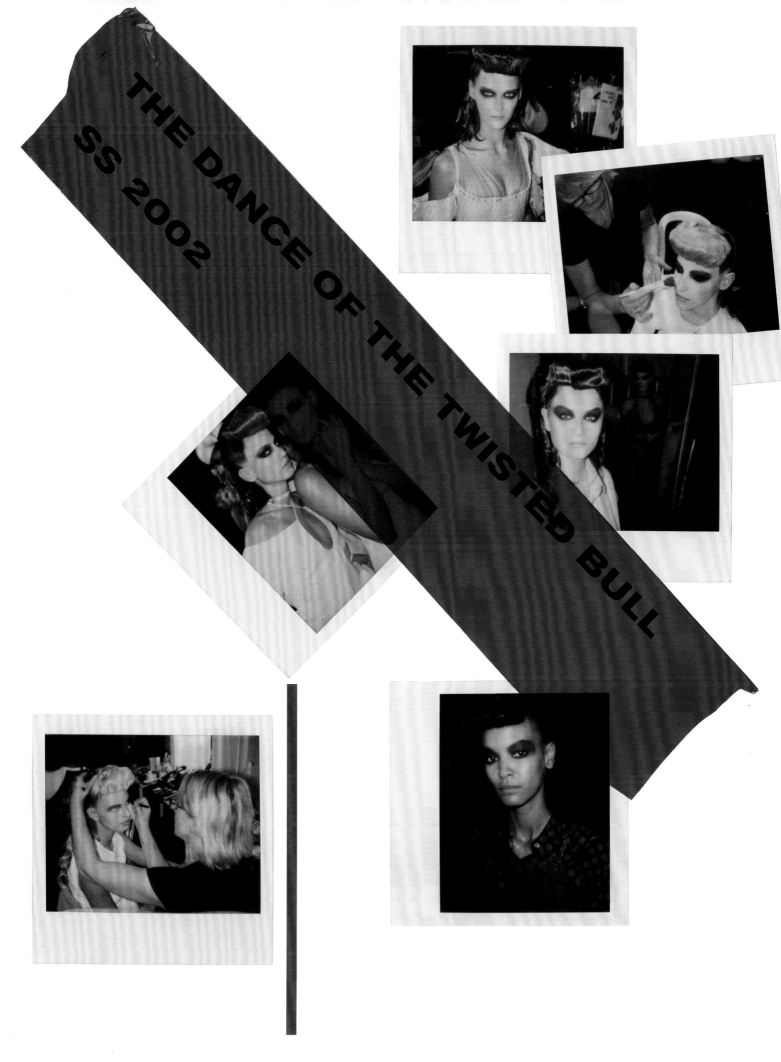

THE DANCE OF THE TWISTED BULL

SS 2002

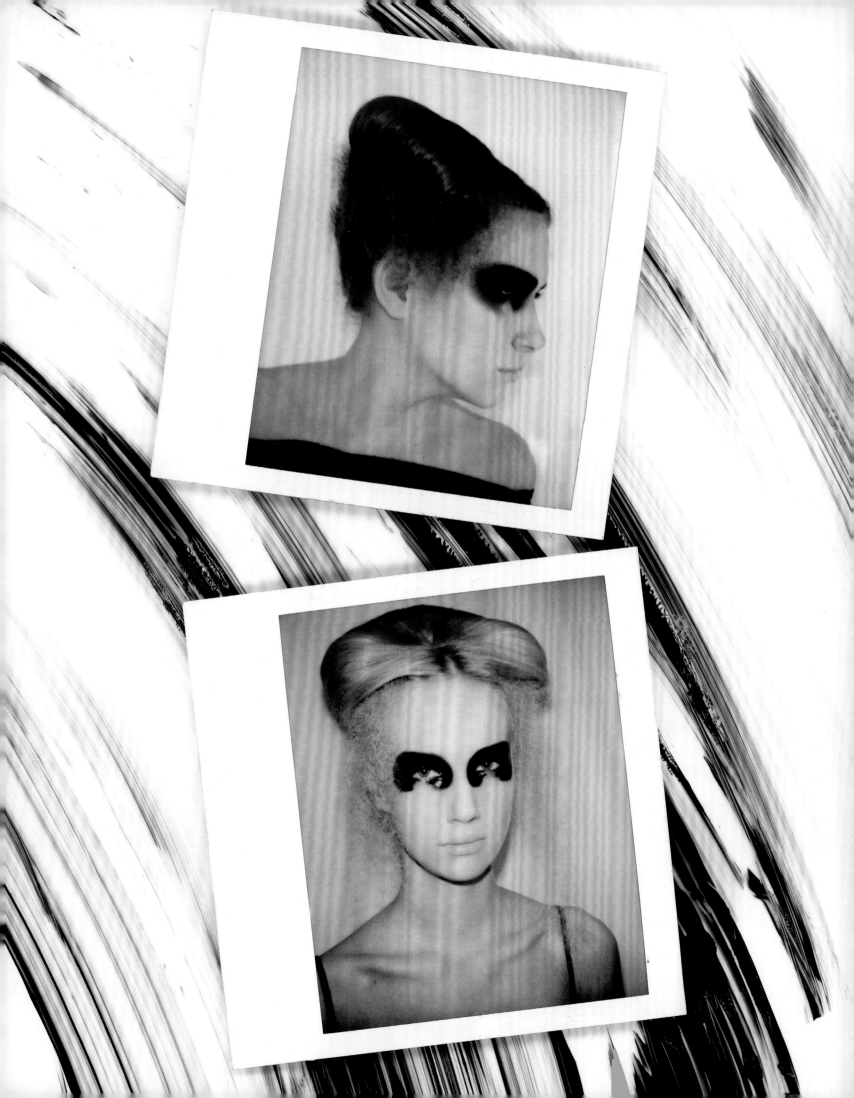

IRERE SS 2003

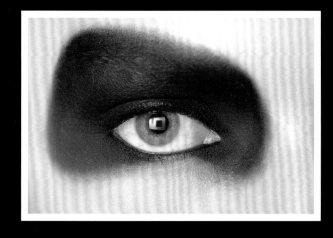

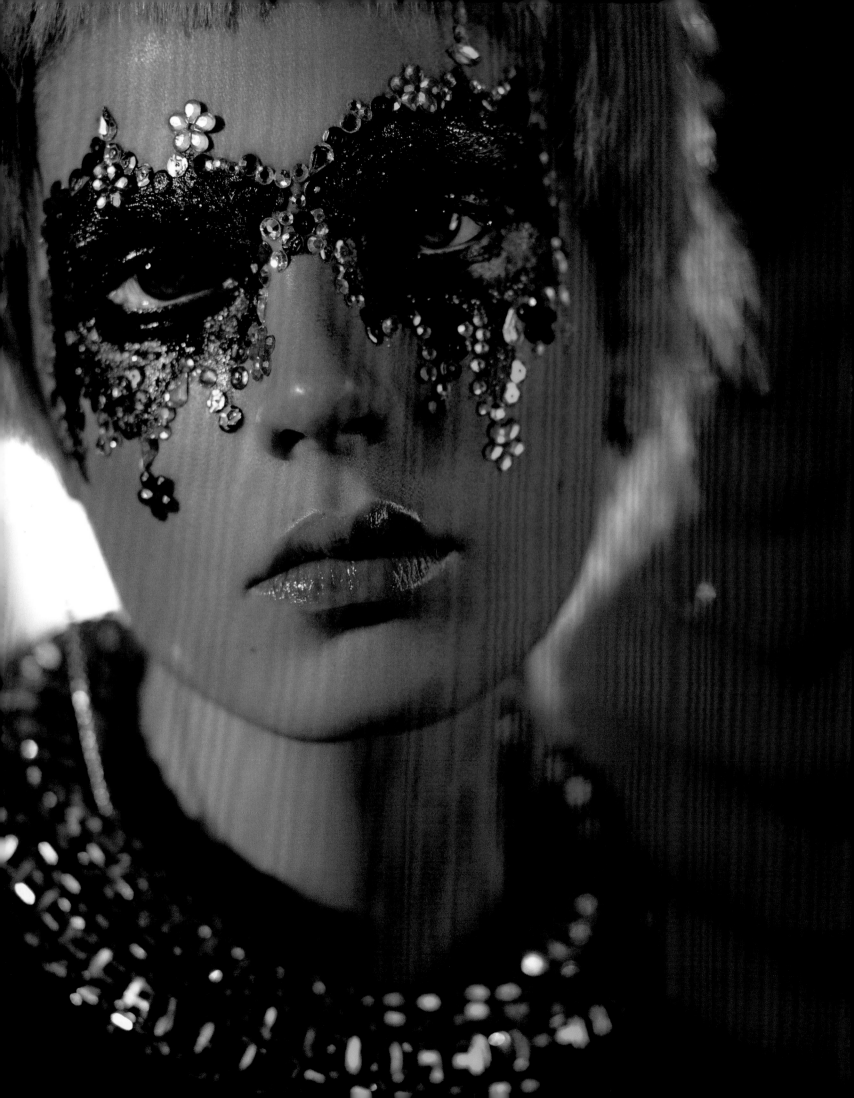

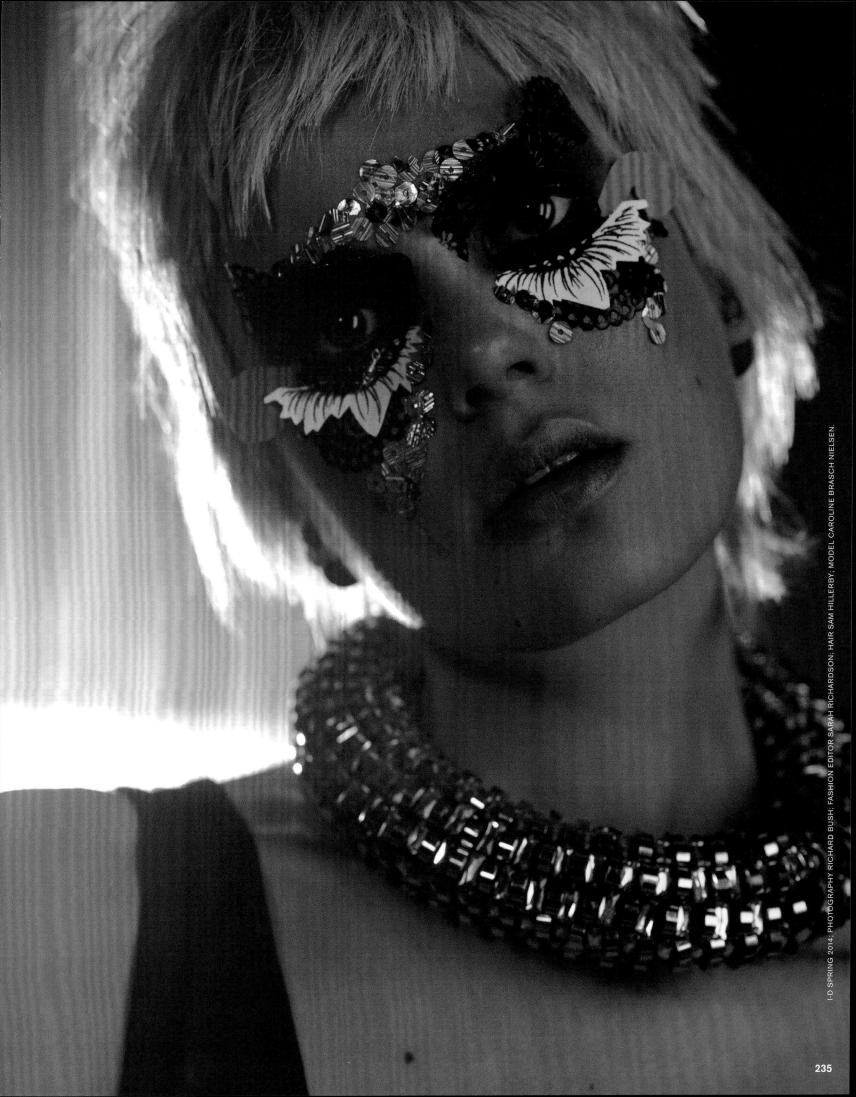

I-D SPRING 2014; PHOTOGRAPHY RICHARD BUSH; FASHION EDITOR SARAH RICHARDSON; HAIR SAM HILLERBY; MODEL CAROLINE BRASCH NIELSEN.

PHOTOGRAPHY MARY MCCARTNEY; FASHION EDITOR CHARLOTTE STOCKDALE; HAIR EUGENE SOULEIMAN/ALAIN PICHON; MANICURIST MARIAN NEWMAN; MODELS BJÖRK WITH KATE LEE AND MELANIE INGLESSIS.

Lee McQueen arrived at Fashion Rocks and asked me to do Björk's makeup, she was performing at the show. He said 'I've got these Swarovski crystals and I want you to stick them all over her face.'

She looked like an otherworldly being.

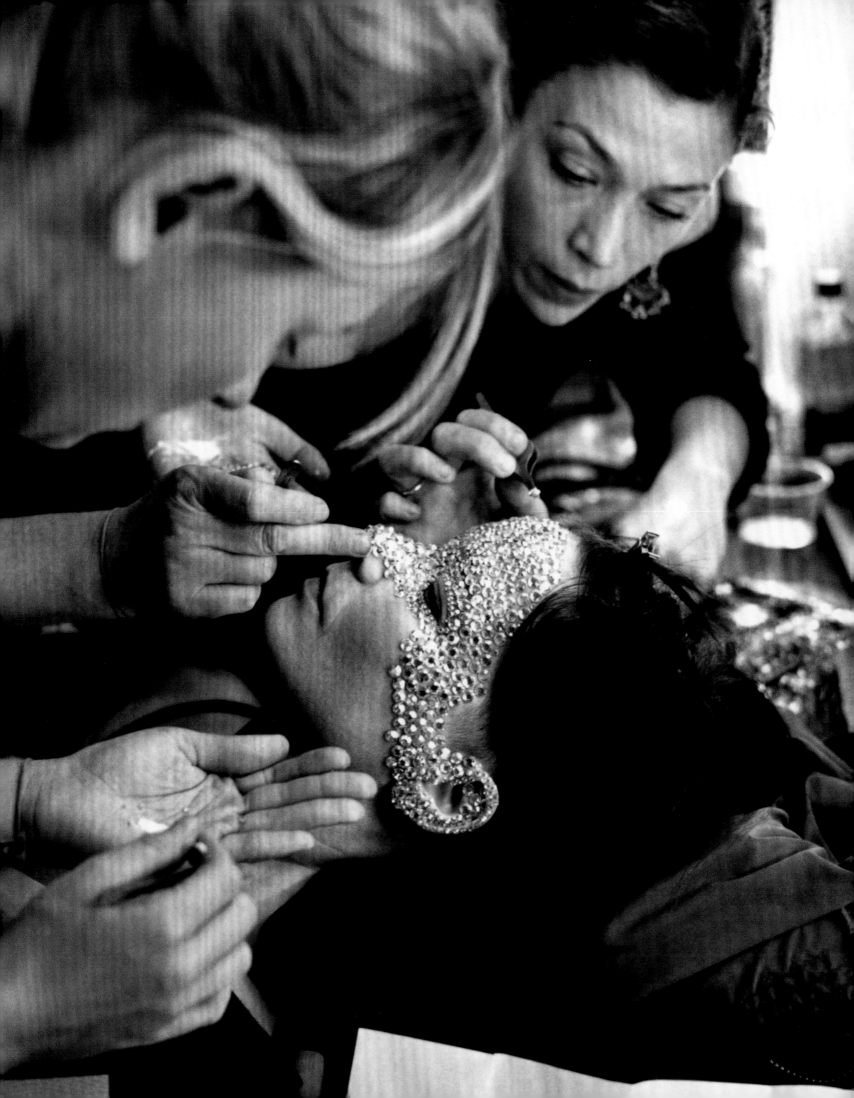

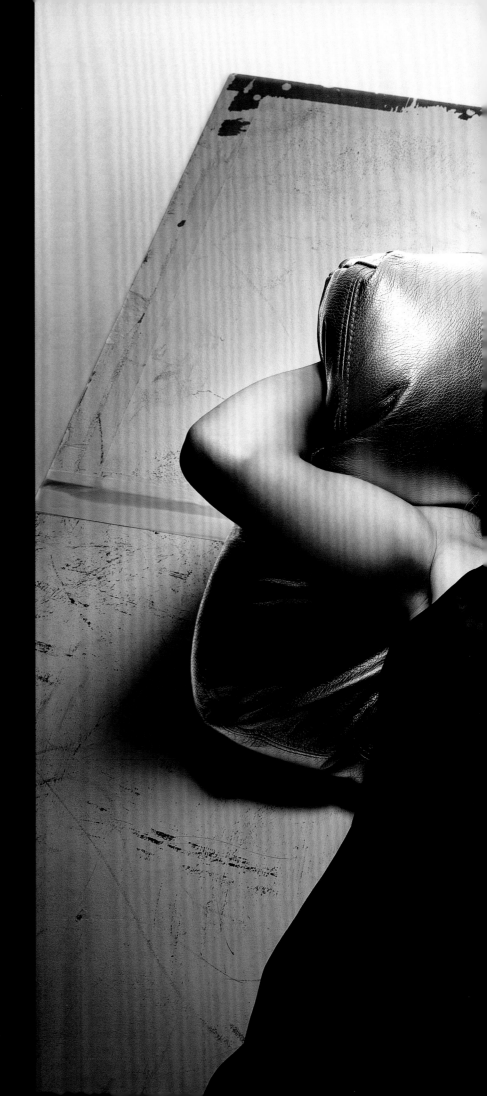

W MAGAZINE OCTOBER 2001; PHOTOGRAPHY NICK KNIGHT; FASHION EDITORS JONATHAN KAYE AND SIMON FOXTON; HAIR SAM MCKNIGHT; MANICURIST MARIAN NEWMAN; MODEL VIVIEN SOLARI.

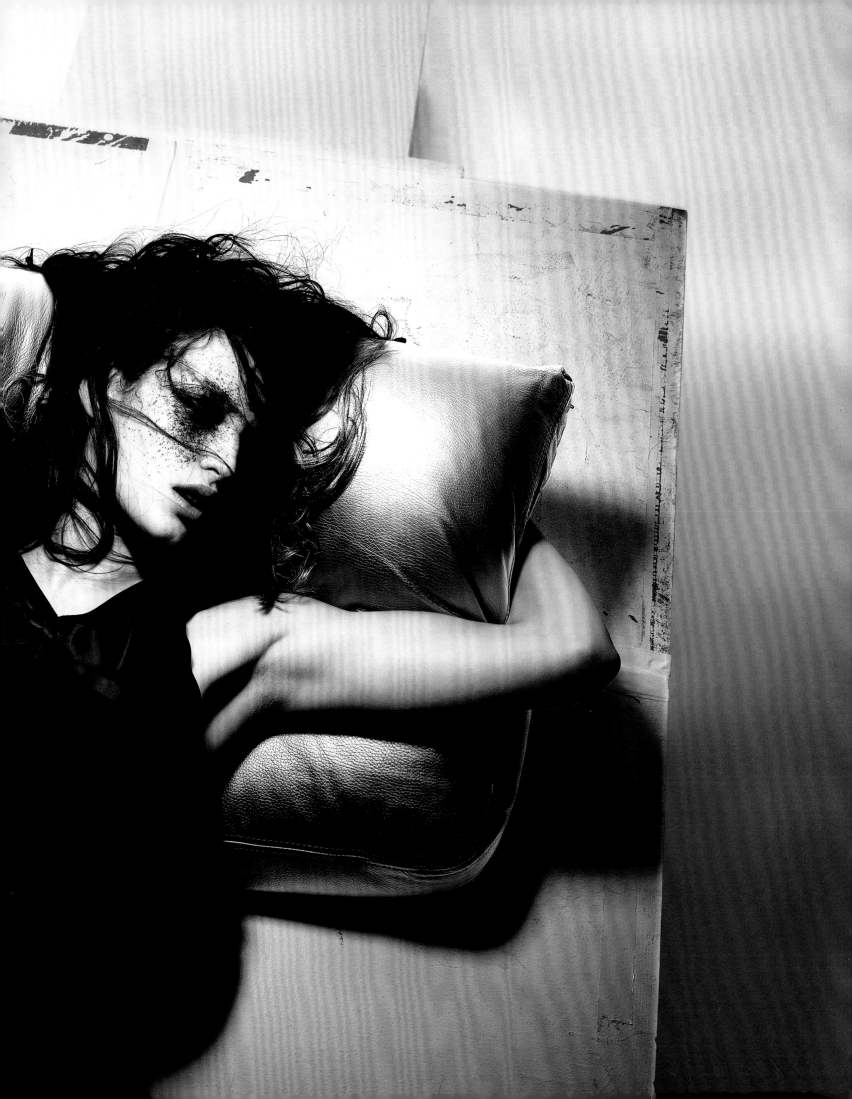

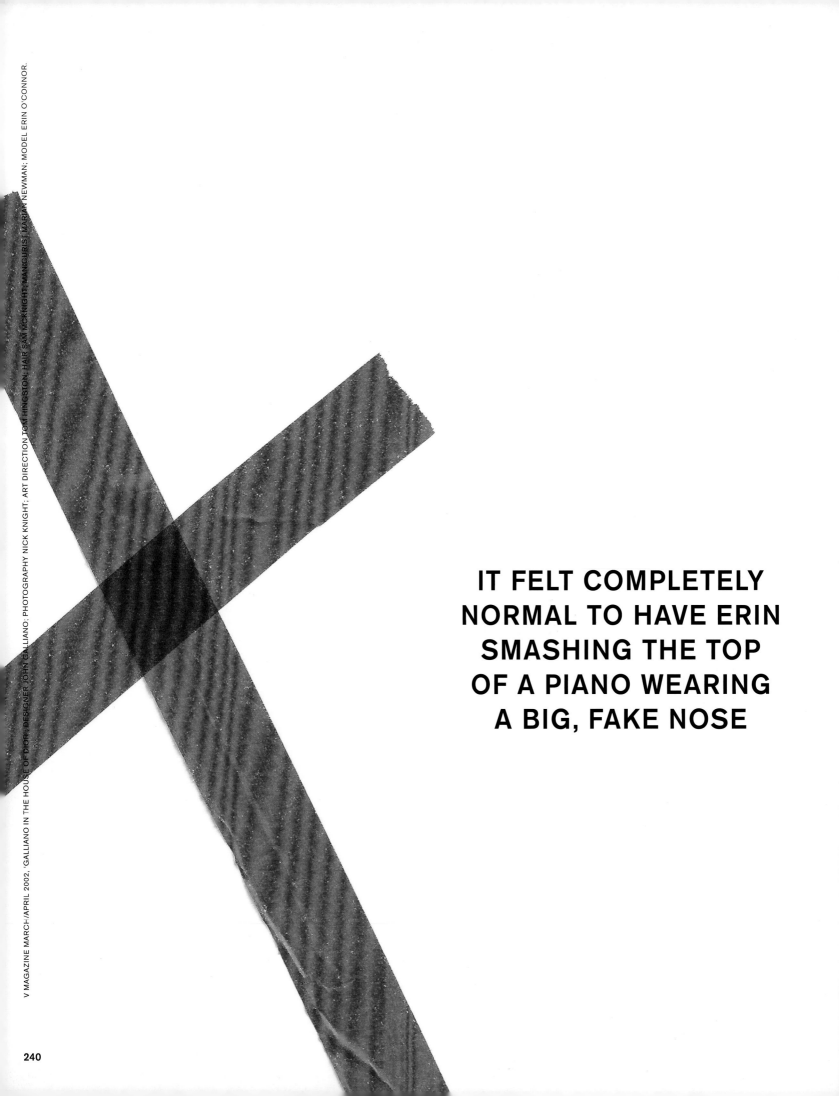

V MAGAZINE MARCH/APRIL 2002; 'GALLIANO IN THE HOUSE OF DIOR'; DESIGNER JOHN GALLIANO; PHOTOGRAPHY NICK KNIGHT; ART DIRECTION TOM HINGSTON; HAIR SAM MCKNIGHT; MANICURIST MARIAN NEWMAN; MODEL ERIN O'CONNOR.

IT FELT COMPLETELY
NORMAL TO HAVE ERIN
SMASHING THE TOP
OF A PIANO WEARING
A BIG, FAKE NOSE

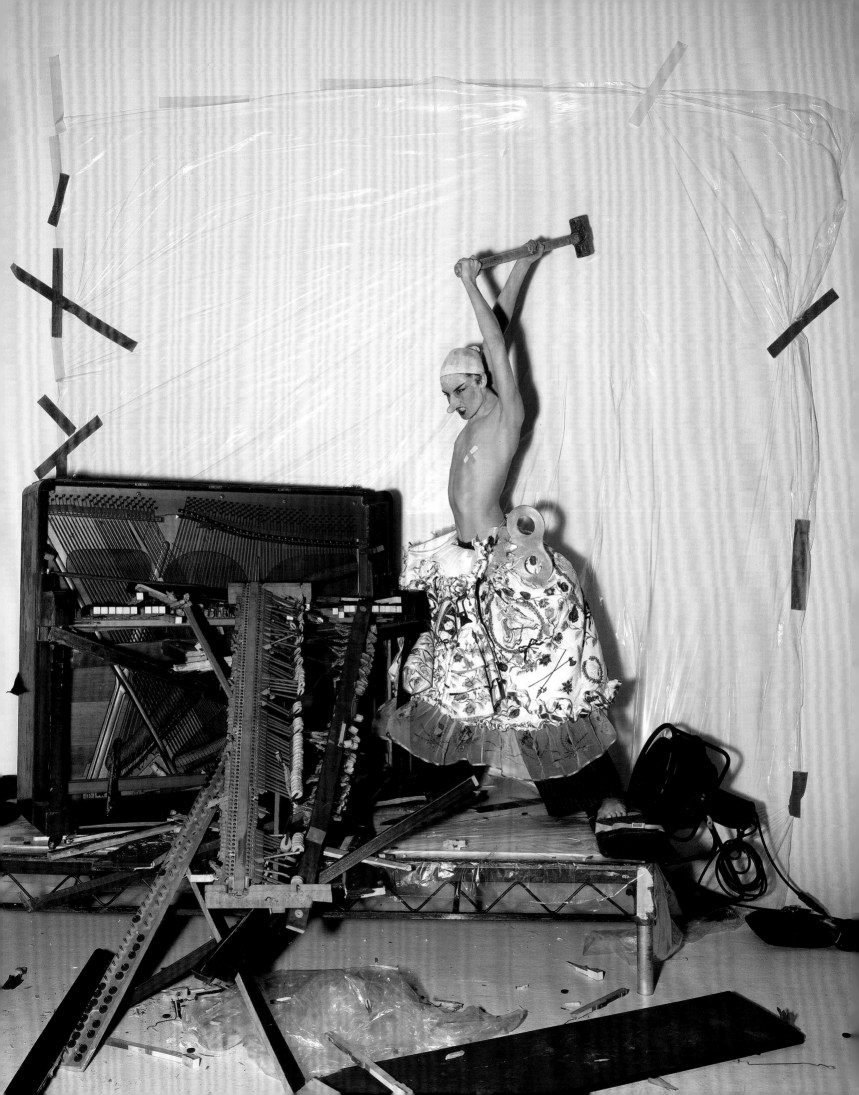

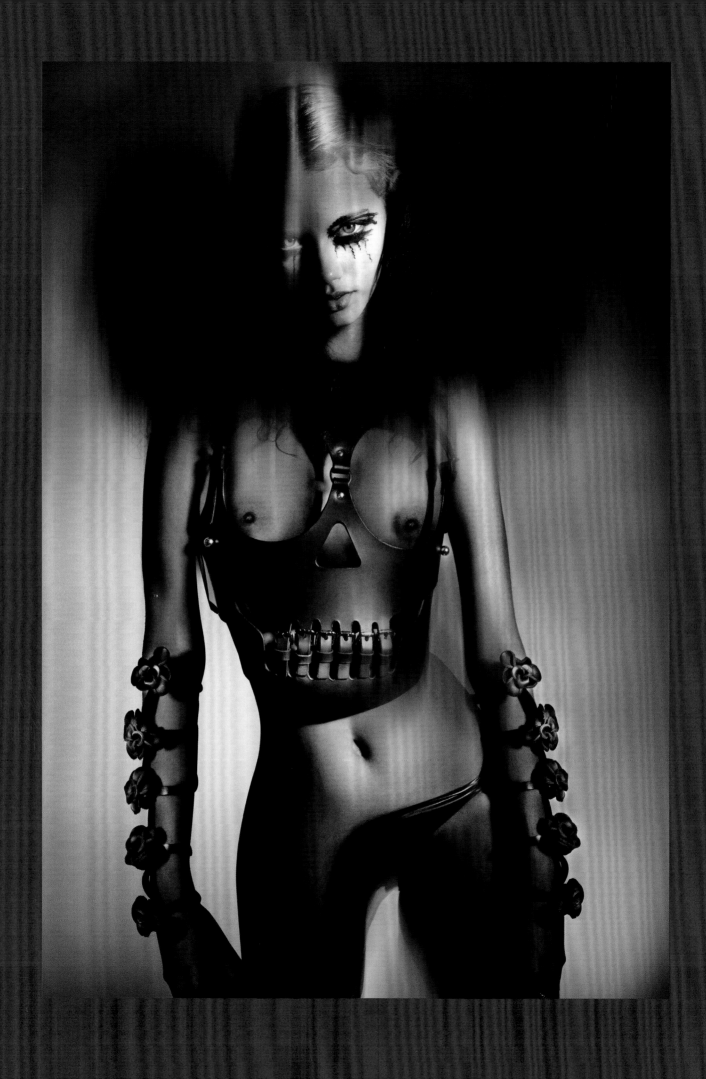

GARAGE MAGAZINE. PHOTOGRAPHY NICK KNIGHT. FASHION EDITOR CHARLOTTE STOCKDALE. HAIR SAM MCKNIGHT. MANICURIST MARIAN NEWMAN. MODEL KARLIE KLOSS

GARAGE MAGAZINE SS 2014. PHOTOGRAPHY NICK KNIGHT. FASHION EDITOR CHARLOTTE STOCKDALE. HAIR SAM MCKNIGHT. MANICURIST MARIAN NEWMAN, MODEL KARLIE KLOSS

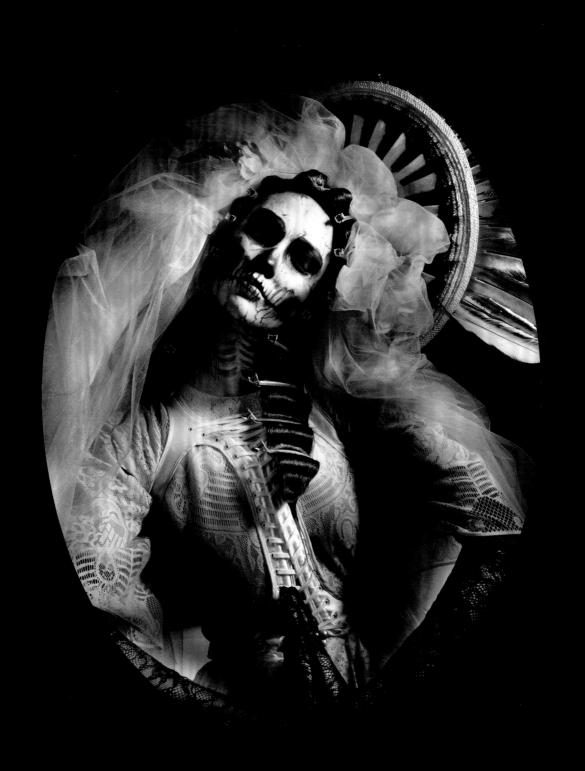

A JOURNALIST ONCE SAID TO ME, 'PEOPLE DON'T EXPECT YOU TO DO GORGEOUS MAKEUP. YOU DO EXTREME'. AND I THOUGHT, I CAN DO THAT AND I DO DO BEAUTIFUL MAKEUP, BUT I LIKE THE UNEXPECTED – SOMETHING CHALLENGING THAT MAKES YOU QUESTION SOMETHING OR STOP TO LOOK. THAT'S MORE INTERESTING TO ME.

· AMERICAN VOGUE SEPTEMBER 2012; PHOTOGRAPHY STEVEN KLEIN; FASHION EDITOR TONNE GOODMAN; HAIR GARREN; MODEL KAREN ELSON.

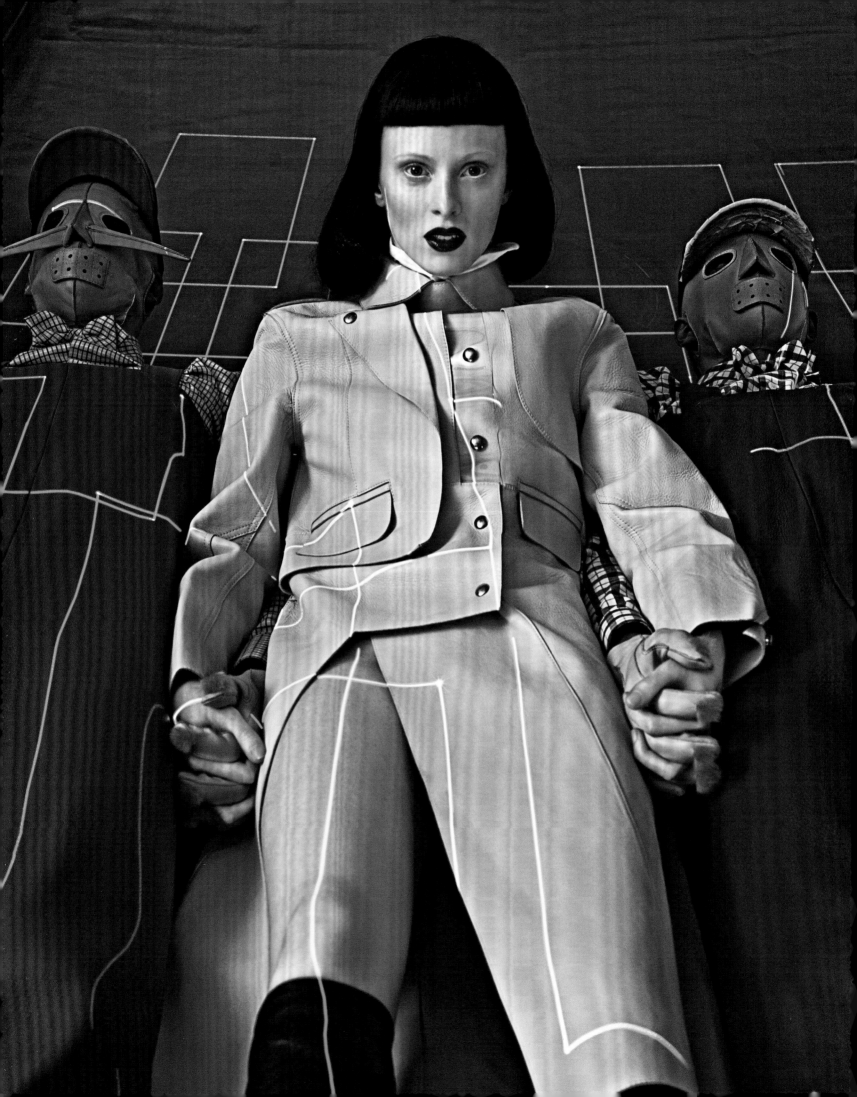

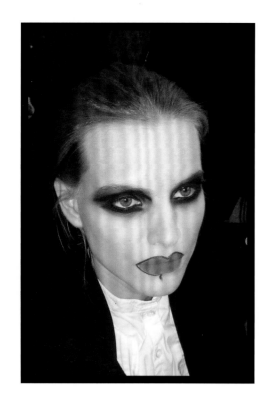

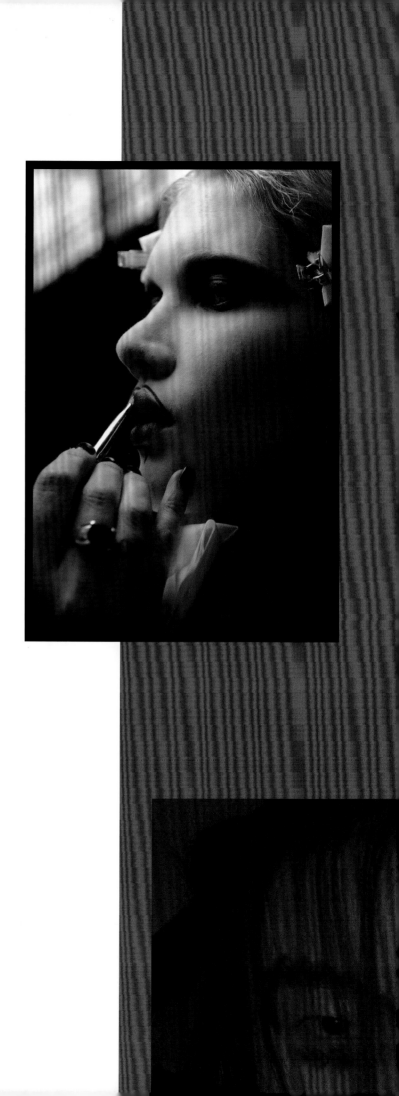

VIVIENNE WESTWOOD GOLD LABEL AW10; PHOTOGRAPHY LUCA CANNONIERI.

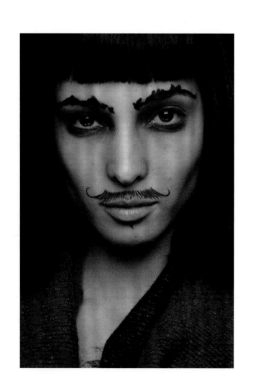

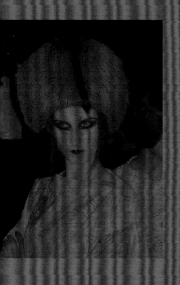

'I CAN'T JUST SAY "WELL, SHE'S THE BEST", BECAUSE THAT WOULDN'T BE FAIR ON OTHER PEOPLE. BUT SHE IS. AND WHAT I FIND REALLY REMARKABLE IS THAT I SUSPECT SHE'S MORE CRAZY THAN I AM.'

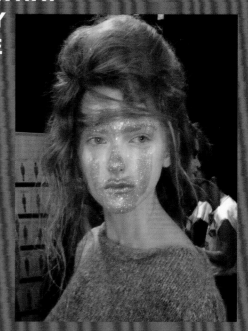

VIVIENNE WESTWOOD

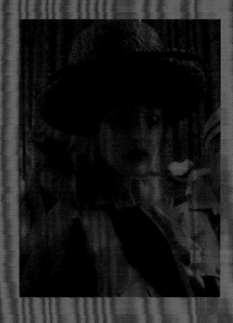

'I CAN'T JUST SAY "WELL, SHE'S THE BEST", BECAUSE THAT WOULDN'T BE FAIR ON

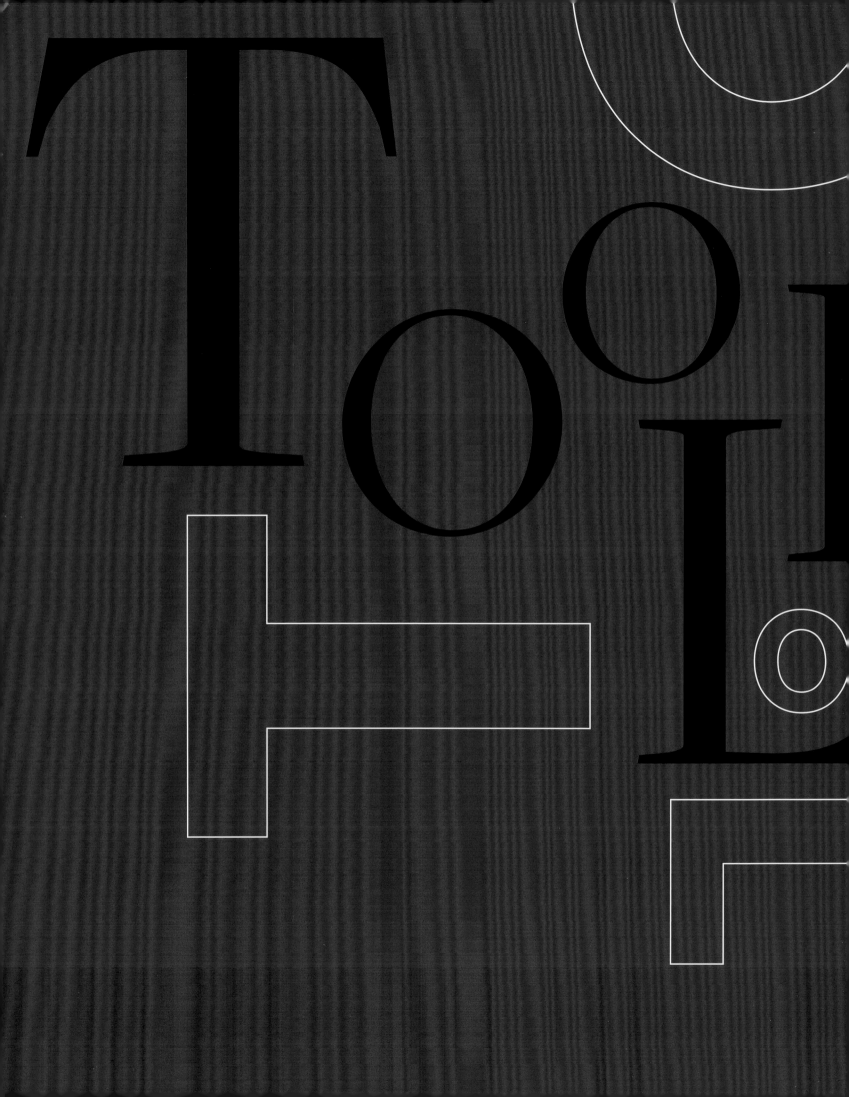

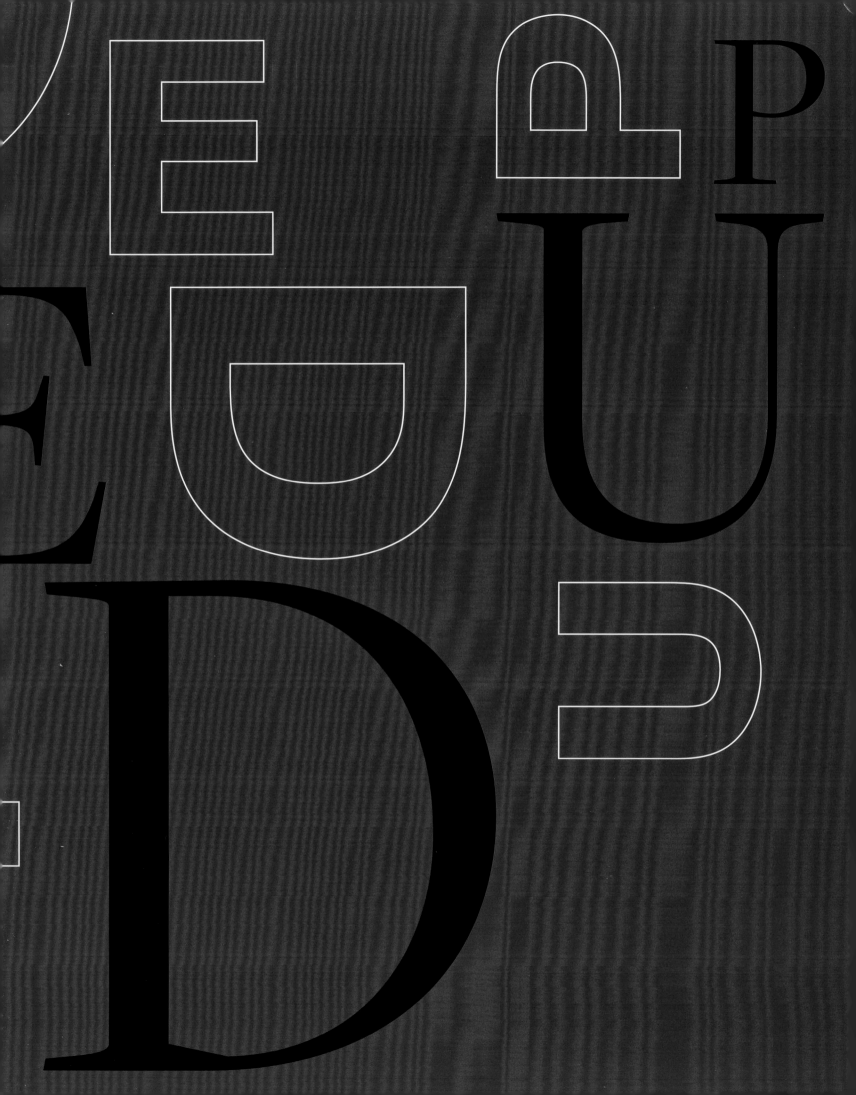

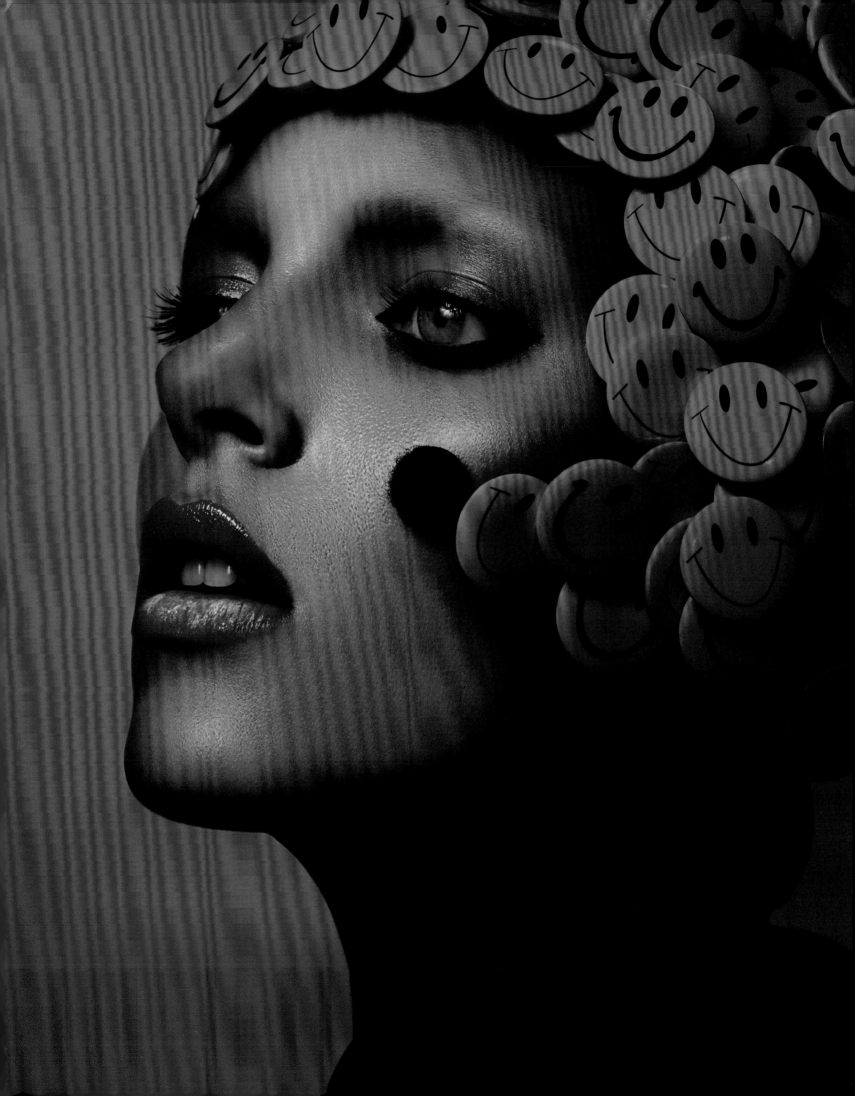

THINKING

THE
MAKEUP
BOX

OUTSIDE

Leave any preconceived ideas you may have about makeup at the door. This final section is about the more unusual tools of Val's trade. The inventive ways in which she has incorporated these unorthodox items into her art shows us how she quite literally thinks outside of the makeup box.

Val never wanted to be seen as a makeup artist in the traditional sense, and since her early days as a makeup rookie in the nineties she has cultivated what she calls her 'sticky-back plastic bag' – named in homage to her childhood love of the television show *Blue Peter*, renowned for its inventive lessons in arts and crafts.

Delve into Val's kit and you will discover all manner of items that have enabled her to create truly astonishing images, including writing icing used to give a filigree-like three-dimensional aspect to a model's features; pencil shavings in place of false eyelashes; ingeniously placed elastic bands to provide a parody of Juvéderm-plumped cheeks; seaweed wetted and patted onto cheeks to mimic a woodgrain veneer; a common or garden potato utilized to stamp Lichtenstein-esque polka dots onto the flesh of a world-famous recording artist.

Like many creatives, Val is never content to conform – in fact, the idea of utilizing only cosmetics in her work is anathema to her. So, from the mundanity of the paint roller to the sparkling allure of Swarovski crystals, Val's 'tools of the trade' continue to evolve, and their possibilities appear infinite. If a bad workman always quarrels with his tools, Val has quite the opposite relationship with hers; she can credit them with enabling some of her most outré and unconventional work to date, while showing us how invention in art can begin with the humblest ingredients.

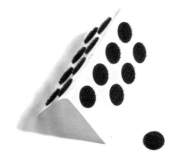

NUMÉRO 108, NOVEMBER 2009; PHOTOGRAPHY MIGUEL REVERIEGO; FASHION EDITOR CAPUCINE SAFYURTLU; HAIR KEN O'ROURKE; MANICURIST MIKE POCOCK; MODEL ANJA RUBIK. PRODUCT SHOTS THROUGHOUT BY JAMES STOPFORTH.

Potato

This was a shoot I did with the beautiful Beth Ditto. Beth was known at that time for wearing strong eyeliner and the client wanted that look, but I wanted to bring something else to it. I was looking at the backdrop that Andy Hillman, the set designer, had made and it had all these huge spots on it. So I thought, 'Let's carry that on!'

Beth was a lot of fun, but because she's an artist I knew that we'd have to work quickly and apply the spots on set to maintain the momentum of the shoot. I was wondering how to get dots all over her in different sizes quite quickly, and then it occurred to me to do it kiddie-style. I said to my assistant, 'Get me some potatoes!' I needed a stamp and I couldn't find the right one in my kit. I would probably use something different now, like a little round sponge, but potatoes are great because you can cut them into all kinds of shapes. Sometimes you just go inside your head and see what's in there and what you can use. And in my head, it was a potato!

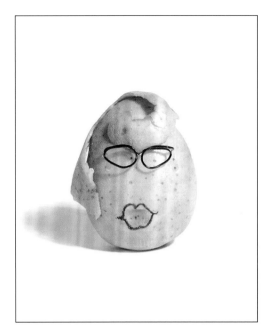 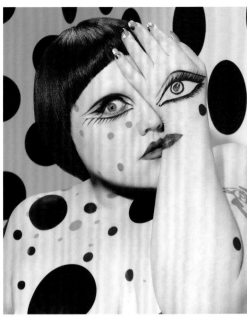

PHOTOGRAPHY MILES ALDRIDGE; HAIR LYNDELL MANSFIELD; SET DESIGN ANDY HILLMAN; MODEL BETH DITTO.

Writing Icing

I wanted to do something three-dimensional with the eye makeup here. I'd used writing icing before with Richard, but in a different way. Sometimes you will find a technique that works and there's nothing wrong with doing that idea again.

This shoot was on 10x8 film, which can take some time. I was panicking, thinking the makeup won't last, it's going to melt and run all over her face, but Richard got the shot. The funny thing is, most people would test out these ideas, but I don't do dress rehearsals – I'm straight in. Just do it! I might even have liked it running. Sometimes what isn't supposed to happen turns out to be the best thing.

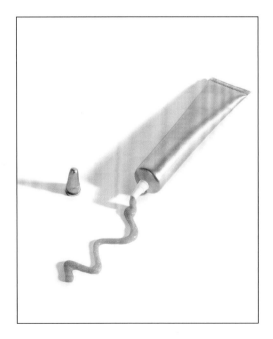 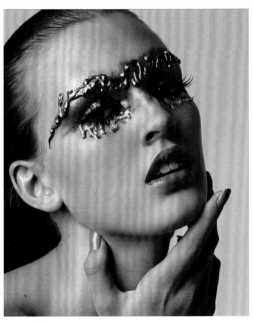

10 MAGAZINE, WINTER 2008; PHOTOGRAPHY RICHARD BUSH; FASHION EDITOR SOPHIA NEOPHITOU-APOSTOLOU; MODEL ALI STEPHENS.

Pantyhose

This was my first ever show with Gareth Pugh, and the theme was Donna Summer, Lindsay Kemp, dark Soho nightclubs. I felt I had to do more than makeup, I needed to create a character. I found some pantyhose in my kit and that sparked an idea. I put them over the model's face and then drew the face over the top. Malcolm put the hair on and it was one of those 'eureka!' moments. Everyone loved the idea, but I needed to figure out how it was going to work in the show.

Malcolm thought there should be a bald cap and we would have to colour it to each girl's skin tone. Basically, the process was this: the hair had to be contained before the bald cap could go on, which takes time, then the cap had to be bled into the forehead and into the nape. Then the wig had to go on top and each wig had to be cut to fit each girl, which takes more time. I realized that once I had done the makeup, the girls wouldn't be able to speak, eat or drink, so the makeup would all have to happen in the last half hour before the show. Talk about cutting it fine!

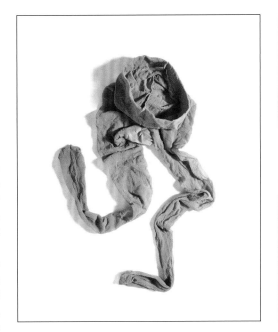

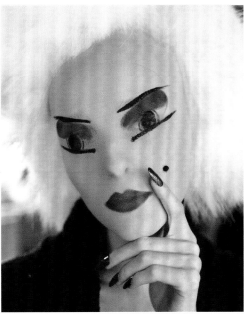

GARETH PUGH SS16; PHOTOGRAPHY LUCA CANNONIERI; HAIR MALCOLM EDWARDS; MANICURIST MARIAN NEWMAN.

Icing Sugar

I needed a theme for an unconventional beauty story so I decided to make the makeup out of icing sugar. For this shot I basically dusted icing sugar onto the model's face using a cake doily as a stencil. The detail made for an incredible image.

For another image on this shoot I stencilled a rose in icing sugar so that it looked like a white tattoo. And there was another where I decided to make a skirt out of the icing sugar, with a pleated peplum at the bottom. Somewhere in my deranged mind I was thinking about sieving the icing sugar so it looked as though it had never been touched, and as the girl lay on the floor I was going to literally sculpt the skirt on to her. Then I realized I didn't have nearly enough icing sugar, but I did just happen to have a car full of sand. So these huge bags of sand had to be carried into the studio, while I sat with a ruler and a brush trying to get the sand into the shape of a skirt so I could then cover it with a layer of icing sugar.

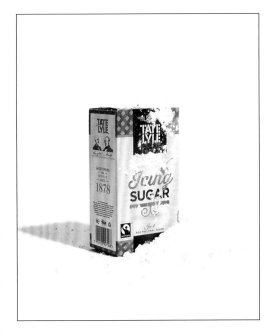

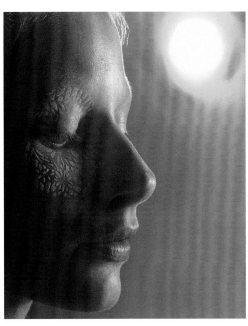

PHOTOGRAPHY HORST DIEKGERDES; FASHION EDITOR CAMILLE BIDOULT-WADDINGTON; HAIR MALCOLM EDWARDS; MODEL RAE.

Seaweed

I love an Asian supermarket, it's a place I often go to for ideas, and I'd recently bought a packet of seaweed. I liked it because it kind of looks like wood and I thought it would be great to give skin a wood-grain effect.

Because the seaweed was so stiff I wasn't sure how I could make it work, I didn't think I could put it on the face – it was just too unyielding. Then I dampened it to see what would happen and it became like one of those sheet face-masks. It was kind of wet and slimy, and I just pressed it into Anouck's skin. It also became quite see-through – all you could really see were the line markings. It had grain to it. I just sort of placed the seaweed there and said, 'Shoot it now, we don't know how long it's going to last.'

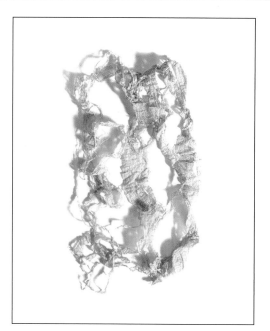 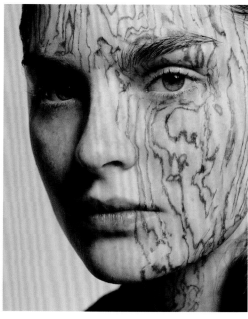

I-D MAGAZINE; PHOTOGRAPHY RICHARD BUSH; HAIR EUGENE SOULEIMAN; MODEL ANOUCK LEPERE.

Pencil Shavings

The inspiration behind this shoot was *Stepford Wives* meets *Women on the Verge of a Nervous Breakdown* – she's a bit agoraphobic and stays at home a lot, and I was thinking: unapproachable, neurotic, suburbia.

For this particular picture, the hair was done in a very fifties-style, gorgeous and glamorous, so I started with a lip. But, although the colours were unusual, it still felt too conventional to me. As I was sharpening the lip liner the shavings hit the table and I said to my assistants, 'start sharpening the pencils and collect all the shavings!' They probably thought I'd lost my mind, but I wanted to use them as lashes.

So it's essentially a very conventional beauty story, but she's mad, on the edge, thinking about ending it all. So why wouldn't she have pencil shavings on her eyes? Because the clothing and the hair on this shoot were very nice and straight laced, something had to be a bit unconventionally crazy, and I thought, 'That's got to be me'.

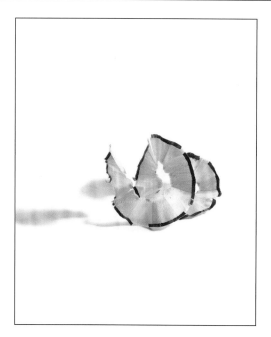 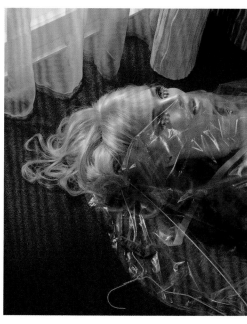

SUNDAY TIMES STYLE MAGAZINE, JANUARY 2014; PHOTOGRAPHY MILES ALDRIDGE; FASHION EDITOR CATHY EDWARDS; HAIR KERRY WARN; MODEL MELISSA TAMMERJIN.

Sunbed Goggles

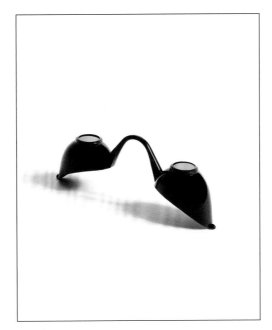

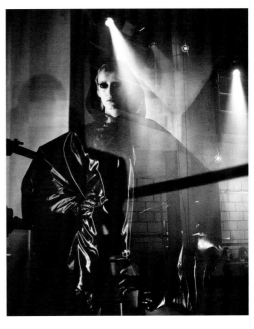

There are all manner of things inside my sticky-back plastic bag. Many have been in there for years but I haven't found a use for them yet. One time I reached in and pulled out the goggles and it was the birth of an idea that I used for Gareth Pugh's AW17 show.

Gareth wanted the women to feel very strong, like soldiers – it was very *The Night Porter*. I always challenge myself to try to bring Gareth something that he hasn't seen before. When I showed him the goggles he thought they looked amazing and wanted to get some specially designed so they were a bit more fierce. What I liked was how the goggles made the models look robotic. We also put a dark, inky-green shadow behind the goggles so you weren't sure if it was a big smoky black eyeball. I called them 'insectoid eyes'. They gave another dimension to the face in profile, and when the light hit them you could see the lids blinking behind. It was very weird, like a moth caught inside a jar.

GARETH PUGH AW17; PHOTOGRAPHY AMBRA VERNUCCIO.

Pom-poms

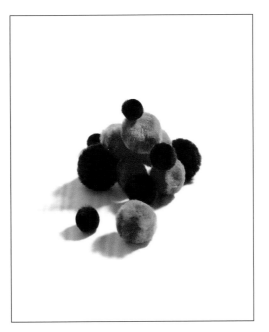

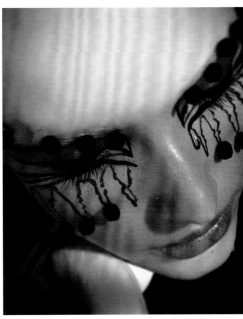

This was for a show I did at Australian Fashion Week for Romance Was Born, who are like Australia's answer to John Galliano. They're wild, outrageous, and they always want something quite theatrical. I wanted to give them something really interesting so I did fluoro makeup, and because that kind of makeup doesn't stay on very well – it sort of cakes and breaks – I thought I'd do really gorgeous, innocent young skin, a little bit of a dolly blush, keeping the lips real and then making the eyes look really graphic. The hair was brightly coloured wigs and the clothes were psychedelic, so it was a case of 'We can go there; the louder the better!'

I thought I had to make it less of a flower-power seventies thing and give it more of a contemporary festival vibe. So I delved in the sticky-back plastic bag and found all these brightly coloured pom-poms. I hadn't done this idea before, and as it's for a runway show you just have to hope and pray the pom-poms stay on. But they did, thankfully!

ROMANCE WAS BORN, AUSTRALIAN FASHION WEEK 2015; HAIR ALAN WHITE.

Elastic Bands

There are often things I've used before, but I'll use them again in a different way. I had used elastic bands in a shoot where I wanted the girls to look like they had dolly limbs, and I also used them in Nick Knight's SHOWstudio film.

For Gareth Pugh's show, the fitting had a forties feeling and Malcolm was doing strong hair – a victory roll with a cartoon edge. Gareth wanted the girls to look severe, so I thought about doing a classic forties-style makeup, strong brow, dark lip and fierce eyeliner. But this felt too ordinary – I had to find a way to make it look fresh. I went back to an idea I often go to, and that's super-perfection, botox beauty – like fillers in the skin and very exaggerated cheeks.

I brushed the eyebrows upwards and asked Malcolm to make the hair as tight as possible to give a stretched effect. To pronounce the cheeks I put gloss on the cheekbone and, where you would normally put contour or sculpt, stretched elastic bands under the cheekbone.

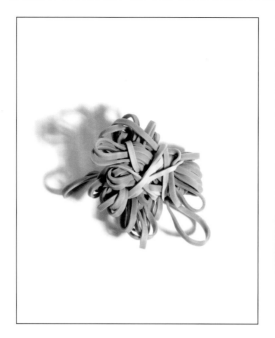

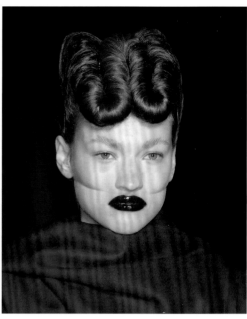

GARETH PUGH AW16; PHOTOGRAPHY LUCA CANNONIERI; HAIR MALCOLM EDWARDS.

Feather

This was a feather I'd used in a quite theatrical Westwood show. There were a lot of pale faces and it was very painterly, and I was wondering how I could get the makeup on, without using a makeup brush. So I was thinking quills, ink ... let's use a feather! And, you know, the actual execution of it looked great. When I was talking to Vivienne and Andreas Kronthaler I remember thinking, 'a beautiful nightmare', like she's a ghost with everything decayed. There's also a sense of Chinese theatre in the way it looked.

It never occurs to me to get approval. I mean, I'm always crossing my fingers, especially when we go into the rehearsal, because that's when I'll know if people are going to like the makeup or not. But I believe there is never any point in selling your idea, because the moment you have to defend the makeup and say, 'I think this is right because of this', they don't want it. They don't like it. Take it off and do something else. But it's all part of the journey.

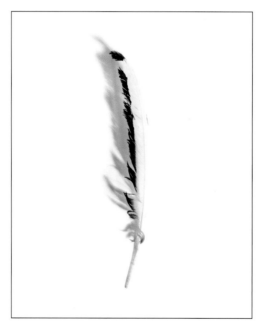

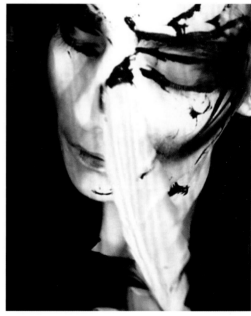

VIVIENNE WESTWOOD RED LABEL SS14.

Paint Roller

The paint roller is super ordinary, it's just a tool for getting colour from one place to another. Just an application tool. This shoot was in Paris, and the story was called 'The Little Prince', so we kind of made Cate Blanchett look like a character from that book. She had this short, blonde wig on and very ruddy cheeks, just like the Little Prince. Then we came to this shot, in which she was wearing a very big Yohji Yamamoto dress. Julien did this amazing headpiece and she wasn't really wearing any makeup. I told Tim what I wanted to do, I had my paint roller and the colour on a paper plate, and Tim said, 'OK, off you go.'

So I went onto the set and said to Cate, 'I'm going to be honest with you Cate – most people bring out the best of your beauty, but I'm going to attack you with a paint roller.' And she said, 'Great! Do it!' So I just put the roller in the paint and rolled it up her, just like you would if you were doing a wall. Everyone was a bit anxious, like the publicist, but it took five seconds to do and that was it. I walked away. And the truly great thing about Cate is that she's such a good sport. I think she wanted to do something different, something a bit edgy. I mean, it was for *W* magazine so why not?

W MAGAZINE, DECEMBER 2015; PHOTOGRAPHY TIM WALKER; FASHION EDITOR JACOB K; HAIR JULIEN D'YS; MODEL CATE BLANCHETT.

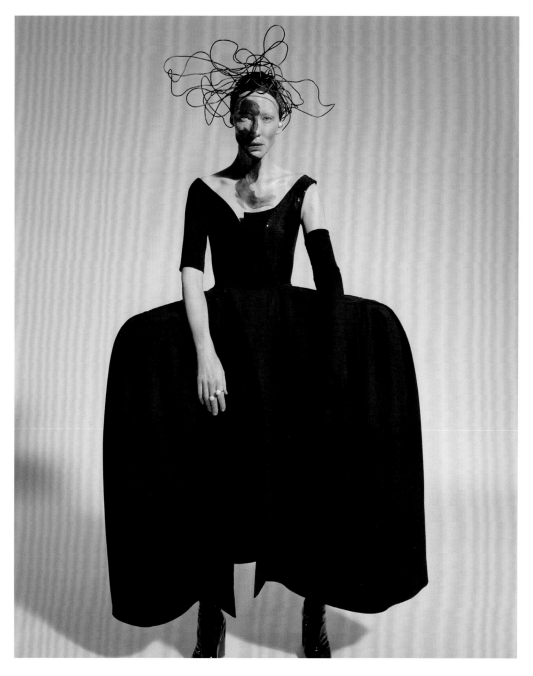

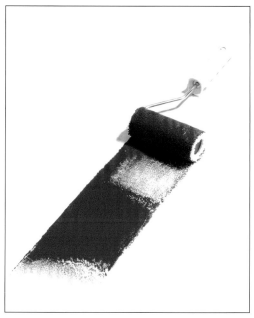

I'M GOING TO ATTACK YOU WITH A PAINT ROLLER

Crystals

We gave Caroline, the model, this beautiful skin texture and I wanted to do a lip that looked like she was magnetized with jewels. Some of them were Swarovski crystals and some were from the bead shop in London's Covent Garden.

This was actually for a beauty shoot based on the futuristic movie *Bladerunner*, so I chose to do incredible skin, but everything else would be an embellishment, whether it was on the eye or the cheek or the mouth. It was like 'Diamonds are a Girl's Best Friend', but the cyber version. It felt like it was the right thing to do at the time because, while other people had been doing sequins on the lips, it was usually with a perfect lip line, so I wanted to do something different.

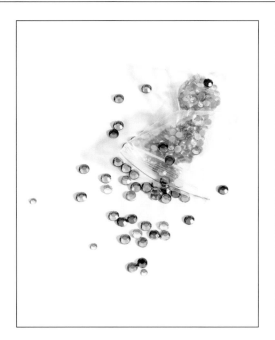

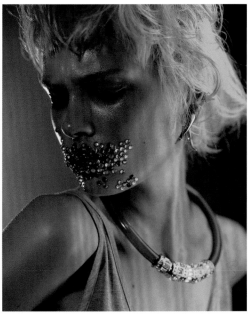

I-D SPRING 2014; PHOTOGRAPHY RICHARD BUSH; FASHION EDITOR SARAH RICHARDSON; HAIR SAM HILLERBY; MODEL CAROLINE BRASCH NIELSEN.

Gilding Brush

Often I find fake lashes really boring. They've looked the same since the sixties. I've experimented with all sorts over the years to get a different lash look, from paper to feathers. This was another idea I had for getting a super-sized flutter, and I used it in a story I did with Sophia Neophitou for *the Independent* magazine. It's modelled here by my wonderful assistant, Joey.

I have a huge array of brushes in my kit, some are custom brushes for applying makeup but I also have loads of others, like this gilding brush. I did once actually use this for its intended purpose, which is applying gold leaf.

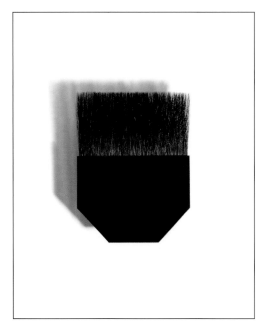

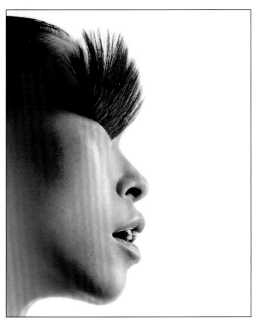

PHOTOGRAPHY JAMES STOPFORTH; MODEL JOEY CHOY.

Paper

This was a beauty story about eyelashes. But how do you make eyelashes interesting and different? And it was six to eight pages. But just because it's an eyelash story it doesn't mean you've got to use false eyelashes. Why not make eyelashes out of another medium?

I carry lots of stationery in my kit and I said to my assistant, 'Let's get some black paper and concertina it'. So we did that, then shredded it, then pulled apart the paper to stick on the eyes. This was more of a collage, rather than just putting on standard fake eyelashes. Michelangelo is great with angles, and the lighting was amazing. I crunched the 'lashes' to look a bit like mosquitoes.

VOGUE ITALIA JUNE 2009; PHOTOGRAPHY MICHELANGELO DI BATTISTA; FASHION EDITOR ALICE GENTILUCCI; HAIR STÉPHANE LANCIEN; MODEL ALEK ALEXEYEVA.

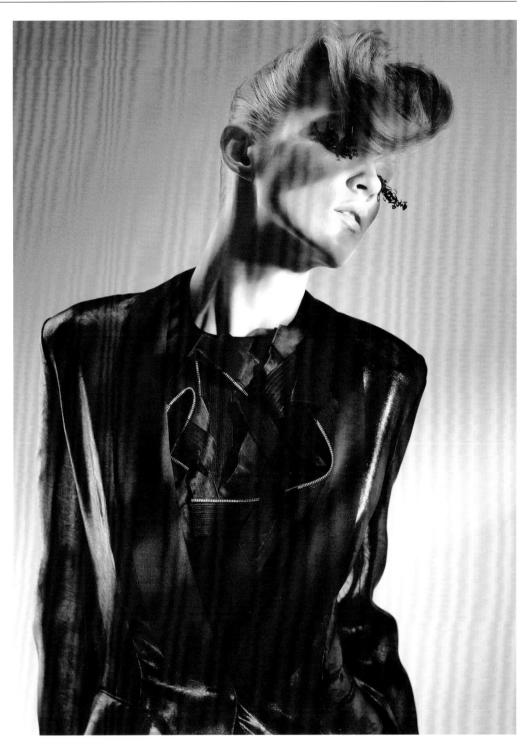

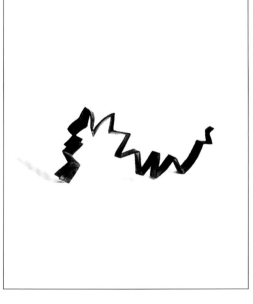

IT DOESN'T MEAN YOU'VE GOT TO USE FALSE LASHES

PICTURE CREDITS

The author and publisher would like to thank the following
individuals and organizations for permission to reproduce images
in this book. In all cases; every effort has been made to credit
the copyright holders and contributors; but should there be
any omissions or errors the publisher would be pleased to insert
the appropriate acknowledgment in any subsequent edition
of this book.

COVER

(front and back) Sølve Sundsbø/Art+Commerce

INTRODUCTION

4 © Ann Ray; 6 © James Stopforth; 8 © James Stopforth;
10 © James Stopforth

RAW

14 Sølve Sundsbø/Art+Commerce; 18 © Mario Testino, Cara
Delevingne and Kate Moss, London, Burberry 2014; 19 Mario
Testino/Vogue © The Condé Nast Publications Ltd.; 20 Nick
Knight/Vogue © The Condé Nast Publications Ltd.; 21 Nick Knight/
Vogue © The Condé Nast Publications Ltd.; 23 © Nick Knight;
25 © Nick Knight; 26 © Tim Walker; 27 © Tim Walker; 28 © Tim
Walker; 29 © Tim Walker; 30 Luca Cannonieri/Gorunway.com;
31 Luca Cannonieri/Gorunway.com; 32 Luca Cannonieri/Gorunway.
com; 34 Sølve Sundsbø/Art+Commerce; 37 Alasdair McLellan/Art
Partner; 38 © Tim Walker; 39 © Tim Walker; 40 Sølve Sundsbø/
Art+Commerce; 41 Sølve Sundsbø/Art+Commerce; 42 Photographer
Richard Bush; 43 Photographer Richard Bush; 44 Steven Klein/W,
November 2012 © Condé Nast; 45 Steven Klein/W, March 2012 ©
Condé Nast; 46 Steven Klein/W, November 2012 © Condé Nast

GRAPHIC

50 Miguel Reveriego/Art Partner; 54 ©Mario Testino, London,
British Vogue 2009; 56 ©Mario Testino, London, British Vogue
2009; 58 Sølve Sundsbø/Art+Commerce; 59 Sølve Sundsbø/
Art+Commerce; 60 Craig McDean/Art+Commerce; 61 Val Garland;
62 Ruth Hogben; 64 Luca Cannonieri/Gorunway.com; 65 Liz
Collins/Trunk Archive; 66 Photographer Richard Bush;
68 Photographer Richard Bush; 69 Photographer Richard Bush;
71 Miguel Reveriego/Art Partner; 72 Backstage photograph Val
Garland; Background image © James Stopforth; 73 Backstage
photograph Val Garland; Background image © James Stopforth;
74 (top) Val Garland; 74 (bottom) © Nick Knight; 75 © Nick Knight;
76 Michelangelo di Battista/Management + Artists/AUGUST;
77 Michelangelo di Battista/Management + Artists/AUGUST;
78 Photographer Richard Bush; 80 Sølve Sundsbø/Art+Commerce;
81 Sølve Sundsbø/Art+Commerce; 82 Bauer Media; 83 Bauer
Media; 85 John Akehurst; 86 Sølve Sundsbø/Art+Commerce;
88 Photographer Richard Bush; 89 Photographer Richard Bush;
90 Alasdair McLellan/Art Partner; 91 Alasdair McLellan/Art Partner;
92 Luca Cannonieri/Gorunway.com; 93 Luca Cannonieri/Gorunway.
com; 94 Luca Cannonieri/Gorunway.com; 95 Luca Cannonieri/
Gorunway.com; 96 © Phil Poynter

COLOUR CHAOS

100 Photography by Norbert Schoerner; 102 © Nick Knight;
103 © Nick Knight; 104 © Mario Testino, Catherine McNeil,
London, V Magazine 2007; 107 © Nick Knight; 108 Photographer
Richard Bush; 109 Photographer Richard Bush; 110 Corinne Day/
Vogue © The Condé Nast Publications Ltd.; 113 Photograph by Inez
and Vinoodh; 114 Sølve Sundsbø/Art+Commerce; 115 Sølve Sundsbø/
Art+Commerce; 116 Craig McDean/Art+Commerce; 118 Paolo
Colaiocco; 120 Sølve Sundsbø/Art+Commerce; 122 Sølve Sundsbø/
Art+Commerce; 123 Sølve Sundsbø/Art+Commerce; 124 Sølve
Sundsbø/Art+Commerce; 126 © Nick Knight; 127 Backstage image
Val Garland; Background © James Stopforth; 128 Sølve Sundsbø/
Art+Commerce; 129 Sølve Sundsbø/Art+Commerce; 130 Sølve
Sundsbø/Art+Commerce

DOLLY MIXTURE

134 © Tim Walker; 136 © Tim Walker; 137 © Tim Walker;
138 Val Garland; 139 Val Garland; 140 Val Garland; 141 © Tim
Walker; 142 Sølve Sundsbø/Art+Commerce; 143 Sølve Sundsbø/
Art+Commerce; 145 Patrick Demarchelier/W, May 2013 © Condé
Nast; 147 © Tim Walker; 148 © Tim Walker; 149 © Tim Walker;
150 © Nick Knight; 151 © Nick Knight; 153 © Tim Walker; 154 © Tim
Walker; 155 © Tim Walker; 156 © Tim Walker; 157 © Tim Walker;
158 © Tim Walker; 160 Luca Cannonieri/Gorunway.com;
161 Luca Cannonieri/Gorunway.com

STICKY SEXY

164 Craig McDean/Art+Commerce; 167–169 Sølve Sundsbø/
Art+Commerce; 170–172 © Nick Knight; 174 © Nick Knight;
176 Miguel Reveriego/Art Partner; 177 Sølve Sundsbø Art+Commerce;
179 Nick Knight/Vogue © The Condé Nast Publications Ltd.;
181 © Tim Walker; 182 Inez and Vinoodh; 185 © Nick Knight;
186 Steven Klein/Art Partner; 187 Steven Klein/Art Partner; 188 Val
Garland; 189 © Nick Knight; 190 ©Mario Testino. Imaan Hamman,
Los Angeles, Vogue Paris, 2015; 192–201 Photographs are from
Pirelli Calendar 2004, photographer Nick Knight, art director Peter
Saville, stylist Katy England, hair Sam McKnight, models Frankie
Rayder, Natalia Vodianova, Karolína Kurková, Mariacarla Boscono,
Alister Mackie, Alek Wek, Liberty Ross, Esther De Jong

AUTHOR'S ACKNOWLEDGMENTS

Special thanks go to Karl Plewka for his brilliant mind, wit and words, to Glenn Crouch for always being there, and to Maureen Vivian for being keeper of the coinage. A very special thank you to Joey Choy, who I love more than garlic. To Paula Jenner, my agent, and all at Streeters London. To Camilla Morton, Gaynor Sermon and Tory Turk for making this book happen. To Angus Hyland and Amira Prescott, for your incredible attention to detail, DING DONG!

I would also like to thank the following artists that I have had the good fortune to work with in my career, and whose contributions feature throughout this book:

PHOTOGRAPHERS/FILM DIRECTORS

Alasdair McLellan, Ambra Vernuccio, Ann Ray, Corinne Day, Craig McDean, Emma Summerton, Horst Diekgerdes, Inez and Vinoodh, James Cochrane, James Stopforth, John Akehurst, Jonathan Evans, Liz Collins, Luca Cannonieri, Mario Testino, Mark Alesky, Mary McCartney, Matt Lever, Michelangelo Di Battista, Miguel Reveriego, Miles Aldridge, Nick Knight, Norbert Schoerner, Paolo Colaiocco, Patrick Demarchelier, Phil Poynter, Richard Bush, Ruth Hogben, Sølve Sundsbø, Steven Klein, Tim Walker, Vincent Peters

FASHION DIRECTORS

Aleksandra Woroniecka, Alice Gentilucci, Alister Mackie, Beat Bolliger, Camile Bedoult, Capucine Safyurtlu, Cathy Edwards, Cathy Kasterine, Charlotte Stockdale, Edward Enninful, Elliott Smedley, Emmanuelle Alt, Francesca Burns, Frank Benhamou, Jacob K, Jane How, Jillian Davison, Jonathan Kaye, Kate Phelan, Katie Grand, Katie Lyall, Katie Shillingford, Katy England, Lucinda Chambers, Marie Amelie Sauve, Nicola Formichetti, Phyllis Posnick, Sabrina Schreder, Sarah Richardson, Simon Foxton, Simon Robins, Sophia Neophitou-Apostolou, Tabitha Simmons, Tonne Goodman

HAIR STYLISTS

Adam Bryant, Alain Pichon, Alan White, Angelo Seminara, Anthony Turner, Christiaan, Duffy, Eamonn Hughes, Eugene Souleiman, Garren, Gary Gill, Guido Palau, James Pecis, Julien D'ys, Ken O'Rouke, Kerry Warn, Luigi Murenu, Lyndell Mansfield, Malcolm Edwards, Marc Lopez, Neil Moodie, Odile Gilbert, Orlando Pita, Paul Hanlon, Peter Gray, Rudi Lewis, Sam Hillerby, Sam McKnight, Scott Ade, Shay Ashaul, Stéphane Lancien, Ward

NAIL ARTISTS

Anatole Rainey, Bernadette Thompson, Debbie Knight, Elsa Durrens, Glenis Baptiste, Honey, Lorraine Griffin, Marian Newman, Mike Pocock, Nichola Joss, Sophy Robson, Trish Lomax, Yuko Tsuchihashi, Yuna Park

MODELS

Aaron Lewins, Alek Alexeyeva, Alek Wek, Aleksandra T, Ali Stephens, Alla Kostromichova, Amy Wesson, Angela Lindvall, Anja Rubik, Anna Ewers (@ Women NY), Anna V, Anouck Lepere, Ariana London, Ashleigh Good, Audrey Marnay, Aya Jones, Barbara Palvin, Beth Ditto, Björk, Cara Delevingne, Carmen Kass, Caroline (Westwood show), Caroline Brasch Nielsen, Cate Blanchett, Catherine McNeil, Chen Li, Chris Belcher, Clarice Vitakauskas, Coco Rocha (Nomad Mgmt), Dana Lucia Lopez, Dasha Malevich, Debra Shaw, Devon Aoki, Dewi Driegen (Paparazzi Model Management), Diana Khalitova, DJ Funghi, Dustin Phil, Ed King, Edita Vilkeviciute, Eliza, Emma Watson, Erin O'Connor, Esther De Jong, Fernanda Tavares, Frankie Rayder, Frog, Gemma Ward, Ginta Lapina, Gisele Bundchen, Guillaume Babouin, Han Hye Jin, He Cong, Indie, Imaan Hammam, Imogen, Isabella Emmack, Jack Corradi, Jay Wright, Joan Smalls, Johnny Epstein, Jordan Matheson, Juana Burga, Julia Hafstrom, Karen Elson, Karina T, Karlie Kloss, Karolin Wolter, Karolína Kurková, Kate Moss, Keira Knightley, Kim Iglinsky, King Edward (potato), Kirsi Pyrhonen, Kristen McMenamy, Lady Gaga, Lara Stone, Liberty Ross, Lina Hoss (PMA), Lindsey Wixson, Linnea Ahlman, Liya Kebede, Lorena Randi, Lorna Foran (The Hive Management), Louis, Mariacarla Boscono (@ Women NY), Marina Nery, Marta Ortiz, Melissa Tammerjin, Michael Clark, Minnie, Natalia Vodianova (Viva London), Nataša Vojnović (@ Women NY), Nicole Kidman, Nika Cole, Nykhor, Onya, Polina Kuklina, Pollyanna McIntosh, Rachel Kirby, Raica Oliveira, Raquel Zimmermann (Viva London), Rikki Smut, Rie Rasmussen, Ruth Crilly, Scarlett Johansson, Shirley Mallmann, Sofie Hemnet, Stella Lucia (Viva London), Stina Olsson, Sung Hee Kim (Nomad Mgmt), Sylvester Ulv Heriksen, Thea, Tiiuk Kuik, Toby, Tom Pearce, Vivien Solari, Xiao Wen Ju, Zoe Colivas, Zora Star

FASHION DESIGNERS

Andreas Kronthaler, Carson McColl, Christopher Bailey, Gareth Pugh, John Galliano, Lee McQueen, Mary Katrantzou, Phoebe Philo, Preen, Romance Was Born, Shaun Leane, Stella McCartney, Vivienne Westwood

SET DESIGNERS

Andrew Tomlinson, Andy Hillman, Shona Heath, Gideon Ponte, Jack Flanagan, Michael Howells, Rhea Thierstein

ART DIRECTORS
Peter Saville, Sam Alex Wiederin, Stephen Gan, Tom Hingston

MAKEUP ARTISTS
A big thank you to the incredible teams of makeup artists that
I have worked with, past and present.

Akari Sugino, Alena Moiseeva, Alexis Day, Aliana Moss, Anastasia
Hess, Andrea Gomez Anzola, Aneesha Sangha, Anja Detobon,
Ariane Jaksch, Ashley O'Connor, Ashley Rudder, Azra Red,
Baltasar González Pinel, Bea Sweet, Campbell Ritchie, Carla
Francesa, Carlos Saidel, Carly Utting, Carol Mackie, Caroline
Hernandez, Caroline Sims, Cat Smith, Chantel Miller, Charlene
McGreene, Charlotta Pichon, Charlotte Day, Charlotte Reid,
Cher Webb, Chiara Guizetti, Christian McCulloch, Christine
Du Puys, Christopher Ardoff, Claire Mulleady, Claire Urqhart,
Cynthia Rivas, Dean Rudd, Debbie Finnegan, Denis Hilly,
Denny Richards, Dominic Skinner, Elaine Lynskey, Elizabeth
Hsieh, Emma Miles, Fabianna Gomes, Famida Pathan, Fatima
Thomas, Fiona Rookley, Florence Teerlinck, Francesca Etu-
Menson, Gemma Smith Edhouse, Gilbert Soliz, Gregory Arlt,
Hadeel El-Tal, Hannah Maestranzi, Hiroyo Iwaki, Irena Rodgers,
Irena Rubens, James Molloy, James O'Reily, Jane Harwood
Charity, Jay Kwan, Jeta Bujupi, Jo Leversuch, Joey Choy, John
Stapleton, Jordan King, Julia Carmus, Kana Nagashima, Karina
Constantine, Karl Berndsen, Karoline Traktina, Kate Lee, Kate
Romanoff, Katerina Brans, Katrin Rees, Katy Nixon, Kenneth
Soh, Keri Blair, Kristina Vidic, Kumiko Hirose, Laisum Fung,
Laura Dominique, Laura Noben, Lee Pearson, Lesley Keane,
Linda Anderson, Liset Garza, Liz Martins, Lois Moorcroft, Lou
Copperwaite, Louise Bryan, Louise Zizzo, Lydia Bredl, Lydsey
Alexander, Macky Pratayot, Maki Ihara, Maria Comparetto,
Maria Gomez, Marina Keri, Marisol Garcia, Mathias van Hooff,
Meekyung Kim, Melanie Inglessis, Melissa Gibson, Michael
Patterson, Michele Magnani, Michelle Campbell, Miguel Ramos,
Miki Matsunaga, Mirijana Vasovic, Momo Rauch, Mona Leanne,
Naoko Scintu, Naomi Nakamura, Neil Young, Nicky Weir, Nicole
Wittman, Nina Lackson, Nina Sagri, Pablo Rodriguez, Peter
Pisani, Petros Petrohilos, Phoebe Walters, Porsche Poon, Rachel
O'Donnell, Rebecca Butterworth, Rebecca Muir, Regan Rabanal,
Rhea le Riche, Romero Jennings, Sam Bryant, Samantha Lau, Sara

Mencattelli, Sharon Dowsett, Siobahn Huckie, Susy Carducci,
Sylvie Mainville, Takako Noborio, Tami Shirey, Tarryn-Lee
Kelley, Tashi Honnery, Terry Barber, Tiffany Johnson, Tiffany
Patton, Tom Sapin, Tonee Roberio, Vass Theotokis, Veronica
Martinez, Veronique Boumaza, Victor Cembellin, Victoria Baron,
Vimi Joshi, Vinton Gordon, Yayoi Sasaki, Yulia Bondarenko

**ADDITIONAL THANKS GO TO THE FOLLOWING INDIVIDUALS
AND ORGANIZATIONS:**
Aimee Frost, Charlotte Knight, Fiona Scott, Georgina Billingham,
Gordon Espinet, Hayley Roughton, Issima Oniangue, James
Gager, Kat Davey, Lucy Baxter, Remy Averna, Samy Cheddadi, Zak
Yopp, 42 West, Absolutely Fashion, Arizona Model Management,
Art Partner, Art+Commerce, August, Bauer Media, Brand
Model Management, City Models, Code Management, Condé
Nast, D' Management Group, D1 Models, DNA, Dominique
Models, Elite Model Management London, Esteem, Forward
Artists, Getty Images, Hardland Management, Haus of Gaga,
Icon Model Management, IMG, Insurge Entertainment, Jonathan
Sanders, Kate Moss Agency, KCD Worldwide, Line Up Model
Management, Mario Testino+, Michael Clark Company,
Models 1, Mother Model Management, Muse Management,
Nevs London, New Blood Agency, New York Models, Next
Model Management, Nomad Management, One Little
Indian, One Management, Paparazzi Model Management,
Pirelli, Promod Model Agency (PMA), RPD Models, Saoirse
Kennelly, SHOWstudio, Sight Management Studio, Starsystem,
Starworks Group, Steven Robinson, Storm Artists, Storm
Management, Style International Management, Sun Esee Model
Management, Supreme Management, Tess Management, The
Hive Management, The Lions NYC, The Society Management,
Trino Verkade, True Public Relations, Trunk, United Agents,
Untitled Entertainment, Vision Los Angeles, Viva London
Model Management, VLM Studio, Way Model Management,
Wilhelmina Models, WOLF-KASTELER Public Relations,
Women Management

My profound apologies to anyone who has been unintentionally
omitted from this list. Some of the imagery in this book is more
than 20 years old and, as time has passed, my memory of visuals,
people and places has sometimes unfortunately become blurred!

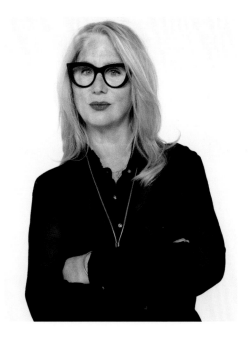

THE AUTHOR

Val Garland is an internationally acclaimed makeup artist who lives in London. Her career spans nearly twenty-five years in the beauty and fashion industries, and in 2017 she was named L'Oréal Paris Global Makeup Director.

Born Valerie Sweeney in Birmingham, UK, Val grew up in Bristol and left school at fifteen to become a hairdresser. She then met her future husband, Terry Garland, and the two young punks, bored with provincial life, emigrated to Australia. In the years that followed they opened the hair salon Garland & Garland – first in Perth and then in Sydney – which would prove to be a hub of individuality and creativity. Val then started working on editorial shoots for several Australian style magazines and, on a 1989 shoot in London, fuelled by the buzz of the city, she called Terry and said that it was time for her to move back. It took her four years to get divorced, close her business and pack just two suitcases (of mostly designer clothes), and a new chapter in her life began.

London in the mid-nineties was vibrating with post-grunge conceptuality and soon Val jettisoned her hairdresser's kit and pursued her true calling as a makeup artist. After a stint of fairly radical shoots for *The London Evening Standard*, working with stylist Katy England, it wasn't long before she began contributing to the revered style bibles of the era, *Dazed & Confused*, *i-D* and *The Face*. But a huge turning point was when Katy England introduced Val to a young designer called Alexander McQueen, and so began a creative union that now forms part of fashion history.

In the following years Val continued to enjoy and explore all aspects of her increasingly prominent position in the industry, most notably her relationship with seminal photographer Nick Knight. Their early collaborations include the ground-breaking nineties campaigns for Christian Dior as well as iconic editorials for *Vogue* and *AnOther* magazine, and avant-garde films for Knight's award-winning fashion website SHOWstudio.

In the decades since, Val Garland's career trajectory has been stellar, with a plethora of designers, brands, photographers, celebrities and magazines now fighting for her time. From runway to editorial to campaign, she is adored by her peers for her radical approach, creative zeal and dedication to a no-nonsense work ethic.

Often referred to as 'the makeup artist's makeup artist', whether she is spontaneously daubing Cate Blanchett's face with a paint roller or painstakingly perfecting a hyper-modern look for a beauty campaign, Val refuses to conform or resort to formula, and her position as one of the world's most prolific image-makers renders the 'artist' suffix to 'makeup' entirely justified.